AGAINST *all* GRAIN

delectable paleo recipes to eat well & feel great

more than 150 gluten-free,
grain-free, and dairy-free
recipes for daily life

written & photographed by

Danielle Walker

www.againstallgrain.com

VICTORY BELT PUBLISHING INC.
Las Vegas

front cover photography and design by Jennifer Skog

First Published in 2013 by Victory Belt Publishing Inc.

ISBN 13: 978-1-936608-36-2

This book is for entertainment purposes. The publisher and author of this cookbook are not responsible in any manner whatsoever for any adverse effects arising directly or indirectly as a result of the information provided in this book.

Printed in Canada

TC 1819

Lifestyle and cover photo team:

Photography—Jennifer Skog

Hair & Makeup—Lindsay Skog

Set Styling—PJ Rude of Milkglass Vintage Rentals

Accessories—Ashley Morgan Designs

This is my invariable advice to people:
Learn how to cook – try new recipes, learn from your mistakes,
be fearless, and above all – have fun!

– JULIA CHILD

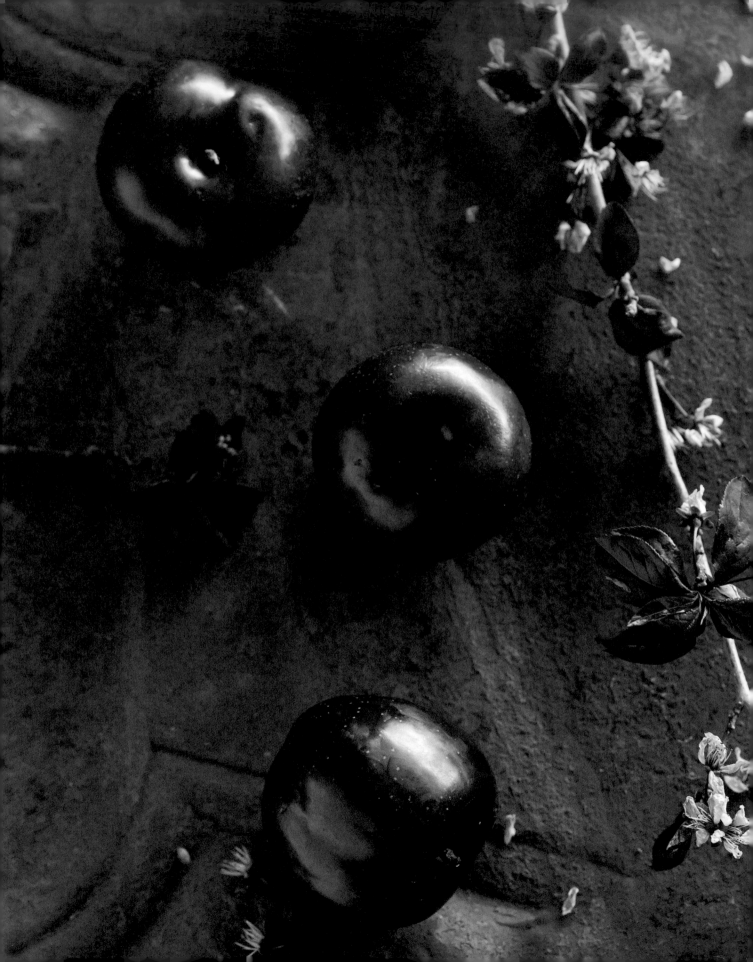

contents

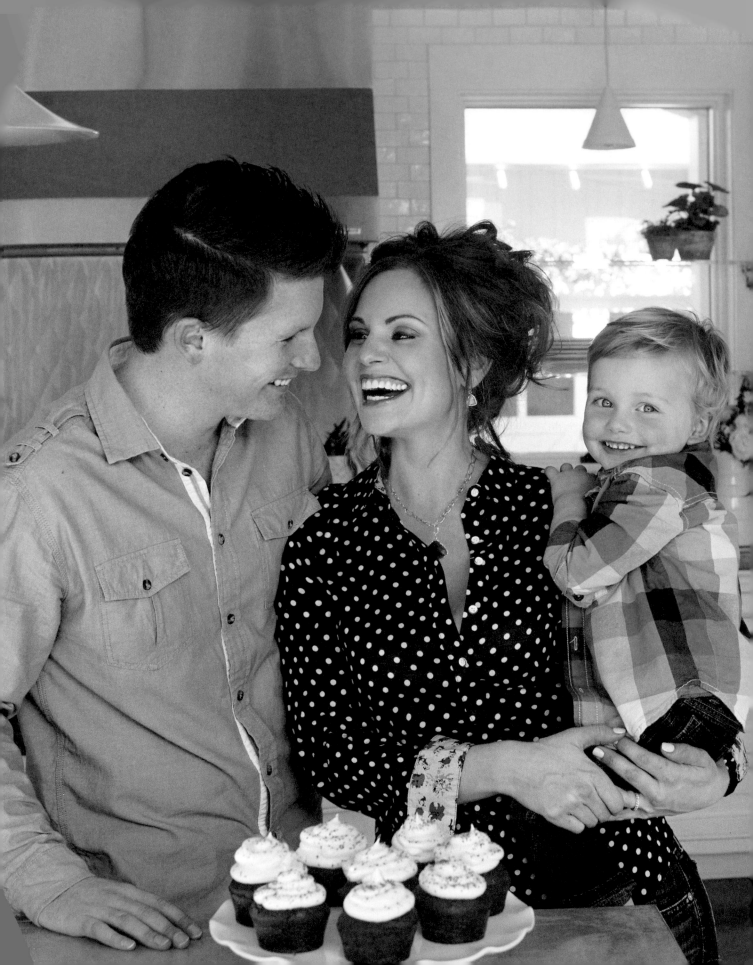

introduction

I can trace my passion for cooking back to a failure in the kitchen when I was in
college. It was my first time attempting a meal totally on my own, and I vividly
remember proudly serving a platter of Chicken Parmigiana to a houseful of college
boys. After anticipating a delicious, home-cooked meal, they cut into their chicken
only to find that it was grossly undercooked. I later learned that the chicken breasts
needed to be pounded into cutlets to ensure even and quick cooking.

That was the first of many culinary failures, but it sparked a hunger in me. The Food
Network became the background to my studies, and cooking magazines smothered
my textbooks. I had a newfound interest in how and why dishes worked or didn't,
but out of fear of poisoning everyone around me, I spent the remainder of my college
years cooking what was familiar and comfortable.

It wasn't until I graduated that I started to actually experiment with new foods. But
not by choice. After a few months of experiencing gastrointestinal upset, fatigue, and
unexplainable anemia, I received a diagnosis of ulcerative colitis—an autoimmune
disease that attacks the intestines. I was prescribed a myriad of harsh medications to
be taken multiple times a day but still experienced terrible symptoms. My various
doctors refused to speak to me about dietary changes and assured me that food could
not cure the disease. Through my own research and reaching out to others in online
communities, I discovered that I could, in fact, drastically change my approach to
eating to alleviate my symptoms.

To my dismay, I learned that I needed to remove grains, lactose, and refined sugars.
Gone were the days of convenience when a meal could come from a jar of spaghetti
sauce, a package of pasta, and frozen hamburger meat. All-purpose flour and white
sugar, which had been staples for me, were no longer options. Whatever I knew about
cooking would no longer serve me. It was back to square one.

After trying a few recipes I found on the Internet and tossing them in the trash because
they were inedible, I came up with a mission: to never again miss the food I once loved.
I set forth to create grain-free, dairy-free dishes that were reminiscent of the standard
American diet, but were wholesome and made from fresh ingredients—things that
would leave a person feeling satisfied rather than deprived.

Danielle Walker

health struggles

But let me backtrack a bit, because it is important to comprehend the gravity of my pain and suffering to understand why this mission became my passion.

In 2007, a mere two months after graduating from college and marrying my high-school sweetheart, I found myself in the emergency room suffering from unbearable pain in my abdomen and a slew of digestive complications. Until then, I had been a perfectly healthy young woman, with no family history of digestive disorders and only the occasional stomach upset as a child. The hospital discharged me without a diagnosis and gave me prescriptions for medication that ultimately intensified my symptoms.

A few agonizing weeks, three specialists, and one lengthy hospital admittance later, I was finally given a diagnosis of ulcerative colitis—a disease similar to Crohn's disease. I was again discharged with a handful of prescriptions and the promise that, while there was no cure for the disease, I could ultimately live a very "normal" life. The doctors didn't discuss the symptoms I might experience or even the side effects the drugs might cause.

About six months later, I found myself in a hospital room in Kampala, Uganda, pleading for my life as I lay precariously near death. My husband and I had been planning for a year to partake in a humanitarian trip to work in the refugee camps in northern Uganda. While I had experienced minor discomfort and symptoms before we left the States, I was in no way aware of the severity of this disease, and so we had decided to follow through with our plans.

In Uganda, I was racked with debilitating pain that forced me into a wheel chair, became severely anemic, and dropped twenty pounds in ten days. I was administered a vast dose of 100mg of intravenous steroids daily, which provoked more side effects than the initial symptoms they were intended to mitigate. After a weeklong stay in the two-room hospital in Kampala, the doctors concluded that the thirty-six-hour journey back to the US for a blood transfusion was imperative: doing so in a country rampant with disease was simply too risky.

That episode was the first of many that landed me in hospitals over and over again and launched me into a world of harsh drug therapies that only exacerbated my condition. It also led to a grave frustration with the lack of awareness the traditional medical establishment had regarding diet and alternative therapies. A mere twenty-five years old, I couldn't fathom the thought of taking immunosuppressant medications and being subjected to frequent flare-ups for the rest of my life. It was at that point that I

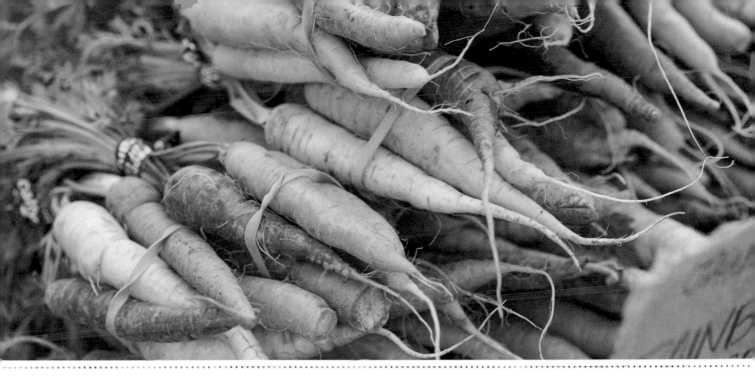

realized I would need to resort to my own research and acquired the tenacity to heal myself through food.

Two years after my initial diagnosis, I was introduced to the Specific Carbohydrate Diet (SCD), which has been used for decades to manage the symptoms of Crohn's disease, ulcerative colitis, celiac disease, and autism. Rather than resigning myself to a life sentence of pain and suffering, I went on the offensive. I implemented the SCD and began to feel minor relief almost immediately. It took a lot of time, and even more discipline, to see drastic changes, but the first inklings of improvement gave me hope. I knew I would have to start over entirely in the kitchen, but it was a small price to pay for my health.

After a few months of eating grain-free and witnessing an upswing in my health, I became pregnant and gave birth to my son, Asher, in the summer of 2010. As is often the case with autoimmune diseases, my symptoms disappeared while I was pregnant. When a woman is pregnant, her immune system essentially shuts down so as not to fight off the new "foreign object" in her body. This is beneficial for someone whose immune system is normally working overtime, falsely attacking otherwise healthy organs. The only problem was that because I felt well, I reverted to eating what had historically been comfort food for me—mainly pizza, ice cream, and French fries!

About nine months after Asher's birth, the hormonal shifts and my food indulgences caught up with me, and I experienced another major flare-up. I was hospitalized yet again, unable to take care of my baby and regretting the bad decisions I'd made while I was pregnant. In order to take care of my family, I had to take care of myself, meaning a strict return to a grain-free diet. With the tastes and textures of those "comfort" foods still fresh on my palate, I embarked on my quest to create versions of the dishes that I could actually enjoy and that my body could tolerate.

Danielle Walker

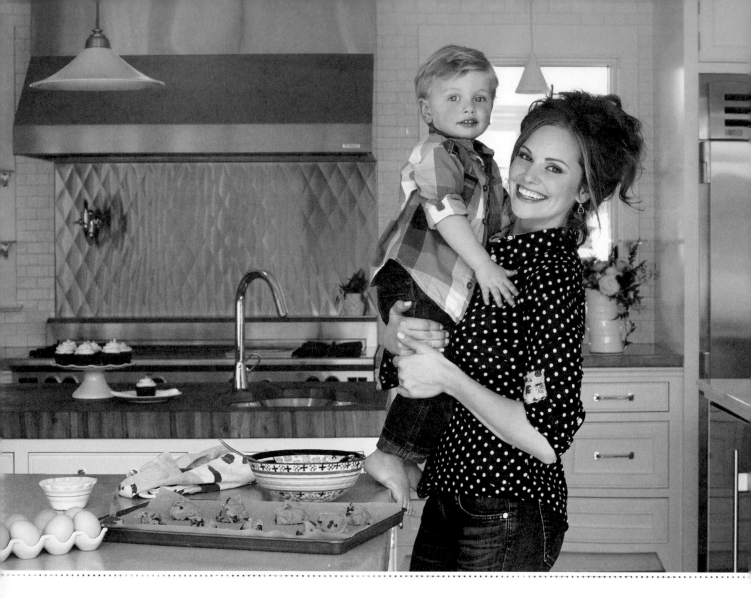

a time for change

As I began my culinary experimentations, I noticed a lack of innovative recipes as well as personal accounts of setbacks and progress, and wanted to document my journey to help others. I decided to combine the power of my acquired culinary skills, my love for food, and my equal love for journalism in an all-out crusade, and started my blog, Against All Grain. I aimed to not only end my own suffering, but also to become a source of hope for others suffering from all types of diseases or allergies.

I transformed my small home kitchen into a formidable command center for culinary operations. I spent, and still spend, countless hours reinventing recipes, converting the taboo and decadent into dishes that those who suffer from digestive disorders or autoimmune diseases can eat and enjoy. My goal was to banish the feeling of deprivation, to feel not just satisfied but exhilarated with each and every bite.

Because my disease was never fully in remission while on the SCD, I realized that I might still be consuming foods that were in fact hurting me. Over time, and with the help of a naturopath, I began to modify the SCD to fit my particular food sensitivities and started a supplement regimen to aid in healing my gut. Through trial and error, and health advances and setbacks, I discovered what my body could process and what it couldn't. I learned that each body may have different nuances and that there is not one diet that necessarily solves everyone's problems.

I also came to the realization that the way food is grown or raised (grass-fed versus grain-fed meat, for instance) was affecting my health. With these findings, I continued my research and discovered the Paleo diet, which excludes grains, legumes, refined sugars, and most dairy. This way of eating mimicked the direction I was already heading, and I embraced it wholeheartedly. Almost immediately, the remaining health issues I continued to experience while on the SCD began to dissipate.

My symptoms have continued to abate since making the transition to Paleo, and I have not experienced a flare-up since the summer of 2011. Like any human, though, I still struggle daily with making the right choices and my yearning to eat what everyone else does. What keeps me pressing onward is the knowledge that the Paleo diet allowed for such a drastic personal health transformation and how much it can benefit those with digestive and autoimmune disorders. I initially perceived this way of eating as a solution for my particular disease, but now continue to learn of the plethora of ailments it can also alleviate like diabetes, autism, and chronic fatigue syndrome, to name a few.

Never in my wildest dreams could I have imagined that my little blog would grow so rapidly in dedicated readership and have the ability to help so many people enjoy eating again, or that it would generate the opportunity to write a cookbook. I hope this book will be a medium to share my healing journey with a greater population than I could ever have reached with my blog, as well as make the transition to a grain-free diet enjoyable.

Within these pages is a collection of my most treasured Paleo recipes, including more than 125 never-before-published recipes that I stashed away especially for this book. There are also a few reader-favorites from my blog, many of which have been slightly altered, as my culinary skills and point of view are constantly evolving. It has been difficult keeping such savory secrets all to myself, so I am thrilled to finally share them with you!

Danielle Walker

paleo and the SCD guidelines

Paleo is not so much a diet as a way of life. In time, it will come naturally and you won't have to constantly question what you are and are not allowed to eat. For those new to Paleo, here are the basic guidelines of the lifestyle and the recipes in this book. As I still greatly respect the Specific Carbohydrate Diet and the healing it provides for those with gastrointestinal diseases, I am including the general guidelines for this protocol as well. You will see that they overlap in many areas.

Paleo is defined as "ancient or prehistoric." The Paleolithic, put simply, means reverting to the foods that our bodies were intended to consume and process.

eat

- Fish
- Grass-fed, pasture-raised meats
- Vegetables, including root vegetables
- Fruit
- Nuts and seeds
- Healthy oils and fats

avoid

- Grains (including corn and soy)
- Legumes
- Dairy
- Refined sugars
- Refined or hydrogenated oils
- Processed foods

suggested reading:

- *Practical Paleo* by Diane Sanfilippo
- *The Paleo Solution* by Robb Wolf

SCD is based on the theory that eliminating complex carbohydrates (those carbohydrates that require minimal digestion are still allowed) can reduce inflammation, restore a healthy gut ecosystem, and make eating enjoyable once again for people with gastrointestinal disorders.

eat

- Fish
- Meats
- Cooked vegetables and fruits
- Cultured cheeses
- 24-hour fermented yogurt
- Nuts and seeds in moderation
- Properly soaked legumes

avoid

- Grains
- Lactose
- Refined sugars
- Starchy vegetables
- Chocolate
- Processed and canned foods

suggested reading:

- *Breaking the Vicious Cycle: Intestinal Health Through Diet* by Elaine Gloria Gottschall

let's get cooking!

My best advice for people just starting out in the grain-free world is to experiment. Years of trial and error in the kitchen led me to write this book and my blog, and have also kept our meals lively and fresh. I suggest following each recipe exactly as written when you take your first stab at it. Once you have an idea of the intended flavors, you can let your taste buds be your guide and let your imagination go crazy. Leave out the garlic if you have a hot date, or add an extra pinch of red pepper flakes to spice things up. Swap raisins for cranberries, chicken for beef, kale for spinach, chocolate for currants, or rosemary for thyme.

feel free to play with ingredients and have fun!

The recipes in this book are meant to appeal to all palates, regardless of your medical condition. But there is no one-size-fits-all recipe, so I have created a labeling system that allows you to easily decipher which recipes will fit your personal dietary needs:

EF NF SCD V

EF
egg-free

NF
nut-free

SCD
specific carbohydrate diet

V
vegan

Danielle Walker

achieving maximum results

⑨ I recommend always reading through a recipe in its entirety before getting started. Then, gather the ingredients and tools you will need and set up your *mise en place* (have everything in its place). This will save you time and make the entire process much more enjoyable. You will notice that I sometimes list an ingredient with its preparation method—such as, "1 medium onion, finely diced"—because it is helpful to have these ingredients ready to go before you start to cook. This way, you will not be frantically chopping that onion while your meat is burning in the pan waiting for said onion to be added.

⑨ Many serious bakers will scoff at the lack of weights in my recipes. I wanted this book to be accessible to everyone, whether a novice or seasoned chef, and recognize that not everyone owns a kitchen scale or understands ratios. There are conversion charts in the back of the book for those that prefer to bake by weights or live outside of the United States. In my experiments with grain-free baking, I have found that it is easier to measure rather than weigh. This is because when I am testing recipes I frequently add a teaspoon of coconut flour if the batter is too moist, or increase the fat by a tablespoon the next time if the result came out too dry.

⑨ For the purpose of these recipes, use the scoop-and-sweep method for measuring flour: fluff up the flour in your package with a fork, dip the cup or spoon into the flour to scoop it up, and then sweep the top level with the back of a knife. If you double a recipe that calls for coconut flour, I recommend measuring out the ingredients twice. This may sound tedious, but coconut flour is very finicky, and even an extra half-teaspoon can change the texture of baked goods.

I am brimming with excitement to finally share my heart and soul with you, so let's get to the food shall we? I hope you experience as much joy from the recipes on these pages as I did in creating them for you.

wishing you health and happy cooking!

Danielle

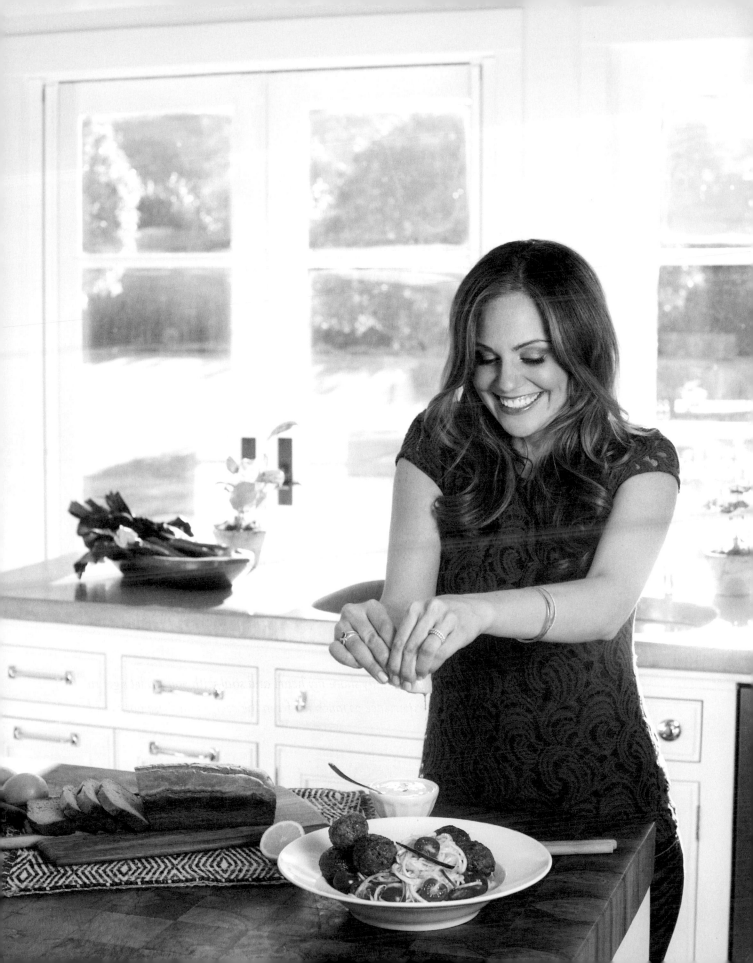

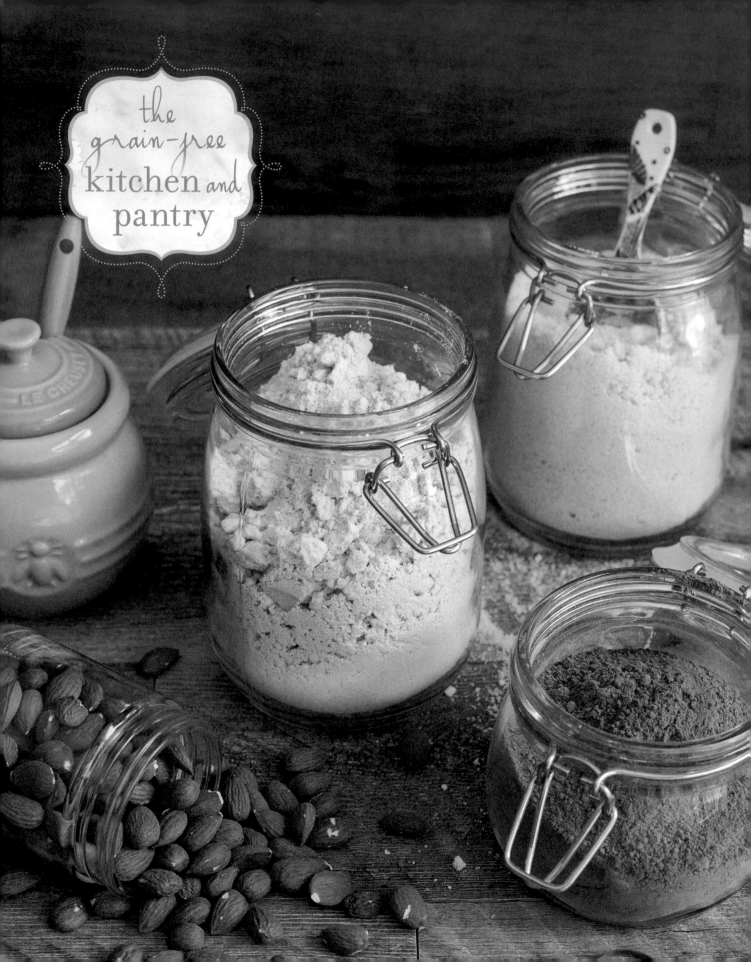

the grain-free
kitchen and
pantry

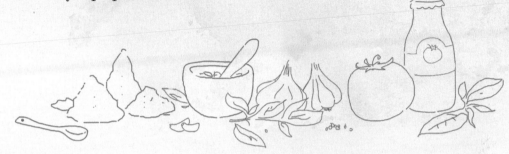

navigating a new lifestyle

If you're new to grain-free, get ready to completely overhaul your pantry, refrigerator, and freezer. Save your all-purpose flour for making play dough and your white sugar for plant food, because they will no longer be of any other use to you. Instead, you will be stocking up on protein-rich almond flour, fiber-rich coconut flour, and immune-boosting honey.

The cost of grain-free ingredients may not be a pleasant surprise if you're just starting out. It is unfortunate that real foods are more expensive than the processed and factory-farmed alternatives, but there's nothing more valuable than your health. Here are a few tips to make your dollar go further.

shop in bulk and online when possible

If you have the space to store excess goods, be it in the garage or an additional closet, buy in bulk. Ingredients like almond flour, coconut milk, coconut flour, and nuts can be found cheaper online, especially when purchased in large quantities. Store half in the freezer or go in on a large order with friends. A lot of sites also offer promotions like discounts or free shipping. Keep an eye out for them, and stock up when you see one.

buy local

How my food is grown and where it comes from is important to me. Fresh and organic produce is not only better for our bodies and the environment, but it also amplifies the flavors of a finished dish. I prefer to use fresh citrus juices and will always choose fresh herbs over dried if the season is right. In fact, if you have the space, planting an herb garden is an inexpensive way to ensure fresh, organic herbs whenever you need them.

Farmers' markets are a great place to purchase local produce, pastured-raised meats, and eggs for many reasons. The produce at these markets is left in the field until it reaches maximum ripeness, then picked at its peak nutrient and flavor state and transported directly to the stands. Most foods in supermarkets are picked when they are under-ripe, travel an average of 1,500 miles, and are then sprayed with gasses to expedite ripening before being placed on the store shelves.

Aside from avoiding chemicals and pesticides, purchasing directly from your local farmers is a great way to give back to your community. Most local farmers are trying to make a living from their crops, and receive a much better return selling it directly than if they were to try to compete with the big-business agriculture monopolies. Because of this, they price their goods closer to wholesale cost. For even deeper discounts, try hitting your market at the end of the day and asking for discounts on mildly bruised or slightly damaged fruits and vegetables. These minimal blemishes will make them look less appealing, but ultimately don't change the quality of the food. The vendor's goal is to sell all of their goods that day and would prefer to not have to pack up or waste any, so they may oblige.

pick and choose

I believe that purchasing grass-fed meat and organic produce is essential, but I know it can add up. To save money on produce, follow the "dirty dozen" rule, always buying organic for the 12 fruits and vegetables that are on the left side of the chart. You can offset the overall cost by occasionally buying conventionally-grown produce as long as it is one that is listed as a lower pesticide food on the right side of the chart.

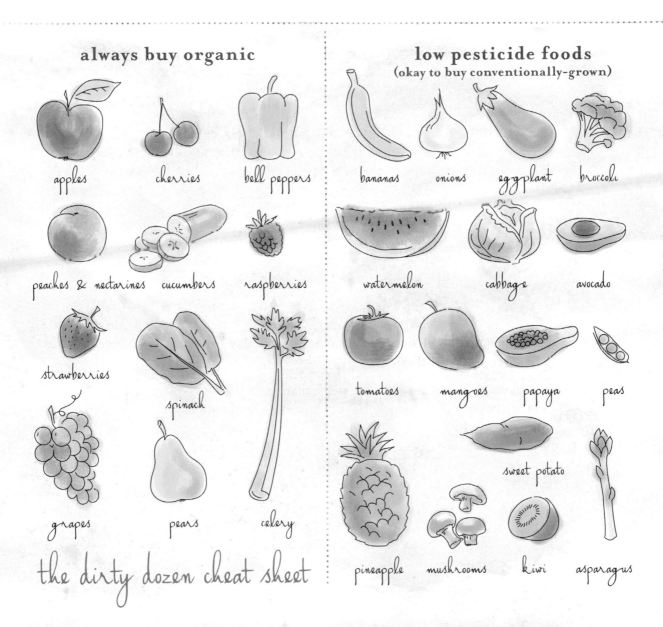

always buy organic

apples   cherries   bell peppers

peaches & nectarines   cucumbers   raspberries

strawberries   spinach

grapes   pears   celery

the dirty dozen cheat sheet

low pesticide foods
(okay to buy conventionally-grown)

bananas   onions   eggplant   broccoli

watermelon   cabbage   avocado

tomatoes   mangoes   papaya   peas

sweet potato

pineapple   mushrooms   kiwi   asparagus

When it comes to meat, avoid purchasing precut pieces if you can. A beef or pork roast will be cheaper than a steak because butchers charge for the labor of slicing and trimming. Cook the whole roast and then slice it, or learn how to butcher your meat online. Purchasing whole animals is always the most economical choice, but most of us do not have the storage space, let alone the know-how, for this. If grass-fed is important to you, but is out of your budget, go for inexpensive cuts of meat. The more expensive cuts tend to be naturally tender and cook quickly with little preparation, but you can purchase less-expensive cuts such as chuck roasts or shanks that still make an exquisite meal. This is especially true if you marinate, braise, or slow cook the meat to tenderize it.

If that is daunting, buying an entire chicken and dividing it up at home is much less intimidating than dealing with an entire cow. Many butchers will segment it for you if asked but will generally not skin or bone it for you. You can learn to do this yourself fairly easily, or opt to work with the whole chicken for better flavor. The feet, head, and neck can be used to make a nutrient-dense bone broth or stock so no part goes unused.

Keep your eyes peeled for sales and stock up when you can. If properly packaged, most meat can be frozen for a year.

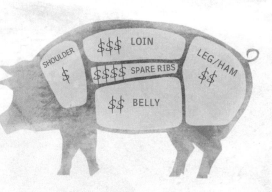

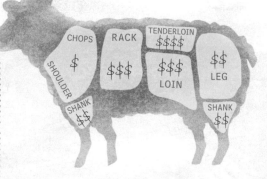

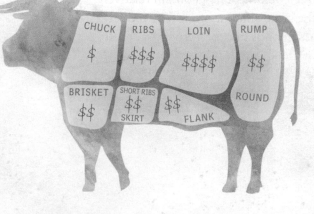

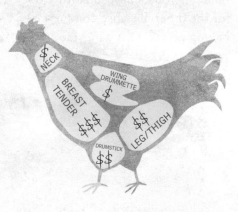

my ingredients

almond flour

is simply blanched, skinless almonds that are finely ground into flour. The finer the grind, the better your baked goods will turn out. Coarsely ground brands such as Bob's Red Mill will result in overly moist products that will sink in the center or have a grainy texture. I recommend purchasing your flour online from Digestive Wellness or Honeyville Farms. For the purpose of this book, I refer to this type of almond flour as "blanched almond flour."

almond meal

is similar to almond flour, but it is coarser and the skins have generally not been removed. It works wonderfully for breading fish or poultry or as a breadcrumb substitute, but does not work well in baked goods.

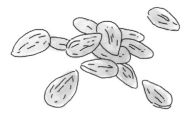

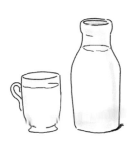

almond milk

is easy to prepare (see page 314) and more delicious when homemade. If using store-bought, always buy the unsweetened original flavor and compare brands to find the one with the fewest ingredients.

baking soda

and baking powder are not one in the same, so you cannot substitute one for the other. Because commercial baking powders contain starch, the recipes in this book call for only baking soda, which is used as a leavening and browning agent.

cashews

are a super food for dairy- and grain-free cooking. They contain relatively the same amount of protein and fat as almonds but their flavor is almost invisible and they add a velvety texture to dishes. I use them a lot as a substitute for cream in soups or sauces. If you cannot tolerate cashews but can handle dairy, you will have good results substituting grass-fed cream. In recipes for baked goods that call for whole raw cashews or raw cashew butter, you may also use macadamia nuts.

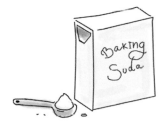

Danielle Walker

chocolate chips

are a sweet addition to baked goods and treats. I try to use unsweetened chocolate and sweeten it naturally as often as possible, but I recognize the convenience of packaged chocolate chips. I typically purchase brands that are free of soy, dairy, and gluten, such as Enjoy Life.

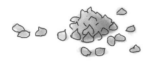

coconut aminos,

made from naturally aged coconut sap blended with sea salt, are a soy- and gluten-free soy sauce substitute. They are low-glycemic but are slightly sweeter than soy sauce.

As this product was not yet available when the SCD was written, there is no concrete answer as to whether they are allowed on this diet. However, they are widely accepted and used throughout the SCD world because they are fermented and made from coconut. I chose to include them in the recipes that are labeled SCD, but please use your own discretion.

coconut crystals,

also known as coconut sugar, or coconut sap sugar, are produced from the sap of the flower buds of the coconut palm tree. They have been used as a traditional sweetener for thousands of years and have a very low glycemic index.

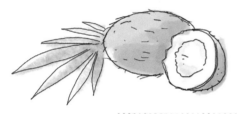

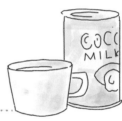

coconut flour

is made by drying and finely grinding the meat of a coconut. It is packed with dietary fiber and protein, and is a naturally gluten-free flour alternative. The high fiber content also keeps sugars from being absorbed into the bloodstream. It is a great alternative for those with nut or wheat allergies, but can be somewhat tricky to bake with. Even an extra teaspoon can yield a different result in baked goods.

coconut milk

is made by puréeing the meat and water from a coconut. Avoid the boxed coconut milk 'beverages' typically sold in the refrigerated section of grocery stores, as they contain additives and stabilizers to retain a liquid consistency. Instead, look for canned coconut milk (in BPA-free cans) that contains only coconut and water and are preferably free of guar gum, which some people may be sensitive to.

coconut oil

is a healthy fat that is extracted from the meat of the coconut. It has many medicinal properties and is used in food as well as skin-care products. It is heat stable, slow to oxidize, and resistant to rancidity, making it suitable for high-temperature cooking or frying. It is solid at room temperature (except when the room has no air-conditioning and it's summer!) and is wonderful to bake with. It is always best to use virgin coconut oil.

fish sauce

is a salty condiment used in Thai and other Asian cuisines. I also use it in recipes that would typically contain worcestershire sauce as it contributes a similar salty flavor. Look for bottles that contain only anchovy and salt, such as Red Boat brand.

gelatin

is my preferred thickener and binder, especially for desserts. I buy the Great Lakes brand gelatin as it is grass-fed. Gelatin offers many health benefits for the gut, hair, and nails. Kosher fish gelatins are also available for those that prefer it for religious or personal reasons.

ghee

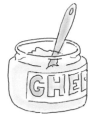

is clarified butter, which means the milk solids have been almost entirely removed, leaving only the healthy butterfat behind. Very pure ghee is 99 percent pure butter oil but may have trace amounts of casein and lactose. Unless you are extremely sensitive, it will normally not cause problems, even if other dairy does. As the recipes in this book are dairy-free, ghee is occasionally recommended as an alternative fat but is never a required ingredient.

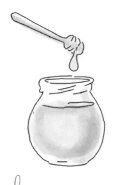

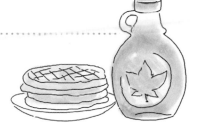

honey

is the most commonly used sweetener in this book. Raw, local, organic honey has incredible health benefits. It is both an energy and immune booster and can greatly help with seasonal allergies if you purchase it locally. Honey contains only monosaccharaides (single sugars), making it easier for the body to absorb and process.

maple syrup

is a natural, unrefined, liquid sweetener that I often use to enhance the flavors of baked goods or savory dishes. Use pure grade B maple syrup or substitute honey if desired.

nuts and seeds

are a good source of protein and are frequently used to mimic grains. I soak and dehydrate all of my whole raw nuts to remove the harmful phytic acid that makes them difficult to digest, but raw and dry-roasted nuts and seeds will also work in my recipes. If you are using soaked and dehydrated nuts and seeds for the "raw nuts" called for in recipes, make sure that they are completely dried and crispy before using.

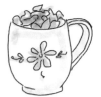

Danielle Walker

olive oil

is a great source of heart-healthy fat and is high in Vitamin E and antioxidants. I'm an Italian girl at heart and use extra-virgin olive oil often for cold foods or foods cooked over moderate heat. Because it can oxidize at high heats, olive oil is not ideal for deep or pan frying.

palm shortening

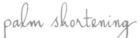

is used as a butter substitute in my baked goods recipes. It has a firm texture and a high melting point, creating fluffy and cakelike delights. Be sure to purchase this oil from sustainable and eco-friendly sources, such as Tropical Traditions. Unsalted grass-fed butter may be used as a substitute if you can tolerate dairy.

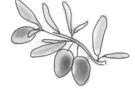

raw cacao butter

is the pure oil extracted from the cacao bean. You can find it on Amazon or at most local health stores.

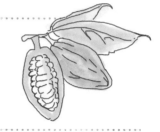

sea salt

brightens the flavor of any dish. I use either Celtic or Himalayan pink sea salt, both of which are unbleached, unrefined, and contain healthy trace minerals. If substituting table salt for the sea salt in my recipes, start with half the amount and adjust to taste.

spices and herbs

add flavor and complexity to any dish. When possible, I use fresh herbs, which provide a more pungent flavor, but will substitute dried if needed. Typically, use half the required measurement when substituting dried herbs and spices for fresh.

tomato products

sold in the United States often contain ingredients besides tomatoes such as citric acid or other stabilizers. I use either Pomi or Bionaturae brands because they have no added ingredients and come in BPA-free containers.

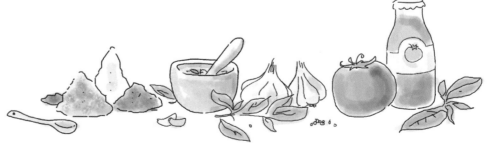

my equipment

blender:

Grain-free and dairy-free cooking requires extra preparation, and a good blender can save you a lot of time. I use mine to create smooth doughs and batters, purée soups, and whip up smoothies. If you can afford one, a Blendtec is a fabulous machine that can pulverize virtually anything. Its twister jar is amazing for nut butters, salad dressings, mayonnaise, and single servings of smoothies.

dehydrator:

I use this machine most often for dried fruit, fruit roll-ups, dehydrating soaked nuts, or my famous granola. It can also be used for beef jerky or even to make homemade Coconut Milk Yogurt (page 46).

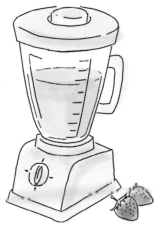

food processor:

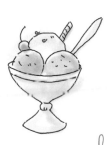

This machine will chop or grate vegetables and fruit, grind whole nuts, and purée cooked vegetables. Most models have a greater capacity than blenders and therefore offer more versatility in food preparation.

ice cream maker:

While not a necessity, an ice cream maker is a great kitchen toy, especially if you have denounced your formerly favorite brands of ice cream for the sake of your health. There are quite a few dairy- and refined-sugar-free ice cream recipes in this book so you and your family can enjoy frozen treats all summer long. You don't have to spend a lot to get a good machine, and if you have a Kitchen Aid mixer you can buy an ice cream bowl attachment to save cupboard space.

parchment paper:

Because it is generally fairly sticky, I always roll grain-free dough out between two pieces of parchment paper. Lining a roasting pan with parchment paper makes for easy clean up, and covering the bottom of cake and loaf pans with a piece means your breads and cakes won't stick.

Danielle Walker

pots and pans:

My all-time favorite pots and pans are Le Creuset. They're made with nontoxic materials, heat quickly and evenly, and are a cinch to clean. Stainless-steel pots are also wonderful, and you can usually find whole sets discounted at stores like Costco or Home Goods. I recommend having at least a 2-quart saucepan, a 9-inch skillet, and a 3.5-quart Dutch oven on hand.

sharp knives:

Eating a whole foods diet entails quite a bit more preparation than a processed foods diet, so a good set of sharp knives is a must. I had to save up and purchase my knives one at a time, but it was well worth it. I use the Japanese brand Shun, but Wusthof and J.A. Henckels are also reputable brands. I recommend that every home-cook have a paring knife, a 5.5-inch Santoku knife, a carving knife, and a serrated knife in their arsenal. I also recommend that you have your knives professionally sharpened at least twice a year.

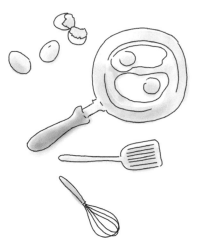

slow cooker:

A slow cooker, or Crock-Pot, is incredibly handy for a busy cook—and who isn't busy these days? There's nothing like coming home after a hectic day at the office or carpooling kids to a gazillion activities to a house full of delectable smells and a complete meal waiting for you.

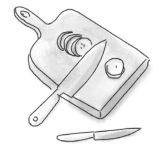

spiralizer:

The winner in the creativity department, this inexpensive gizmo can turn almost any vegetable into a strand of noodles, making meals more exciting for kids and adults alike. You can buy one for as little as $30, but a less expensive julienne slicer will achieve somewhat similar results.

stand or hand mixer:

Electric stand mixers work wonders when it comes to beating frosting, making meringue, or preparing cookie dough. While a stand mixer is convenient and doesn't require any manual labor, an electric hand mixer takes up less kitchen space and will get the job done and at a fraction of the cost.

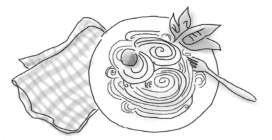

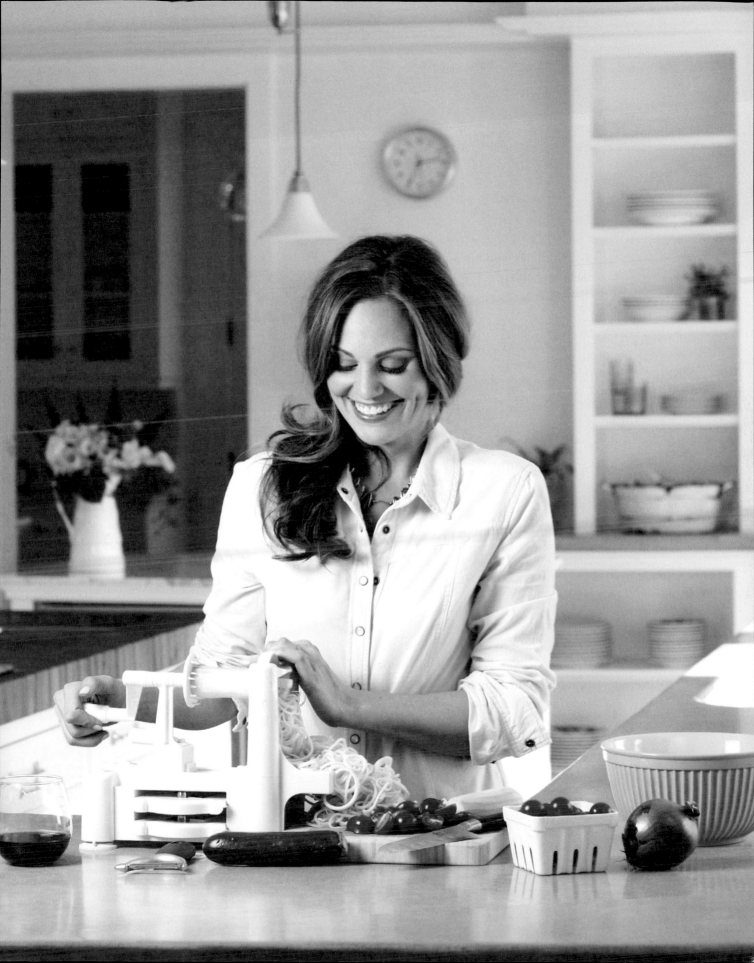

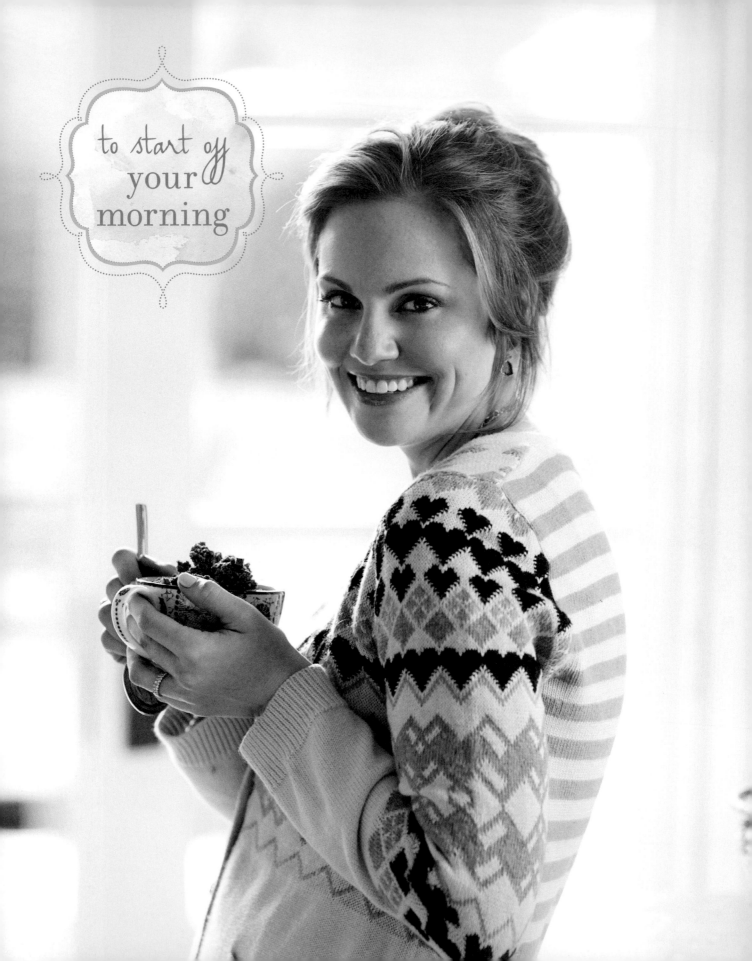

to start off
your
morning

smoked salmon eggs benedict

prep time: 20 minutes   cooking time: 15 minutes   yield: 4 servings

*to start off
your morning*

Hollandaise sauce and poached eggs can appear intimidating to make at first glance. However, with my techniques, you are sure to succeed and will want to make this dish over and over again as your confidence grows. I use palm shortening, rather than coconut oil, because its texture and flavor better mimic butter's. Eggs Benedict is a rich and satisfying morning meal, and I have replaced the traditional Canadian bacon with smoked salmon for its juicy boost of omega-3s.

ingredients

HOLLANDAISE SAUCE

- 2 egg yolks
- 2 teaspoons fresh lemon juice
- ¼ cup palm shortening or ghee, melted
- ¼ teaspoon sea salt
- Dash cayenne pepper or paprika

EVERYTHING ELSE

- 4 eggs
- 1 tablespoon white vinegar
- 4 cups baby spinach
- 8 slices smoked salmon
- 2 teaspoons capers

method

1. Make the hollandaise sauce. Place the egg yolks and lemon juice in a bowl and whisk vigorously. Set the bowl over a pot of boiling water, making sure to keep the bowl from touching the water. Continue whisking over the heat for 5 minutes. Slowly drizzle in the melted shortening, whisking constantly. Whisk until the sauce is thick and doubled in volume. Stir in seasonings and remove from heat. Cover with a towel to keep warm until ready for use.

2. To poach the eggs, bring a deep saucepan with 3 inches of water to a boil. Crack each egg into its own little bowl. Add the vinegar to the water and lower the heat so the water is simmering gently. Carefully slide each egg into the water. Cover the pan and remove from the heat. Poach the eggs for 7 to 8 minutes, or until the whites are cooked. Remove the eggs with a slotted spoon onto a plate lined with a paper towel.

3. **To serve:** Place 1 cup spinach, 2 slices smoked salmon, 1 poached egg, and ½ teaspoon capers on each plate and drizzle with hollandaise sauce.

tidbits:

If the hollandaise starts to separate or curdle, whisk in 1 teaspoon water at a time until the sauce is smooth again. If needed, reheat gently over a pot of simmering water. Do not microwave sauce or heat directly on a burner.

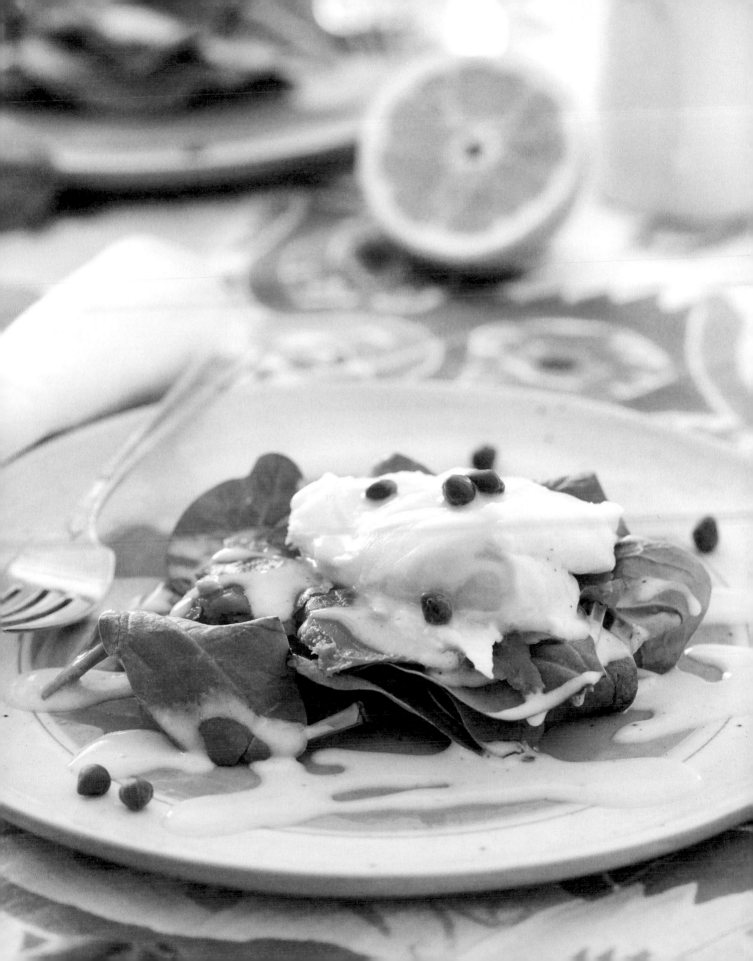

maple sage sausage
with cinnamon apples

prep time: 15 minutes   cooking time: 15 minutes   yield: 4 to 6 servings

This breakfast combination is the perfect marriage of savory and sweet and provides a tasty alternative for those with egg allergies. Making homemade sausage is quite simple, but you can always purchase sage breakfast sausage.

ingredients

- 1 pound ground pork
- 2 teaspoons chopped sage
- 2 teaspoons maple syrup*
- ¾ teaspoon coarse sea salt
- ¼ teaspoon cracked black pepper
- ¼ teaspoon nutmeg
- ⅛ teaspoon crushed red pepper
- ⅛ teaspoon marjoram
- 2 apples, cored, peeled, and sliced
- ½ teaspoon cinnamon

method

1. Heat a skillet over medium-high heat.

2. Place the pork, sage, maple syrup, salt, pepper, nutmeg, red pepper, and marjoram in a bowl and combine well. Form the mixture into patties 2-inches wide and ½-inch thick.

3. Fry the sausage patties in the skillet until cooked through, about 2 to 3 minutes per side. Remove the patties and drain on a plate lined with a paper towel.

4. Sauté the apples and cinnamon in the same skillet for 8 minutes, or until tender. Return the sausage to the skillet and reheat for 2 minutes.

For SCD, substitute honey for the maple syrup.

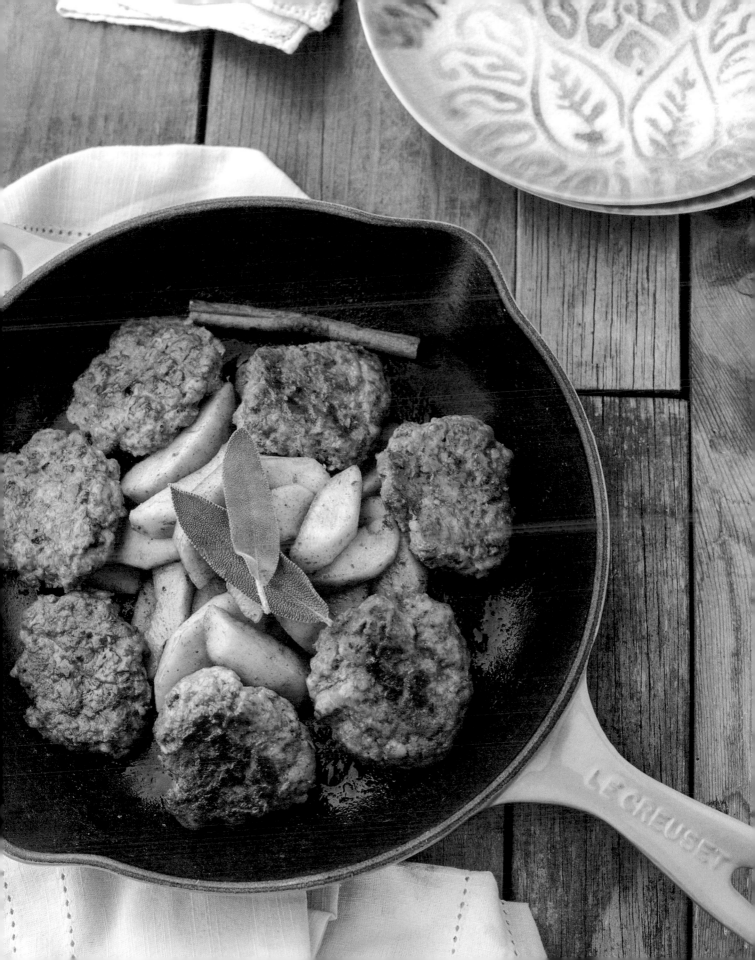

spanish frittata with chorizo

prep time: 15 minutes   cooking time: 18 minutes   yield: 4 servings

A frittata is a gratifying way to use up vegetables and is easy to throw together on a hectic morning. We even make them for dinner on nights when I don't feel like standing over the stove, because the oven does the majority of the work for you—no stirring or flipping of an omelet or scrambled eggs.

ingredients

- 2 tablespoons coconut oil
- ½ pound chorizo sausage, uncooked
- 1 small sweet potato*, scrubbed and shredded (about 1 cup)
- ½ cup sliced yellow bell pepper
- ¼ cup diced yellow onion
- 8 eggs
- 1 teaspoon coconut milk
- ¼ teaspoon sea salt
- 2 Roma tomatoes, sliced
- Garnish: avocado slices and freshly chopped cilantro

method

1. Preheat the oven to 350°F.
2. Heat the oil in an oven-safe skillet over medium heat.
3. Add the sausage, sweet potato, yellow pepper, and onion and sauté for 4 minutes.
4. Beat the eggs with the coconut milk and salt then pour into the skillet and cook for 2 minutes.
5. Arrange the tomato slices in a circular pattern on top of the eggs. Place the frittata in the oven and bake for 12 minutes.
6. Serve with avocado and cilantro.

For SCD, substitute peeled and shredded butternut squash for the sweet potato.

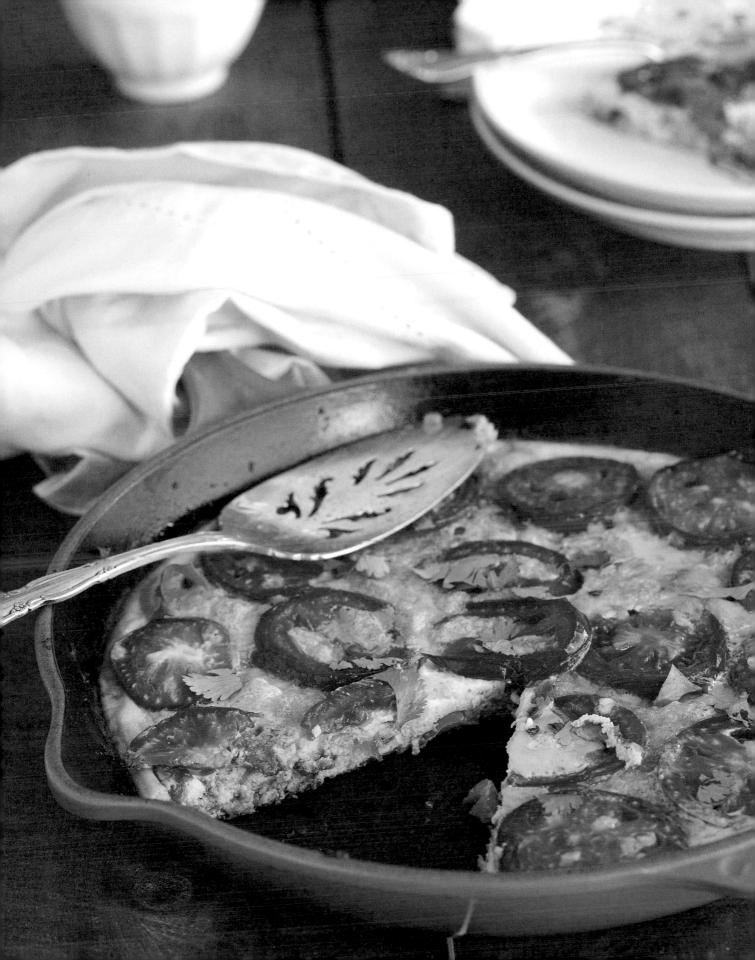

blueberry waffles

prep time: 5 minutes   cooking time: 15 minutes   yield: 4 to 6 servings

*to start off
your morning*

These fluffy waffles are a special weekend treat for us. The first time I made them, my husband Ryan exclaimed that they were the closest things to the real deal I had ever created. They have been a staple in our house for a couple of years, and he would never let it be any other way!

ingredients

- 3 large eggs, at room temperature
- ½ cup coconut milk
- 3 tablespoons honey or maple syrup
- 3 tablespoons coconut oil, melted
- ½ teaspoon pure vanilla extract
- 1 cup raw cashews or macadamia nuts
- 3 tablespoons coconut flour
- ¾ teaspoons baking soda
- ¼ teaspoon sea salt
- ½ cup blueberries

method

1. Preheat a waffle iron to the lowest setting.

2. Place all the ingredients in the order listed, except the blueberries, in a high-speed blender.

3. Blend on low for 30 seconds, then increase to high and continue blending until the batter is completely smooth, about another 30 seconds.

4. Spoon the batter into the waffle iron, filling halfway and spreading evenly. Sprinkle a handful of blueberries over the batter.

5. Close the lid and cook for 45 seconds to 1 minute, until the steam stops rising from the machine and the waffles easily release with a fork. Keep them in a warm oven while you finish making the rest of the waffles.

tidbits:

If you don't have a high-speed blender, grind the nuts in a food processor first. It may take a bit longer to blend, and you may have to use a spatula to scrape the batter down the sides of the jar to mix thoroughly.

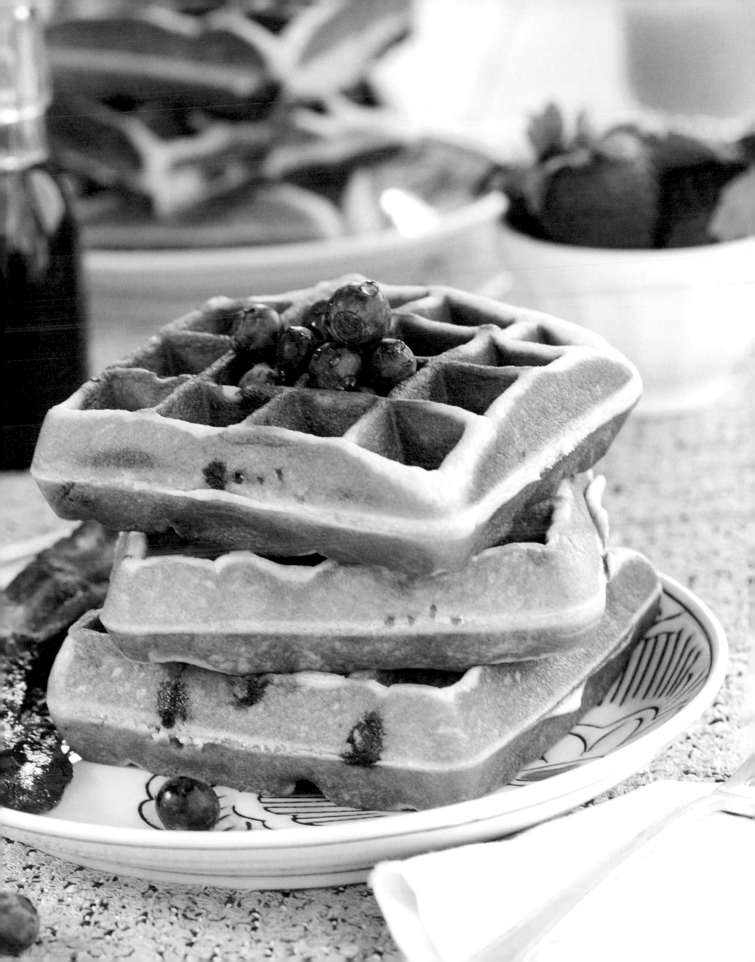

sausage quiche
with sweet potato crust

prep time: 20 minutes   cooking time: 25–30 minutes   yield: 8 servings

Thinly sliced sweet potatoes provide a savory grain-free crust for this piping-hot quiche. You can prepare the whole thing the night before and just pop it into the oven in the morning for an elegant breakfast that is as appealing to the eye as it is to the palate!

ingredients

- Extra-virgin olive oil for greasing pan
- 1 medium sweet potato*
- ½ pound sugar-free breakfast sausage, casings removed and crumbled
- 1 teaspoon chopped fresh rosemary
- 10 eggs
- 3 tablespoons coconut milk
- ½ teaspoon sea salt
- ⅛ teaspoon cracked black pepper

method

1. Preheat the oven to 350°F.

2. Spread a very thin layer of olive oil around the bottom and sides of a pie plate.

3. Scrub the sweet potato and dry it with a towel.

4. Using a mandolin or a sharp knife, thinly slice the potato into ⅛-inch-thick disks.

5. Arrange the sweet potatoes in a concentric pattern, slightly overlapping them so they completely cover the bottom of the pie plate.

6. Spread the sausage in a thin layer over the potatoes, trying to cover the entire surface.

7. Press the rosemary gently into the sausage.

8. Place the eggs, coconut milk, salt, and pepper in a bowl and whisk vigorously.

9. Pour the beaten egg mixture into the dish, gently pressing down any sausage bits that float up.

10. Bake for 25 to 30 minutes, or until the center is set and the eggs have puffed up.

*For SCD, substitute peeled butternut squash
for the sweet potato.*

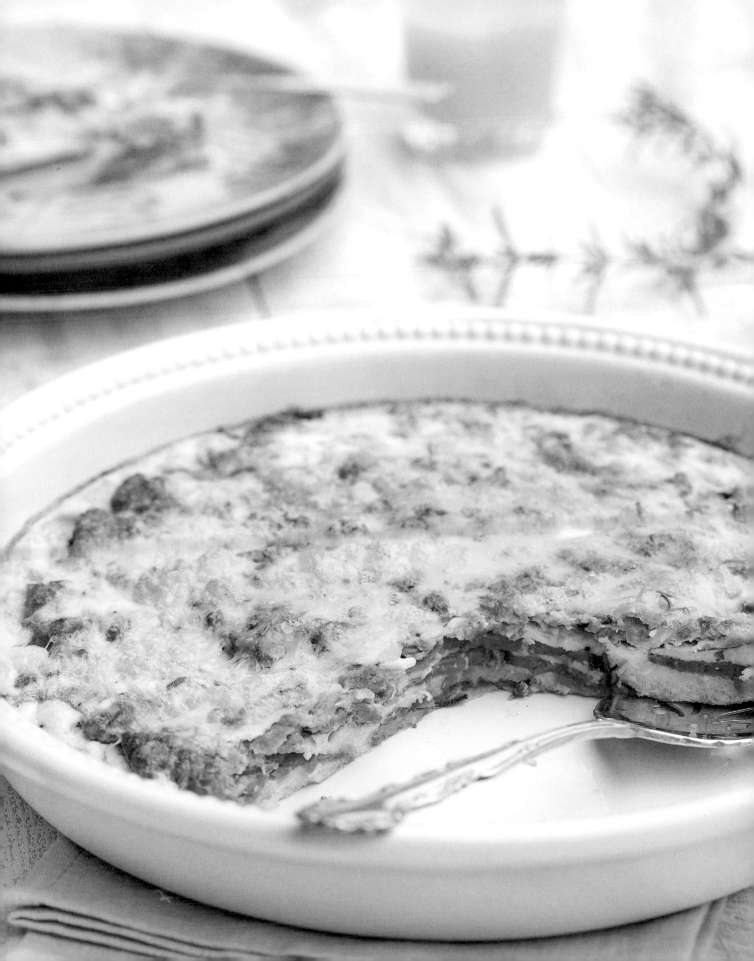

sausage and tomato baked eggs

prep time: 15 minutes   cooking time: 20 minutes   yield: 4 servings

I put an Italian twist on the traditional French dish oeufs en cocotte to create one of our all-time favorite breakfast dishes. The coconut milk tomato sauce ends up tasting like melted cheese (don't ask, just taste!), and the eggs are cooked to perfection with the yolks slightly runny.

ingredients

- ¼ pound sausage, casings removed and crumbled
- 1 cup baby spinach, chopped
- 1 Roma tomato, thinly sliced
- ¼ cup coconut milk
- 1½ teaspoons tomato paste
- 1 heaping teaspoon almond meal
- ¼ teaspoon oregano
- ¼ teaspoon sea salt
- 4 eggs
- Extra-virgin olive oil for greasing

method

1. Preheat the oven to 350°F.

2. Grease 4 shallow individual-size baking dishes with olive oil. Layer each with the sausage, spinach, and tomatoes, dividing the ingredients equally among the 4 dishes.

3. Place the coconut milk, tomato paste, almond meal, oregano, and salt in a small bowl and whisk to combine.

4. Drizzle the sauce over the layered ingredients, dividing evenly among the dishes.

5. Place the dishes on a baking sheet and bake for 15 minutes, then remove from oven and increase the temperature to 400°F.

6. Crack an egg into each dish, being careful not to break the yolk.

7. Return to the tray to the oven and bake 5 to 7 minutes longer, or until the whites are cooked but the yolk is still soft.

tidbits:

Any sausage will work, but my favorite choice for this recipe is mild Italian. Just check the labels carefully: sausage tends to have a lot of unhealthy ingredients, like nitrates and sugars.

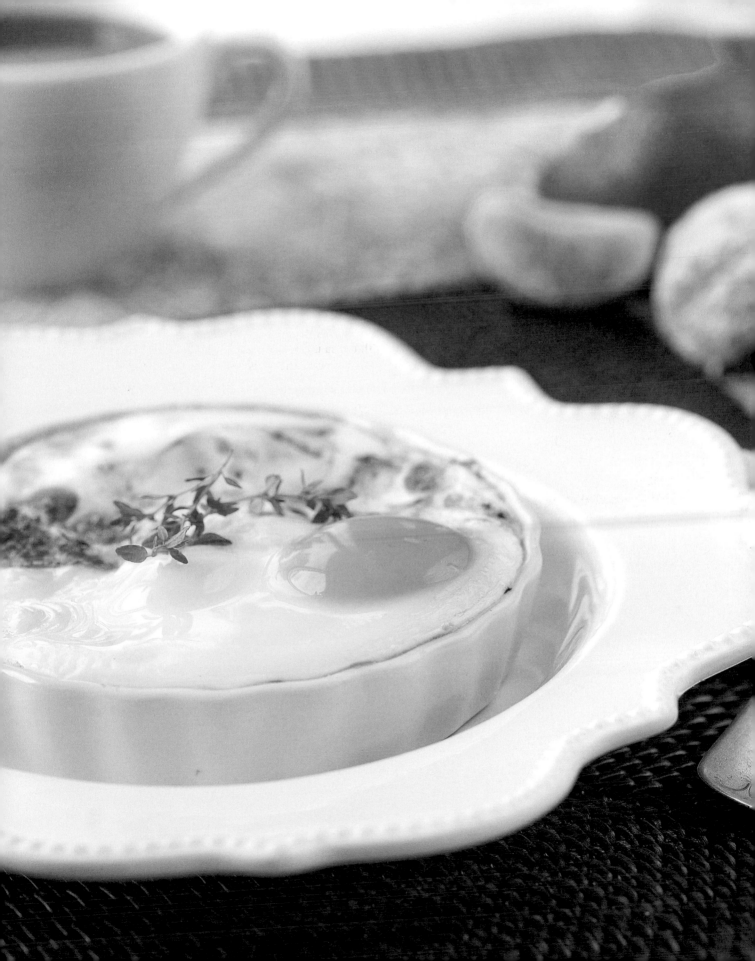

asparagus, leek, and prosciutto quiche

prep time: 20 minutes   cooking time: 55 minutes   yield: 1 9-inch pie

This quiche is sure to impress at your next brunch gathering with its colorful vegetables and briny prosciutto. Its light but full-bodied goodness is encased in a flaky crust made from almond flour, ensuring that the flavors will melt in your mouth like butter.

ingredients

- 1 recipe Pastry Crust, par-baked for 12 minutes (page 310)
- 2 teaspoons extra-virgin olive oil
- 1 leek, thinly sliced (white and light green parts only)
- 1 pound asparagus, stalks trimmed and thinly sliced on the diagonal
- 2 ounces prosciutto, chopped
- 6 eggs
- ¼ cup almond milk
- ½ cup coconut milk
- ½ teaspoon sea salt
- ¼ teaspoon black pepper
- Dash nutmeg

method

1. Preheat the oven to 325°F.

2. Heat the oil in a skillet over medium heat. Add the leek, asparagus, and prosciutto and sauté for 6 to 8 minutes, or until tender.

3. Place the eggs, almond milk, coconut milk, salt, pepper, and nutmeg in a bowl and beat to combine.

4. Cover the edges of the par-baked crust with foil or a pie shield.

5. Spread the vegetable mixture over the bottom of the crust. Pour the egg mixture over it, place in the oven, and bake for 25 to 30 minutes, or until the center jiggles slightly but is not liquid. Cool to room temperature before serving.

tidbits:

If using a tart pan with a removable bottom, place on a rimmed baking sheet to bake the quiche.

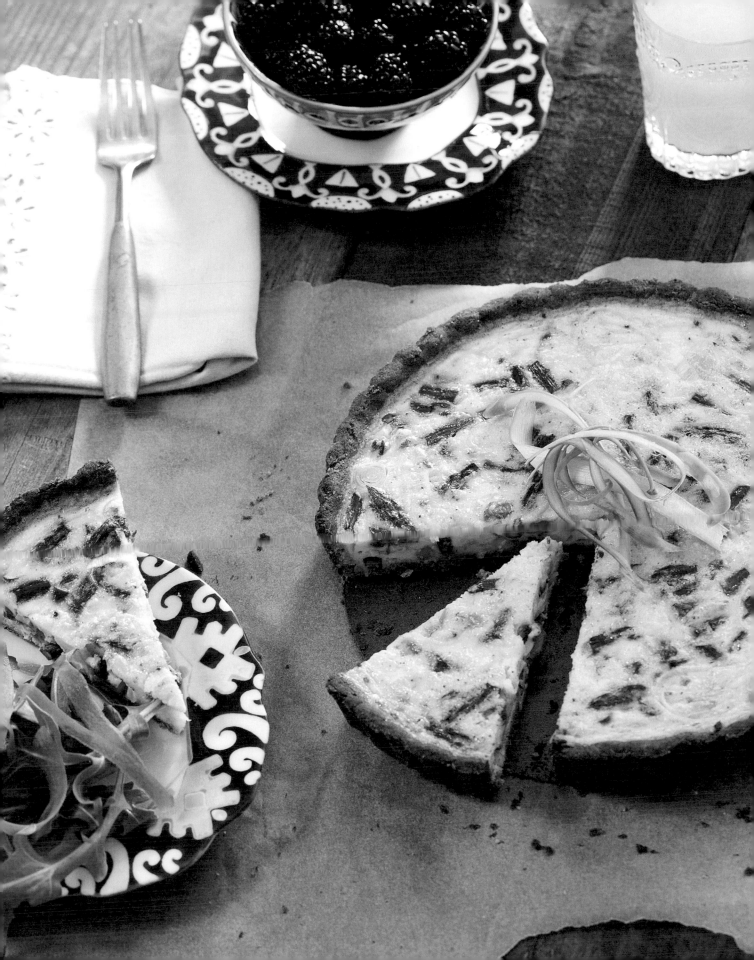

pear-berry crisp

prep time: 20 minutes   cooking time: 35 minutes   yield: 6 to 8 servings

I debated about whether to put this recipe in the treats section or the breakfast section, and decided to place it here as there are so many people who are allergic to eggs looking for an alternative morning meal. Because this crisp is full of various fruits, it's sweet in its natural state and doesn't need anything extra. The crunch of the topping is reminiscent of the typical oat topping you're probably accustomed to, but with a deeper flavor profile that compliments the tart berries. Of course, feel free to dollop with coconut whipped cream, yogurt, or vanilla coconut ice cream as an after-dinner treat!

ingredients

- 3 pounds red pears, cored, peeled, and sliced
- 2 cups blackberries
- 1 cup blueberries
- 1 tablespoon fresh lemon juice
- 2 teaspoons coconut flour
- ¼ teaspoon sea salt
- ¼ teaspoon cinnamon
- ¼ teaspoon allspice

TOPPING

- 2 tablespoons coconut oil, in solid form + ½ teaspoon for greasing pan
- ⅔ cup raw almonds
- ⅔ cup raw pecan halves
- 4 dates, pitted
- 2 tablespoons shredded, unsweetened coconut
- 1½ teaspoons cinnamon
- ¼ teaspoon sea salt

method

1. Preheat the oven to 375°F.

2. Place the pears and berries in a bowl. Add the lemon juice, coconut flour, salt, cinnamon, and allspice and stir to combine.

3. Grease a 1-quart baking dish with ½ teaspoon coconut oil. Place all the topping ingredients in a food processor and pulse until the nuts are chopped and resemble oats.

4. Pour the fruit mixture into the baking dish and spread the topping evenly over it.

5. Bake for 35 minutes, or until the juices are bubbling in the corners of the dish and the crisp is brown and crunchy.

tidbits:

To make this breakfast easier on the tummy and provide an extra crunch, soak and dehydrate the nuts before making the topping.

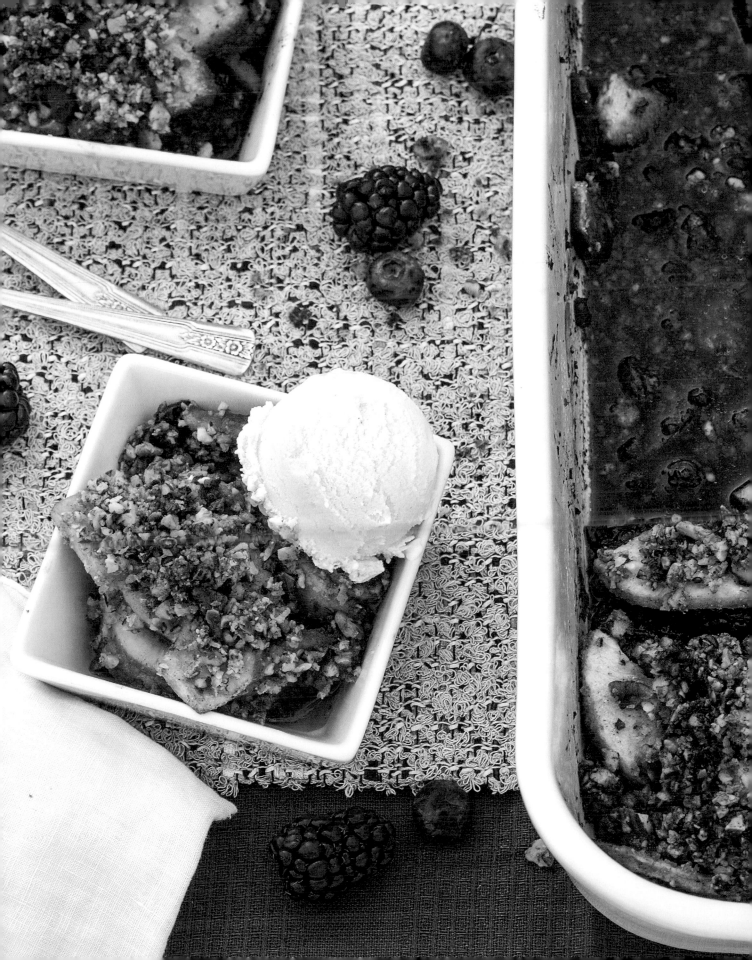

coconut milk yogurt

prep time: 25 minutes cooking time: 10 minutes

fermenting time: 18-24 hours yield: 1 quart

Dairy-free yogurts are readily available at most grocery stores, but they often contain unwelcome additives. Using a dehydrator or yogurt machine is a simple way to make coconut milk yogurt at home with ease and totally control what goes into it. We love ours with fresh berries and granola (page 58). You can use this as a base for anything that calls for yogurt, whether frozen yogurt or savory dips.

ingredients

- 2 13.5-ounce cans unsweetened coconut milk, divided
- 3 teaspoons unflavored gelatin
- 2 tablespoons honey
- 1 50-billion IU probiotic capsule or 1 dairy-free probiotic yogurt starter kit

method

1. Place ¼ cup of the coconut milk in a bowl. Sprinkle the gelatin over it and set aside to bloom for 10 minutes.

2. Heat the remaining coconut milk in a saucepan over medium heat until it reaches 150°F, about 10 minutes.

3. Remove from the heat and whisk in the softened gelatin and the honey until dissolved.

4. Allow milk to cool to 110°F, then whisk in the contents of 1 50-billion IU probiotic capsule or the yogurt starter.

5. Pour the mixture through a mesh sieve into sterilized jars and screw on the lids.

6. Place the jars in a yogurt maker and ferment for 18-24 hours, or ferment in a dehydrator without the trays on 120°F for the same time.

7. The yogurt will still be liquid and the coconut cream may have separated at this point. Place the jars in the refrigerator for 4 hours to allow the gelatin to set and the yogurt to thicken. Once set, whisk vigorously to blend the yogurt or pulse in a blender a few times for an ultra-smooth consistency.

tidbits:

- *The gelatin will solidify as it blooms. Do not be alarmed—it will dissolve once it is mixed with the hot liquid.*

- *Do not skip the honey, as this is what encourages the good bacteria to culture.*

- *Purchase a good quality probiotic from your local health store. Ultimate Flora is free of all allergens and many health stores also carry a generic form.*

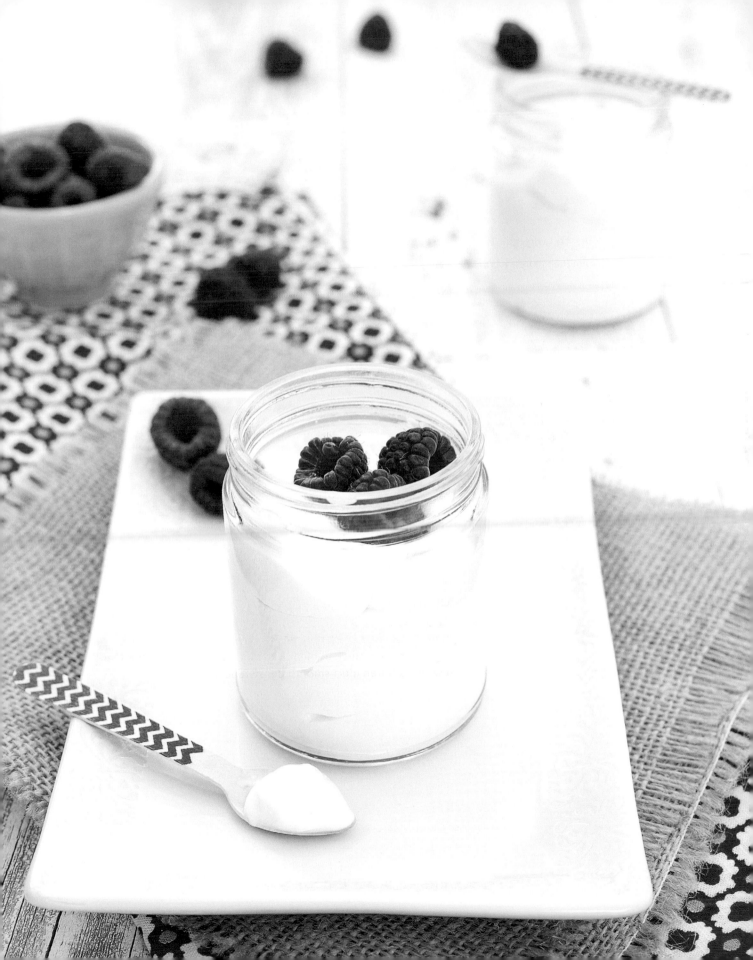

french toast casserole

prep time: 20 minutes   chilling time: 60 minutes   cooking time: 70 minutes

yield: 6 servings

Similar to a bread pudding, this breakfast indulgence consists of cubes of grain–free bread soaked and baked in mildly sweet custard and studded with blueberries that burst with flavor as they bake. You can drizzle with maple syrup for an extra–special treat, but this French toast can fly solo.

ingredients

- 1 loaf **World Famous Sandwich Bread** (page 226), cut into 1-inch cubes
- 1 egg, plus 4 egg yolks
- 1 cup coconut milk
- ½ cup unsweetened almond milk
- ¼ cup honey
- 1 teaspoon pure vanilla extract
- ½ teaspoon cinnamon
- ¼ teaspoon nutmeg
- Coconut oil
- 1 cup blueberries

method

1. Place the bread cubes on a tray and leave to dry overnight. Alternatively, you can toast them for 20 minutes in a 200°F oven.

2. Place the egg, egg yolks, milks, honey, vanilla, cinnamon, and nutmeg in a bowl and whisk to combine.

3. Lightly grease a 2-quart baking dish or a 9-by-13-inch casserole dish with coconut oil. Spread the bread cubes and blueberries evenly around the dish. Pour the custard over them. Cover and refrigerate for 1 hour.

4. Preheat the oven to 325°F.

5. Fill a large pan with 1-inch water. Place the baking dish with the French toast in the water bath. Cover with foil, cut a few holes for venting, and bake for 30 minutes. Remove the foil and bake an additional 40 minutes.

tidbits:

The casserole can be prepared up to step 4 and refrigerated up to 8 hours, which means that you can prepare it the night before and pop it in the oven when you wake up.

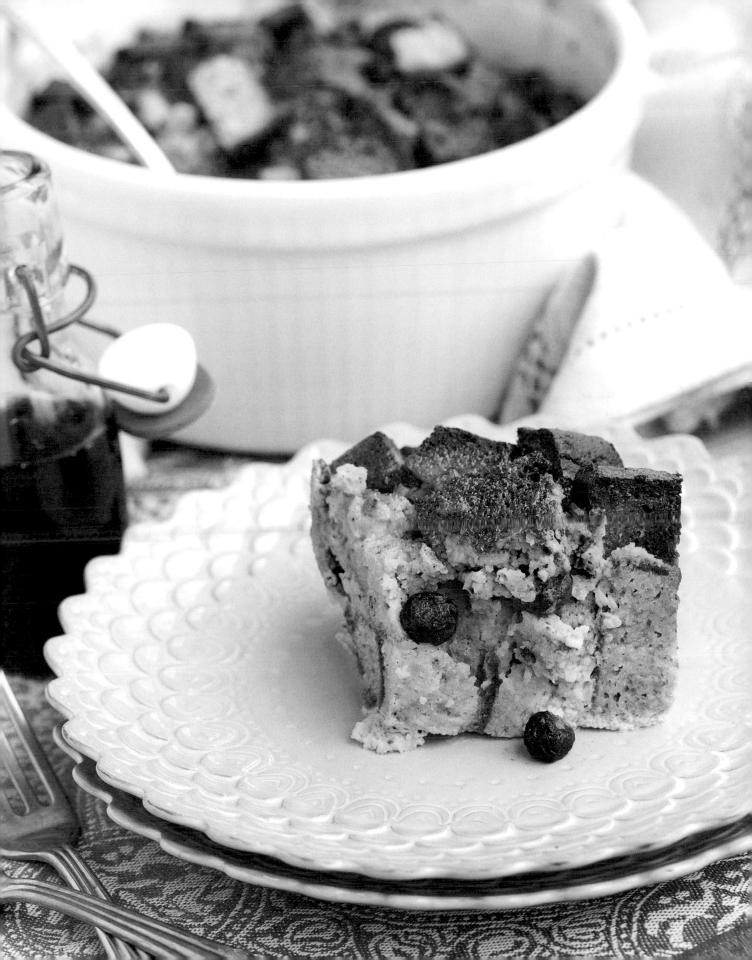

banana porridge

prep time: 10 minutes   soaking time: 8 hours

cooking time: 8 minutes   yield: 4 servings

I tire of eggs easily and also find that my body cannot tolerate them on a daily basis. One of my favorite breakfasts in the past was a warm bowl of steel-cut oatmeal—rich with nutrients and comforting flavors, but unfortunately not so kind to my digestion. This porridge is reminiscent of my old-time favorite and will give you energy and a warm start to the day.

ingredients

- ½ cup raw cashews
- ½ cup raw almonds
- ½ cup raw pecan halves
- Pinch sea salt
- 1 ripe banana
- 2 cups coconut milk
- 2 teaspoons cinnamon

method

1. Place the nuts in a large bowl and sprinkle with the salt. Add enough filtered water to cover the nuts by at least 1 inch. Cover and soak overnight.

2. Drain the nuts and rinse 2 or 3 times, until the water runs clear.

3. Add the nuts to a food processor or high-speed blender. Add the banana, coconut milk, and cinnamon and process until smooth.

4. Pour the porridge into a saucepan and heat over medium-high heat for 8 minutes, or until thick.

tidbits:

This dish will serve 4 small portions, which is more than enough as it is rich and filling. Serve with raisins, chopped nuts, and an extra splash of milk if desired.

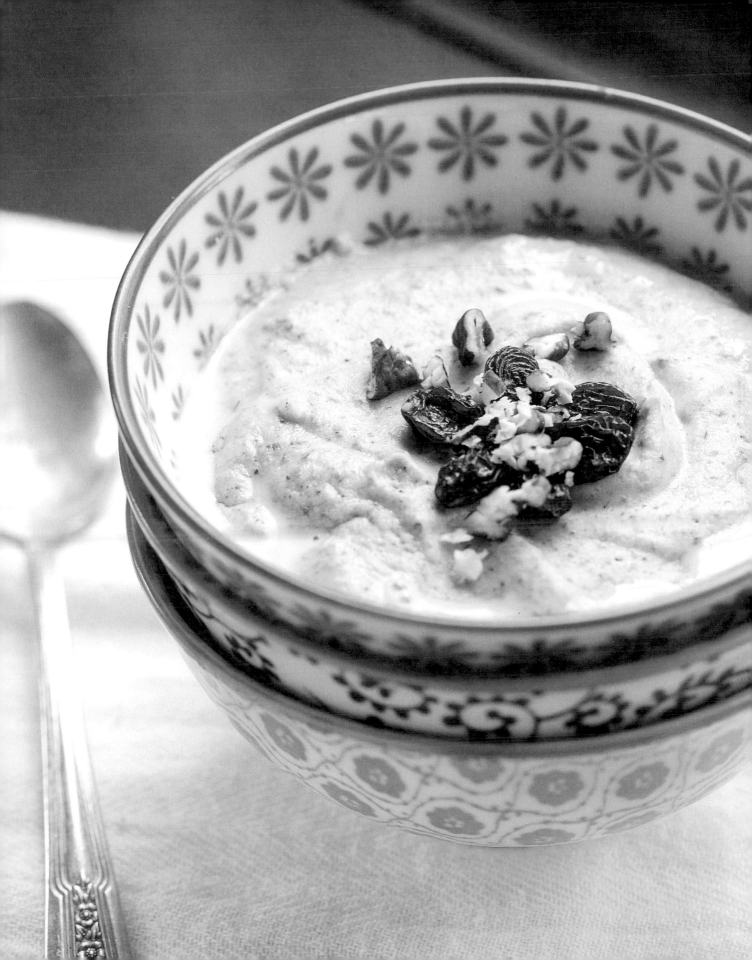

celeriac and sausage hash

prep time: 15 minutes   cooking time: 20 minutes   yield: 4 servings

Celeriac, or celery root, is a fascinating potato substitute and works especially well in breakfast dishes. A hash is a substantial way to start off your day, and you can make it even more substantial by topping each portion with a fried egg.

ingredients

- 1 tablespoon coconut oil or ghee
- 2 cups celeriac, trimmed of roots, peeled, and cubed
- ½ pound breakfast sausage, crumbled (page 32 or store-bought)
- ¾ cup finely diced carrots
- ¼ cup minced yellow onion
- ¾ cup finely diced zucchini
- ½ cup chopped cremini mushrooms
- 1 teaspoon chopped fresh parsley
- 1 teaspoon chopped fresh rosemary
- ¼ teaspoon sea salt
- Cracked black pepper to taste

method

1. Heat the oil in a large skillet over medium heat.

2. Place the celeriac in the skillet and cook for 5 minutes. Add the sausage, carrots, and onion. Continue cooking for 10 minutes, or until the meat is cooked through and the vegetables have softened.

3. Add the remaining ingredients and cook for 6 to 8 minutes longer, or until the mushrooms and zucchini are tender.

tidbits:

To trim and peel a celery root, first slice the bottom off so that there is a flat surface to place on a cutting board. Using a sharp knife, cut the peel and roots off in strips, from top to bottom. If the celeriac is somewhat smooth, a vegetable peeler will also work.

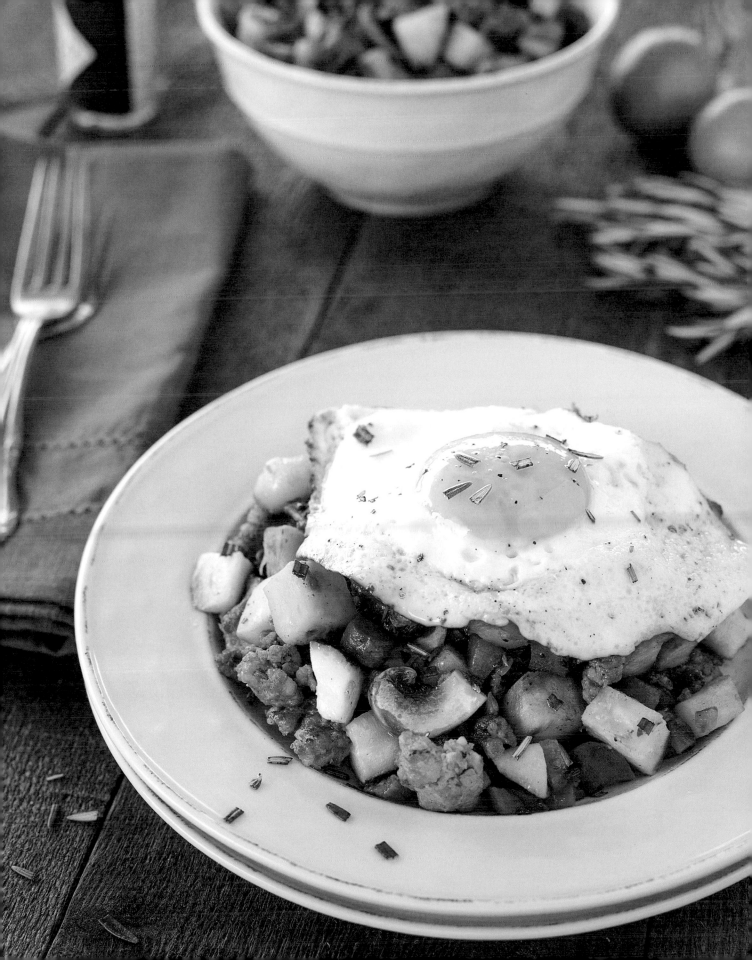

allergy-free breakfast cookies

prep time: 15 minutes   cooking time: 18-20 minutes   yield: 1 dozen cookies

to start off your morning

Fruit-sweetened and made without any of the top 8 allergens, these cookies are an addicting morning treat!

ingredients

- ½ pound ripe bananas (about 1 cup mashed)
- ½ cup unsweetened applesauce
- 2 tablespoons palm shortening
- 2 ounces pitted dates (about 3 or 4)
- ⅓ cup coconut flour
- 2 teaspoons cinnamon
- 1 teaspoon pure vanilla extract
- 1 teaspoon baking soda
- 1½ teaspoons fresh lemon juice
- ½ cup finely shredded unsweetened coconut
- 2 tablespoons chopped dried apricots
- 2 tablespoons dried currants
- 2 tablespoons raisins

method

1. Preheat the oven to 350°F.
2. Place the bananas, applesauce, shortening, and dates in a food processor and purée until smooth, about 30 seconds.
3. Add the coconut flour, cinnamon, vanilla, baking soda and lemon juice and pulse 5 or 6 times to combine.
4. Add the remaining ingredients and pulse twice to incorporate.
5. Spoon golf-ball-size balls of dough onto a baking sheet lined with parchment paper.
6. Flatten the balls slightly with the back of a spatula.
7. Bake for 18 to 20 minutes, until cookies are browned all over and slightly firm to the touch. Cool completely on a wire rack and store in an airtight container in the fridge.

tidbits:

The dough can also be pressed into a greased 8-by-8-inch baking dish, baked for about 17 minutes, and cut into bars when cool.

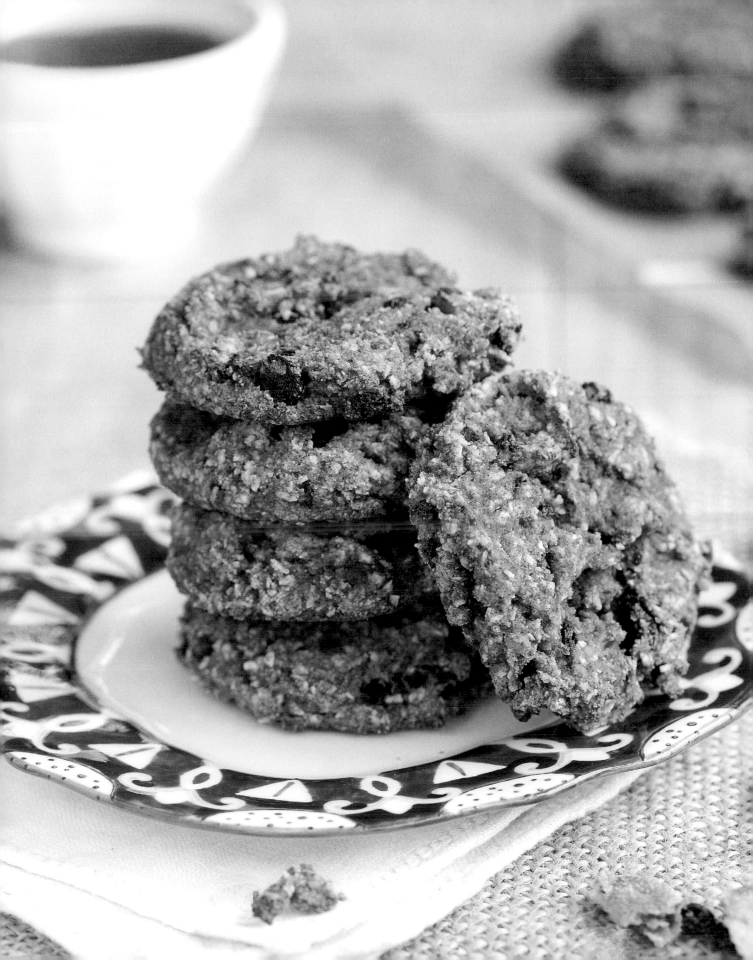

vanilla-almond granola

prep time: 20 minutes   soaking time: 24 hours

dehydrating time: 24 hours   yield: 4 cups

A crunchy and mildly sweet cereal that you can enjoy with cold almond milk or sprinkled over fresh yogurt. It is great to have on hand to eat on the go!

ingredients

- 1 cup raw almonds
- 1 cup raw walnuts
- ½ cup raw pecan halves
- ½ cup raw cashews
- ¼ cup raw sunflower seeds
- 1¾ teaspoons sea salt, divided
- ¾ cup melted honey or maple syrup
- 2 tablespoons coconut oil, melted
- 1½ tablespoons pure vanilla extract
- 1 tablespoon cinnamon
- ½ cup shredded, unsweetened coconut
- ½ cup raisins

method

1. Place all the nuts and seeds in a bowl, add enough water to cover by 1 inch, and stir in 1 teaspoon of the salt. Cover and let soak for 24 hours.

2. Drain the nuts and seeds and place on a paper towel to absorb the remaining water. Transfer to a food processor and process until the nuts are the size of oats. Add the honey, coconut oil, vanilla, cinnamon, and remaining salt. Pulse until combined.

3. Pour the mixture into a bowl, add the coconut, and use a spoon to incorporate. Turn the granola out onto 3 dehydrator trays covered with parchment paper, spreading evenly into thin layers.

4. Dehydrate at 120°F for 24 hours, flipping the granola gently with a spatula once or twice. The granola may feel a little sticky and wet when warm, but will crisp up after cooling.

5. Stir in the raisins, then let cool completely on trays before serving or storing.

tidbits:

To dehydrate in the oven, spread the granola on 3 parchment-lined baking sheets and place in a 170°F oven; use a wooden spoon to keep the oven door open a crack to let the moisture out. After 2 hours, carefully stir the granola. Dry for another hour. Turn the oven off, close the door completely, and dry for 1 more hour.

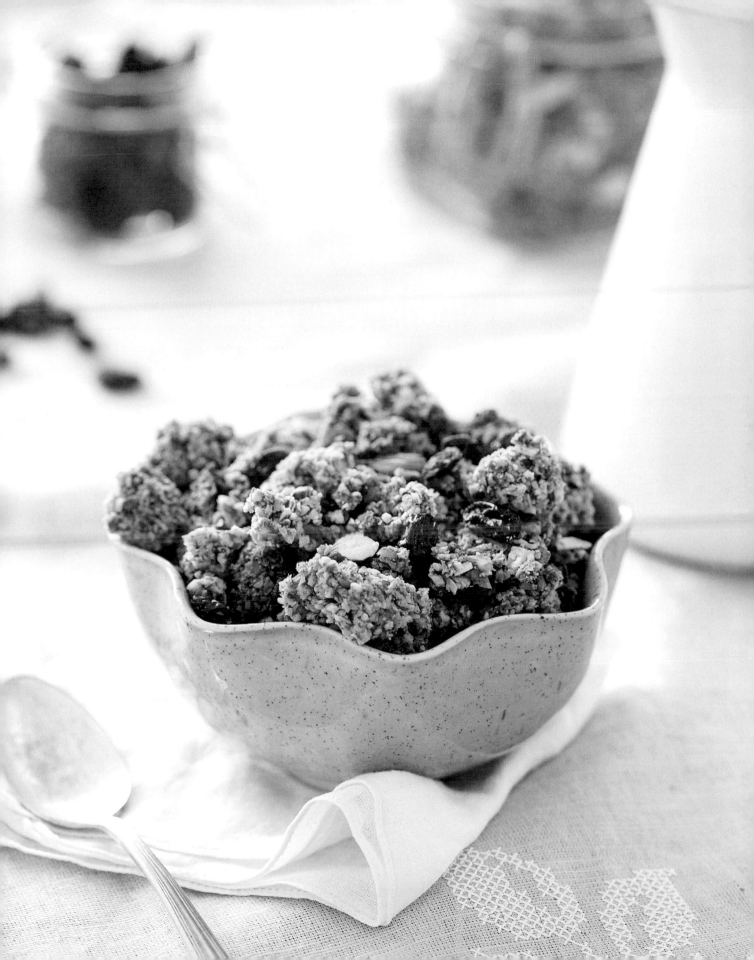

chocolate berry granola

prep time: 20 minutes   soaking time: 24 hours

dehydrating time: 24 hours   yield: 4 cups

Making grain-free granola may seem like a long process when you are craving something crunchy and sweet, but it's worth the wait and requires very little actual work. Soaking the nuts not only makes them easier to digest, but it also gives them an undeniable crunch.

ingredients

- 1 cup raw almonds
- 1 cup raw walnuts
- ½ cup raw pecan halves
- ½ cup raw hazelnuts
- ¼ cup raw sunflower seeds
- 1 tablespoon golden flaxseeds
- 1¾ teaspoons sea salt, divided
- 1 cup honey
- 3 tablespoons coconut oil
- 2 tablespoons raw cacao
- 1½ tablespoons pure vanilla extract
- 1 tablespoon cinnamon
- ½ cup shredded, unsweetened coconut
- ¼ cup dark chocolate chunks
- ½ cup freeze-dried strawberries

method

1. Place all the nuts and seeds in a bowl, add enough water to cover by 1 inch, and stir in 1 teaspoon of the salt. Cover and let soak for 24 hours.

2. Drain the nuts and seeds and place on a paper towel to absorb the remaining water. Transfer to the bowl of a food processor and pulse the nuts until they're the size of oats.

3. Place the honey, coconut oil, cacao, and vanilla in a small saucepan over medium heat until the cacao has dissolved. Add to the food processor with the cinnamon and remaining salt. Pulse twice to combine.

4. Pour the mixture into a bowl and mix in the coconut with a spoon. Turn the mixture out onto 3 parchment-covered dehydrator trays, spreading evenly into thin layers.

5. Dehydrate at 120°F for 24 hours, turning the granola with a spatula twice. The granola may feel a little sticky but will crisp up after cooling.

6. Transfer trays to a wire rack and cool completely. Once cooled, stir in the chocolate and strawberries.

tidbits:

To dehydrate in the oven, place the granola on 3 parchment-lined baking sheets in the oven at 170°F; use a wooden spoon to keep the oven door open a crack to let the moisture out. After 2 hours, carefully stir the granola. Dry for another hour. Turn the oven off, close the door completely, and dry for 1 more hour.

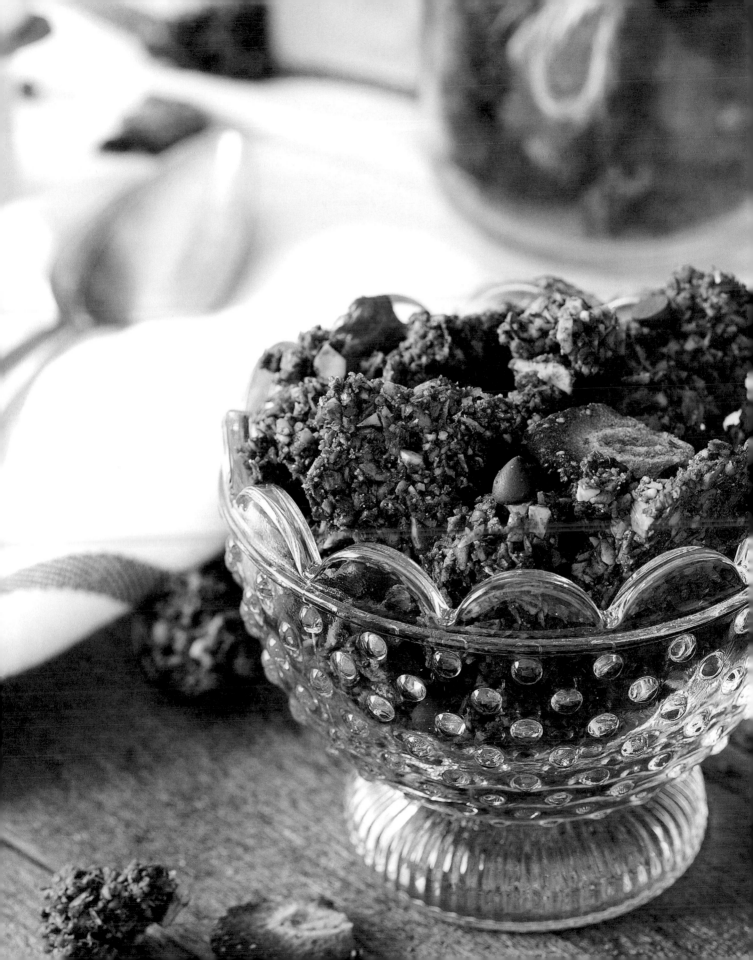

berries and cream

prep time: 5 minutes   yield: 4 servings

to start off
your morning

This simple breakfast choice is great to make when time is short or to simply perk up your usual routine. Just make sure you've always got a can of coconut milk in the fridge!

ingredients

- 2 cups mixed berries
- 1 13.5-ounce can coconut milk, chilled for 24 hours
- 1 teaspoon honey

method

1. Wash and divide the berries evenly among four bowls.

2. Gently open the can of coconut milk and scoop the heavy cream that has risen to the top into a bowl. Save the translucent water underneath for use in shakes or discard. Whisk the honey into the cream. Divide the cream evenly into each bowl of berries.

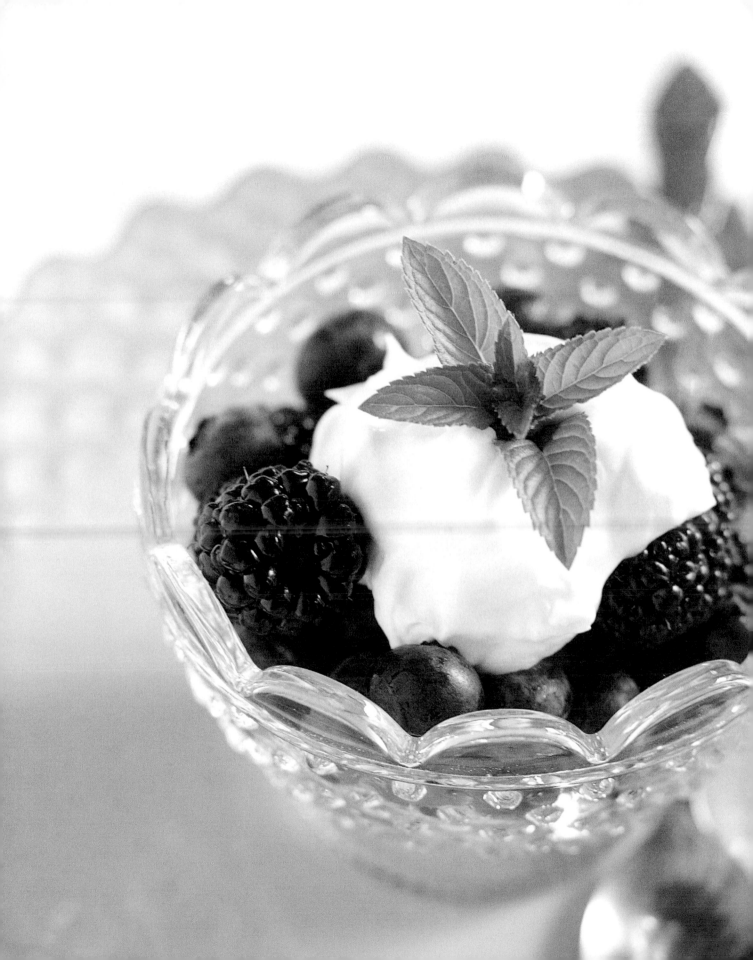

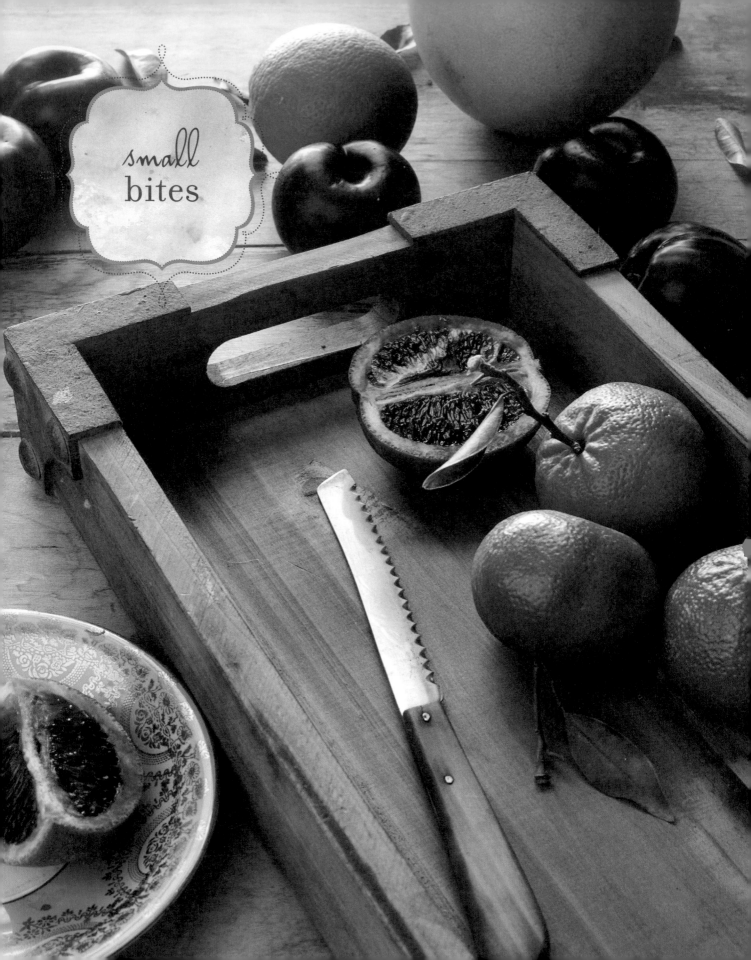

small
bites

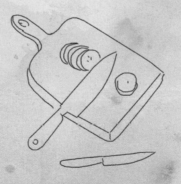

ahi mango poke stack

prep time: 10 minutes   chilling time: 30 minutes   yield: 4 servings

This mildly spicy and tangy ahi salad (poke) is a refreshing appetizer on a hot summer day. The flavors of sesame, ginger, garlic, and lime will trick your taste buds into thinking they've been transported to a Hawaiian beach paradise.

ingredients

- 4 teaspoons finely chopped green onion
- 2 teaspoons coconut aminos
- ½ teaspoon toasted sesame oil
- ½ teaspoon minced garlic
- ½ teaspoon fresh lime juice
- ¼ teaspoon freshly grated ginger
- ¼ teaspoon sea salt
- 1 pound fresh, sushi-grade ahi tuna steak, boneless and skinless
- ½ cup diced avocado
- ¼ cup diced mango
- 2 tablespoons minced poblano pepper, seeded
- Sweet Potato Chips, optional (page 86)

method

1. Place the green onion, coconut aminos, sesame oil, garlic, lime juice, ginger, and salt in a bowl and whisk to combine.
2. Cut the tuna into 1-inch cubes and place in a large bowl.
3. Add the avocado, mango, and pepper. Stir to combine.
4. Pour the marinade over the poke and mix gently to coat.
5. Cover and refrigerate for 30 minutes before serving.
6. Serve stacked between layers of crisp sweet potato chips or in shot glasses.

tidbits:

Because this is a raw dish, purchasing good-quality tuna is essential.

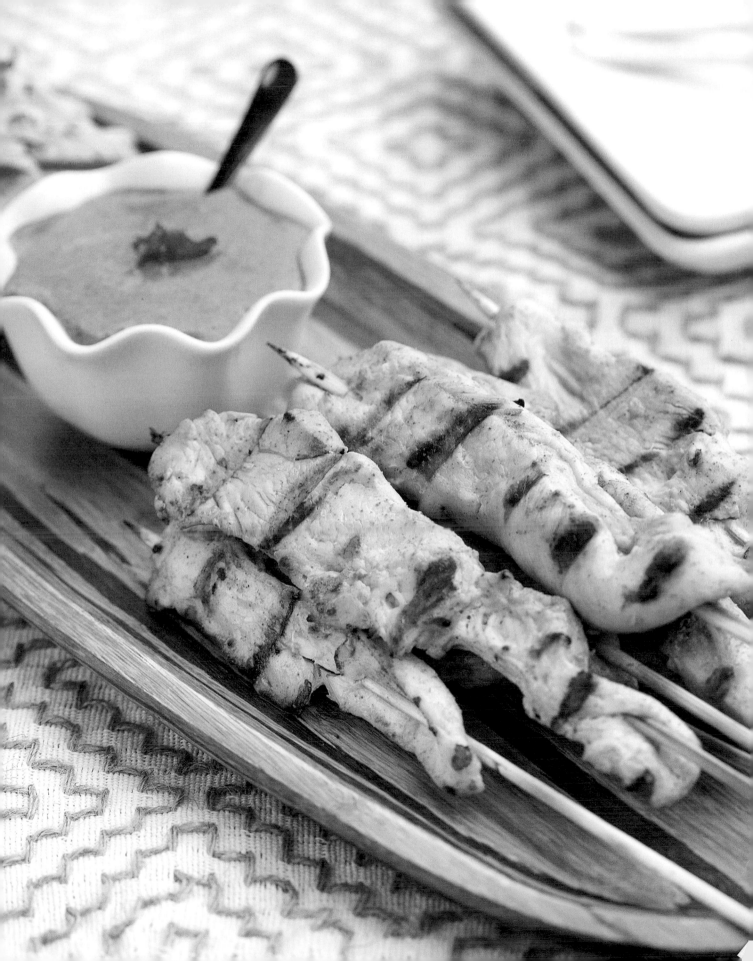

soaked trail mix

prep time: 20 minutes   soaking time: 24 hours

dehydrating time: 24 hours   yield: 3 pounds

I keep this trail mix stocked at all times and like to put out a small bowl when we have guests. Time and time again, the person eating it always asks what I did to the almonds to make them taste so good! The trick is soaking and dehydrating the nuts and tossing them with a small amount of coconut oil and coarse sea salt. Soaking nuts makes them crunchy and crisp and significantly easier to digest. So if you struggle with gut issues, rest assured that this is a snack you will not only enjoy, but one that will also allow you to benefit from the nutrients that nuts provide.

ingredients

- 4 cups raw almonds
- 4 cups raw pecans halves
- 1 teaspoon coarse sea salt, divided
- 2 cups raw cashews
- 1 tablespoon coconut oil, melted
- 1 cup raisins
- ½ cup dried cherries or cranberries
- ½ cup dark chocolate chunks

method

1. Place the almonds and pecans in a large bowl with enough filtered water to cover them by 1-inch and stir in ½ teaspoon of the salt. Cover the bowl and soak at room temperature for 20 hours. Rinse the nuts and return them to the bowl.

2. Add the cashews and fill the bowl with water again, covering the nuts by 1 inch. Cover and soak for 4 more hours.

3. Drain the water and rinse the nuts. Turn them out onto a baking sheet lined with a paper towel and blot off excess water.

4. Line dehydrator sheets or baking sheets with parchment paper and dehydrate the nuts at 150°F for 20 hours.

5. Remove the nuts and pour them into a large bowl. Add the coconut oil and remaining salt, toss well, then return to the dehydrator and continue drying for 4 hours.

6. Let the nuts cool completely on their baking sheets before stirring in the dried fruit and chocolate. Store in an airtight container.

tidbits:

For oven drying, turn the oven to the lowest setting and spread the nuts on baking sheets lined with parchment paper. Dehydrate with the door propped open slightly with a wooden spoon for 8 to 10 hours, or until the nuts are crunchy. Remove from the oven, toss in the coconut oil and remaining salt and then return to the oven to dry for 1 hour longer.

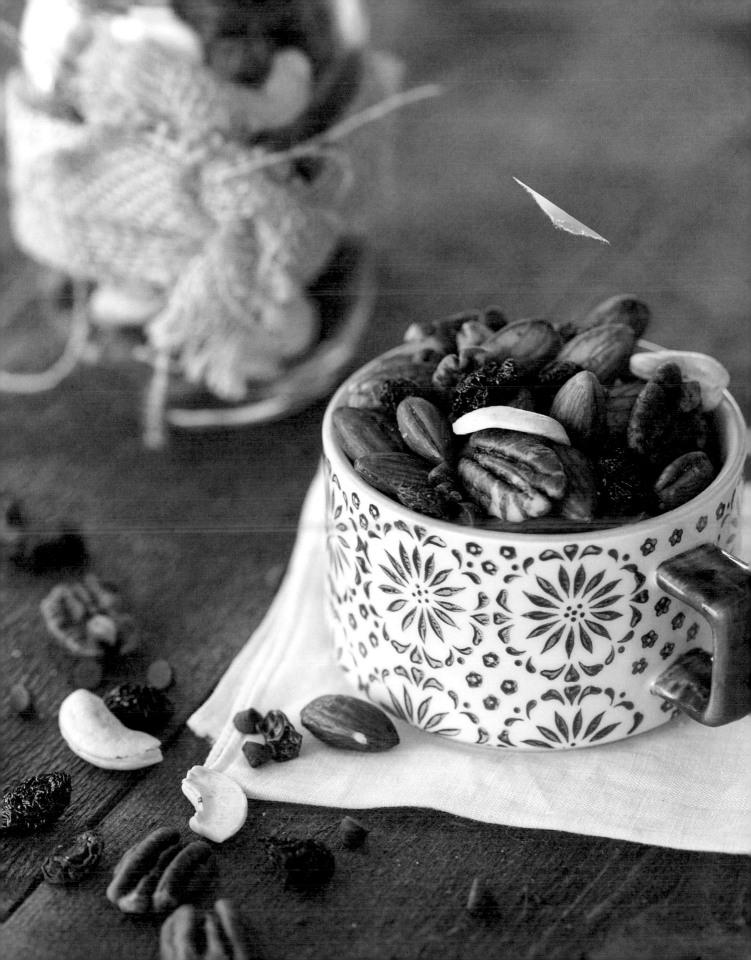

fried brussels sprouts and cauliflower

prep time: 10 minutes   cooking time: 8 minutes   yield: 4 servings

Fried Brussels sprouts are all the rage in the culinary world these days. This dish boasts smoky notes from the fried rosemary and satisfies a craving for salt with a dash of garum, an Italian fermented fish sauce.

ingredients

- 3 cups macadamia oil
- 3 sprigs fresh rosemary
- 1 pound cauliflower, trimmed and cut into florets
- 1 pound Brussels sprouts, trimmed and halved
- 1½ teaspoons garum fish sauce
- ½ teaspoon fresh lemon juice
- ⅛ teaspoon sea salt

method

1. Place the oil in a deep skillet or saucepan and heat to 350°F.

2. Drop the rosemary into the hot oil, then add the cauliflower and Brussels sprouts in batches, frying each batch for 3 to 4 minutes, or until browned and crispy.

3. Remove each batch to a pan lined with paper towels and drain while the next batch cooks.

4. Transfer the vegetables to a mixing bowl. Sprinkle the fried rosemary leaves into the bowl, discarding the stems.

5. Pour in the fish sauce, lemon juice, and salt and stir gently to coat.

6. The dish will soften and lose its crispness as it cools, so serve immediately. Place under the broiler for 2 to 3 minutes to crisp if necessary.

tidbits:

- *You can replace the macadamia oil with palm shortening for a nut-free dish.*
- *Asian fish sauce such as Red Boat may be substituted for garum.*

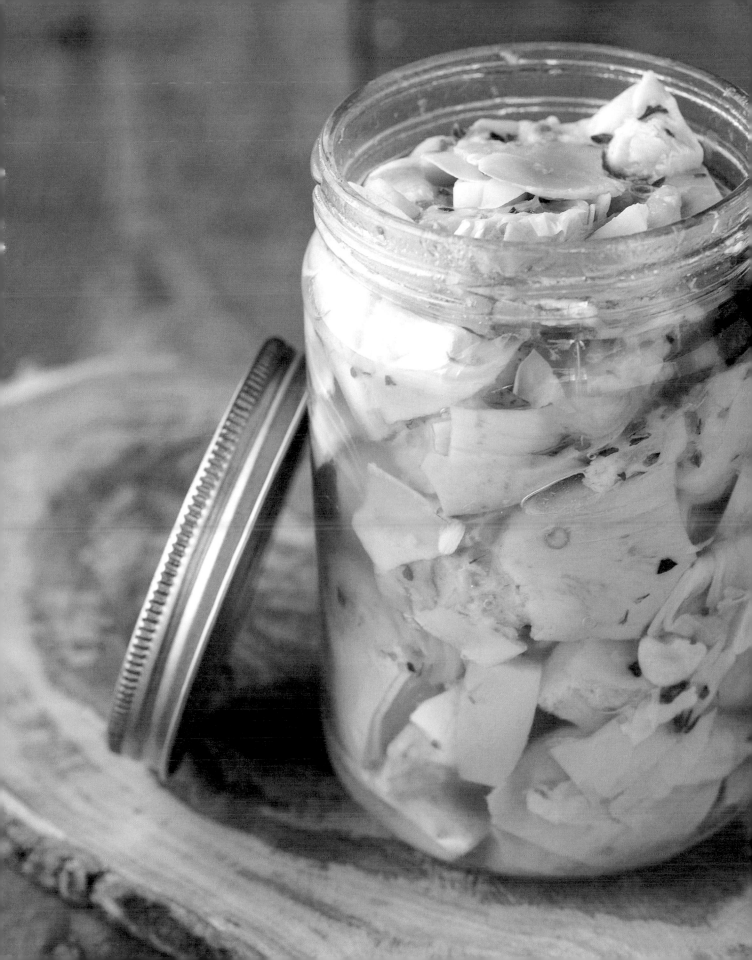

rosemary-raisin crackers

prep time: 15 minutes   cooking time: 15 minutes   yield: 2 dozen crackers

These crackers satisfy both salty and sweet cravings. They will add sophistication to any hors d'oeuvre tray and pair nicely with fig spread, apple or pear slices, or thin slices of prosciutto.

ingredients

- 1 cup blanched almond flour
- 2 tablespoons raisins
- 2 tablespoons cold water
- 1 tablespoon raw sunflower seeds, divided
- 1 sprig fresh rosemary
- 1½ teaspoons extra-virgin olive oil
- ½ teaspoon sea salt

method

1. Preheat the oven to 350°F.

2. Place all the ingredients, except 1 teaspoon of the sunflower seeds, in a food processor. Process for 15 seconds, or until thoroughly combined, with small bits of raisins speckled throughout. Add the remaining teaspoon of sunflower seeds, and pulse once until they are roughly chopped.

3. Form the dough into a ball, then roll it out to a rectangle shape, ⅛-inch thick between 2 sheets of parchment paper.

4. Remove the top sheet of parchment. Use a pizza cutter to cut the dough into 1-inch wide rectangles. Save the end bits and reroll to make more crackers. Carefully transfer the parchment paper to a baking sheet.

5. Bake for 15 minutes, rotating the pan once, until crackers are golden. Let cool on a wire rack for 15 minutes, then carefully break the crackers apart. Cool completely before serving.

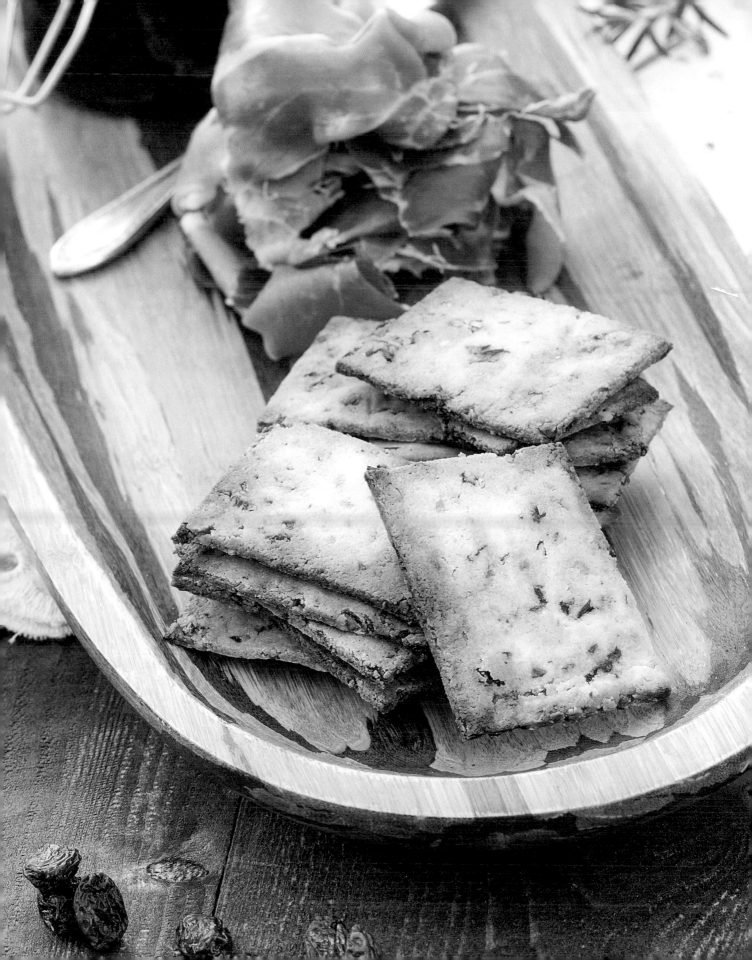

chips and salsa

prep time: 20 minutes   cooking time: 10 minutes   yield: 6 servings

I don't know about you, but Mexican food just doesn't taste as good to me without something crunchy to dip in salsa or guacamole, so I recreated a tortilla chip with almond flour. Make sure to roll the dough very thin to achieve the right crunch. Serve the chips with any of the salsas or the guacamole on page 333.

ingredients

- 1¾ cups blanched almond flour
- 2 teaspoons egg whites
- 2 teaspoons cold water
- 1½ teaspoons coconut oil, melted
- 1 teaspoon chopped fresh cilantro
- ½ teaspoon fresh lime juice
- ¼ teaspoon sea salt
- Coarse sea salt for sprinkling on top
- Salsa (page 332)

method

1. Preheat the oven to 350°F.

2. Place all the ingredients except the coarse salt in the bowl of a stand mixer or food processor and mix until a lose ball of dough forms.

3. Form the dough into 8 small balls and roll them out into thin circles between 2 pieces of parchment paper, about ¹⁄₁₆ -inch thick. Remove the top sheet of parchment.

4. Use a pizza cutter to cut the circles into triangles. Trim off the jagged edges if desired. Sprinkle the chips with coarse salt. Carefully transfer the parchment paper to a baking sheet.

5. Bake for 5 minutes. Flip the chips and gently separate them. Bake for an additional 4 minutes, or until evenly browned. Cool on a wire rack before serving.

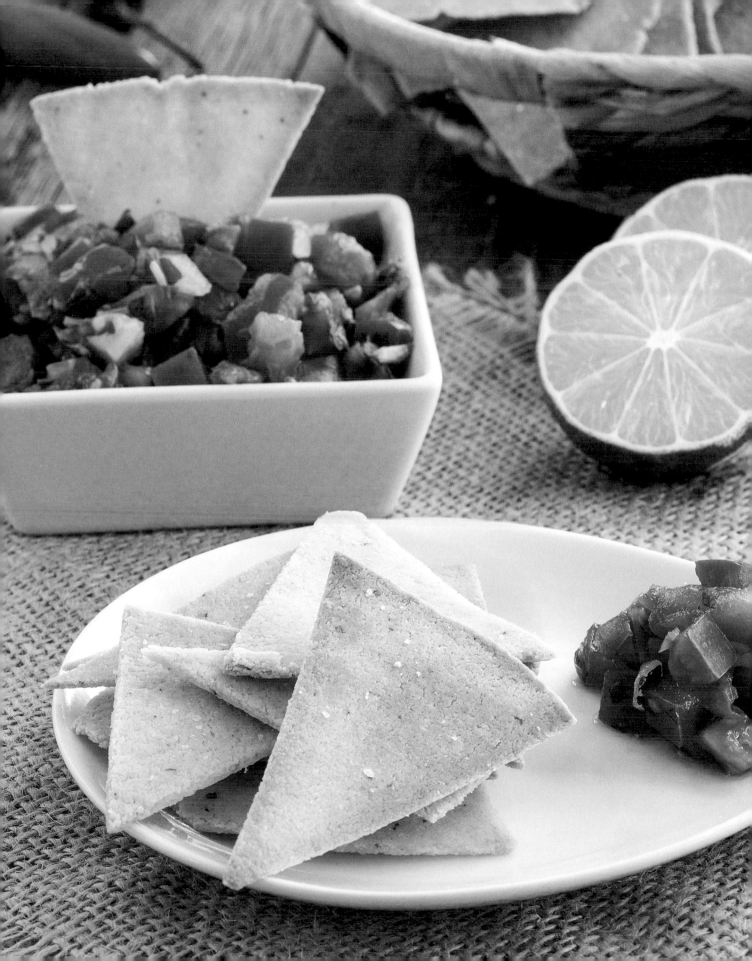

crispy sweet potato fries
with wasabi aioli

prep time: 15 minutes + 1 hour soaking time   cooking time: 20 minutes   yield: 4 servings

Most homemade sweet potato fries go limp after baking or frying and don't crunch the way they do in restaurants. Soaking the potatoes before baking is the key to a perfectly crisp fry: it helps remove much of the starch, which is what makes them get soggy as they cook. This foolproof recipe produces crispy fries at home every time!

ingredients

- 1 pound sweet potatoes, scrubbed clean, with skins on
- 2 tablespoons extra-virgin olive oil
- 2 teaspoons coconut flour
- ½ teaspoon sea salt

WASABI AIOLI

- 2 tablespoons Mayonnaise (page 308)
- 1 teaspoon all-natural wasabi powder
- 1 teaspoon fresh lime juice
- ¾ teaspoon extra-virgin olive oil
- ¼ teaspoon sea salt

method

1. Cut the sweet potatoes into matchsticks, being careful to cut evenly sized pieces. Place in a bowl of ice water to soak for 1 hour.

2. Place the Mayonnaise, wasabi powder, lime juice, olive oil, and ¼ teaspoon of salt in a bowl and whisk to combine. Cover and refrigerate for 30 minutes.

3. Preheat the oven to 425°F and line a baking sheet with parchment paper.

4. Drain the potatoes and place on a paper towel to dry.

5. Place the potatoes, 1 tablespoon of the olive oil, the coconut flour, and the remaining ½ teaspoon of salt in a bowl and toss.

6. Drizzle the remaining oil over 2 parchment-lined baking trays. Scatter the fries evenly on the two trays, being careful not to let any overlap.

7. Bake for 10 minutes, flip, and bake another 10 minutes.

tidbits:

Evenly space fries on the baking sheet and do not let any overlap. Otherwise the fries will bake unevenly and become soggy.

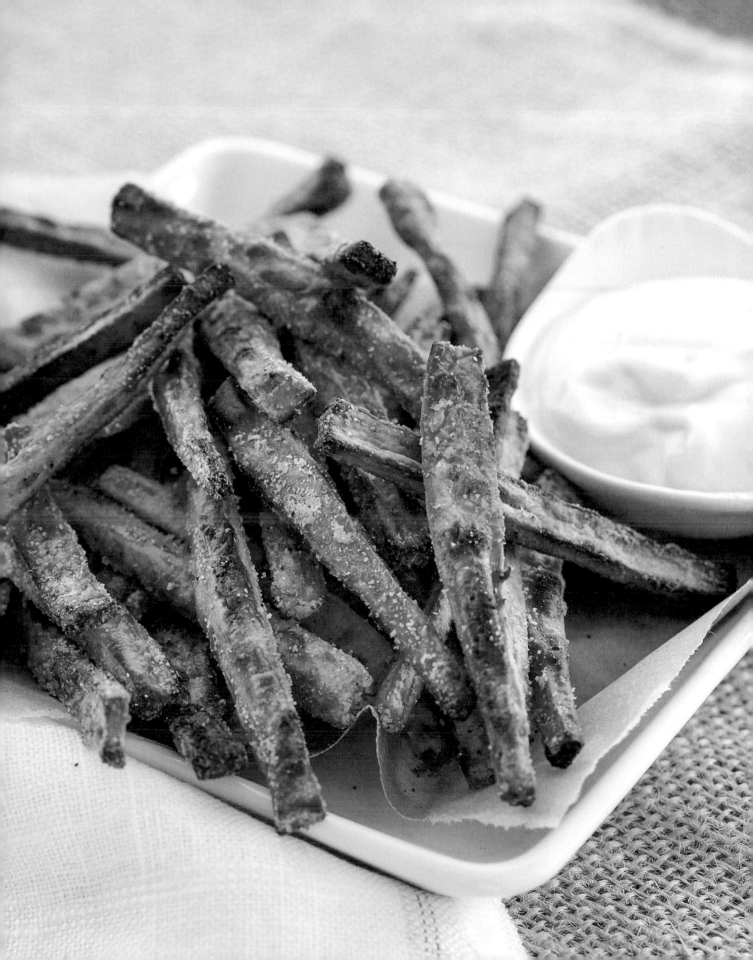

rosemary roasted almonds

prep time: 24 hours   *cooking time:* 35 minutes   *yield:* 2 cups

Crunchy from being soaked and dehydrated, these skinless almonds are smooth and have a full-bodied rosemary flavor.

ingredients

- 1½ cups raw almonds
- ½ teaspoon coarse sea salt, plus a pinch for soaking water
- 2 teaspoons extra-virgin olive oil or ghee
- 1 tablespoon chopped fresh rosemary

method

1. Place nuts in a bowl of enough filtered water to cover by 1 inch, add a pinch of salt, and soak for 24 hours at room temperature.

2. Preheat the oven to 300°F.

3. Remove the skins by squeezing the tip of the almonds and allowing the nut to slide out.

4. Place the almonds in a bowl and toss with the oil, rosemary, and ½ teaspoon salt, then spread them out evenly on a baking sheet.

5. Bake for 35 minutes, turning twice. Increase the temperature to 400° and roast for 10 minutes more.

6. Cool before storing or serving.

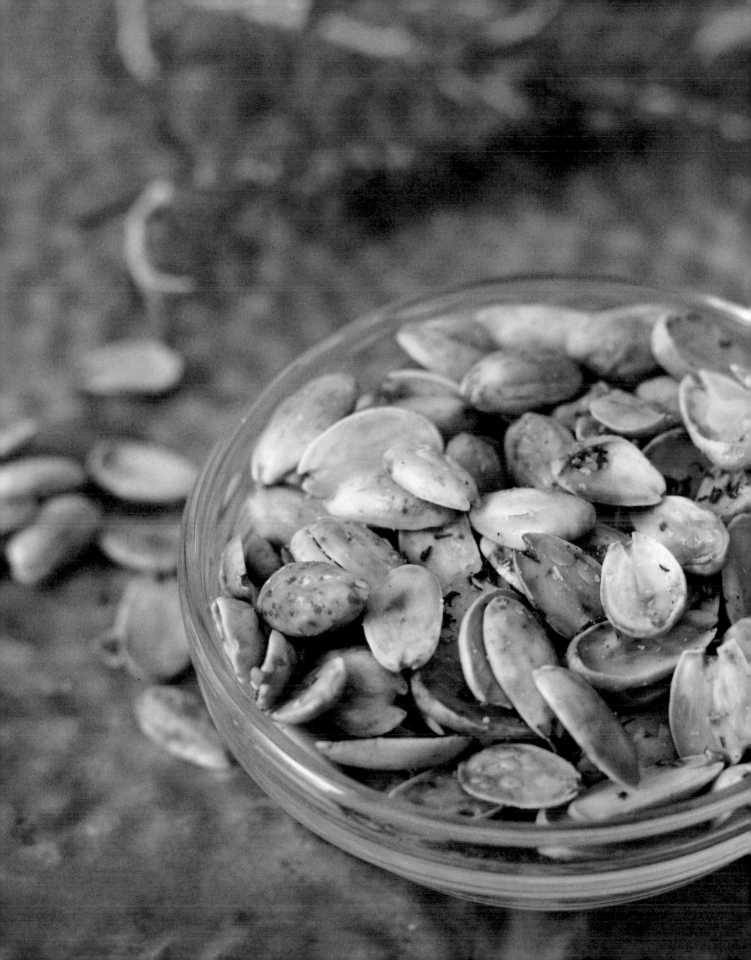

sweet potato chips with creamy cilantro-serrano dipping sauce

prep time: 45 minutes   cooking time: 30 minutes   yield: 4 servings

These chips are baked in just a small amount of oil and sprinkled with a smoky chili sea salt, making them an indulgent but guilt-free snack. Dip them in the tangy sauce for even more flavor and texture.

ingredients

POTATOES

- 2 large sweet potatoes, scrubbed clean, with skins on
- 2 tablespoons melted coconut oil or extra-virgin olive oil
- ¼ teaspoon coarse sea salt
- ⅛ teaspoon chili powder

SAUCE

- ¼ cup whole raw cashews, soaked in warm water for 4 hours
- ¼ cup water
- ½ serrano chili, seeded and minced
- 1 tablespoon cilantro
- ½ teaspoon fresh lime juice
- ½ teaspoon minced garlic
- ¼ teaspoon sea salt

method

1. Use a mandolin or a very sharp knife to cut the potatoes into even ⅛-inch-thick slices. Place the potatoes in a bowl, cover with ice water, and soak for 20 minutes.

2. Preheat the oven to 400°F.

3. Meanwhile, make the sauce. Place all the sauce ingredients in a blender. Blend until very smooth. Cover and refrigerate sauce while you bake the chips.

4. Rinse the chips and pat them dry. Toss them in the oil, then spread them in an even layer on 2 baking sheets lined with parchment paper. Bake for 20 minutes, flipping once.

5. Sprinkle with salt and chili powder.

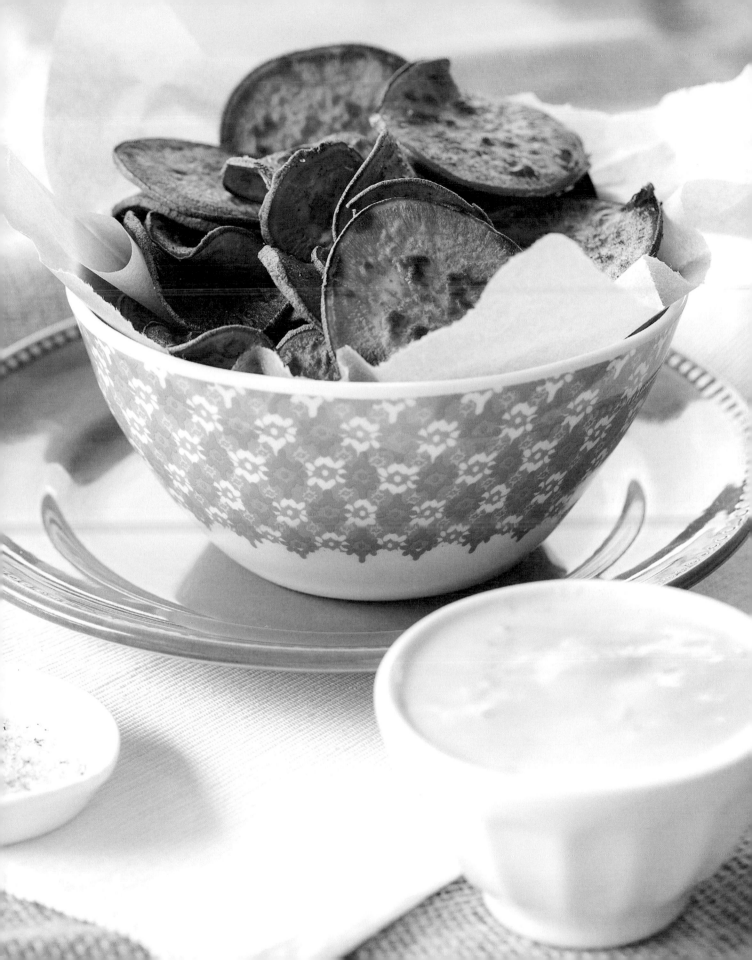

soups,
salads,
and sides

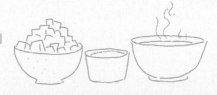

clam chowder

prep time: 30 minutes   soaking time: 4 hours

cooking time: 30 minutes   yield: 6 servings

Creamy soups are my vice and I especially love to indulge in them when I want something comforting. Clam chowder was always one of my favorites growing up, but seeing as it is full of butter, cream, potatoes, and flour, I have missed it terribly over the past few years. If you're in the same boat, get ready to be reunited with your favorite because this version will pass for the original.

ingredients

- 2 cups raw cashews, soaked in water for 4 hours
- 4 slices bacon, chopped
- 1 cup chopped yellow onion
- ½ cup chopped celery
- 1 cup peeled cubed celery root, or celeriac
- 4 cups water
- 16 ounces bottled clam juice
- 1 sprig fresh thyme
- 1 bay leaf
- ½ teaspoon sea salt
- 3 6.5-ounce cans minced clams, drained and rinsed

method

1. Place the bacon in a Dutch oven or deep stockpot and cook over medium-high heat until most of the fat has rendered, about 2-3 minutes.

2. Stir in the onions, celery, and celery root and sauté for 10 minutes, or until the vegetables are cooked but still firm.

3. Add the water, clam juice, thyme, bay leaf, and salt. Cover and simmer for 20 minutes.

4. Remove 2 cups of soup from the pot and place in a blender.

5. Drain and rinse the cashews, then add them to the blender and blend for 30 seconds, until smooth.

6. Return the cream mixture to the pot and stir to incorporate.

7. Stir in the clams and simmer for 5 minutes, until the clams are warm. Remove from the heat and allow the soup to thicken for 10 minutes before serving.

tidbits:

Fresh clams take a bit more work, but if they are available near you, they will amplify the flavor of this soup.

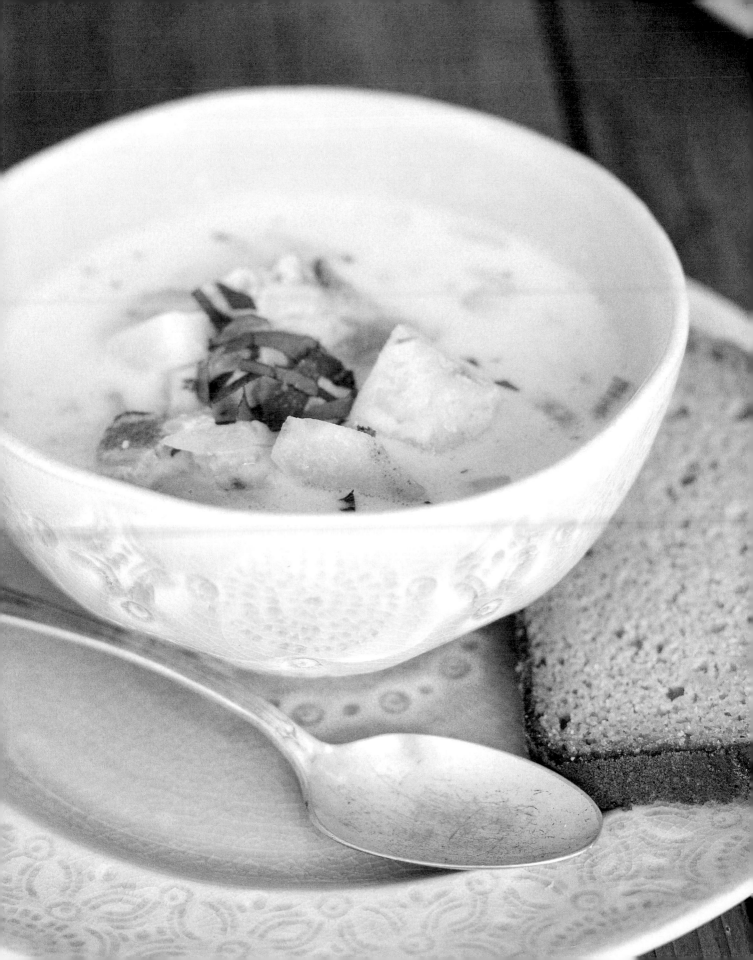

mexican chicken chowder

prep time: 15 minutes   cooking time: 70 minutes   yield: 6 servings

This creamy soup is full of intense Mexican flavors and gets its spice from a Roasted Tomatillo Salsa. Store-bought salsa saves time and allows you to purchase your preferred level of spice, but you can just as easily use the recipe on page 333.

ingredients

- 2 pounds chicken thighs, bone in, trimmed of fat and skin
- 2 cups Roasted-Tomatillo Salsa (page 333)
- 4 cups Chicken Broth (page 316)
- 3 cups peeled and cubed sweet potatoes*
- 2 cups peeled and sliced carrots
- 2 teaspoons fresh lime juice
- 1 teaspoon minced garlic
- ½ teaspoon sea salt
- 2 cups chopped spinach
- Garnish: chopped fresh cilantro and avocado slices

method

1. Place the chicken, Salsa, broth, sweet potatoes, carrots, lime juice, garlic, and salt in a stockpot over medium-high heat.

2. Bring to a boil, then cover and simmer for 1 hour over medium-low heat.

3. Remove the chicken from the pot, and using 2 forks, pull the meat away from the bones and shred it. Set aside.

4. Scoop 2 cups of vegetables from the soup and place in a blender with ¼ cup of the broth. Purée the vegetables for 15 seconds and then incorporate back into the soup.

5. Add the chicken and spinach to the pot and simmer for 10 minutes, until the spinach is slightly wilted.

6. Serve hot, garnished with sliced avocado and fresh cilantro.

*For SCD, substitute butternut squash for the sweet potatoes.

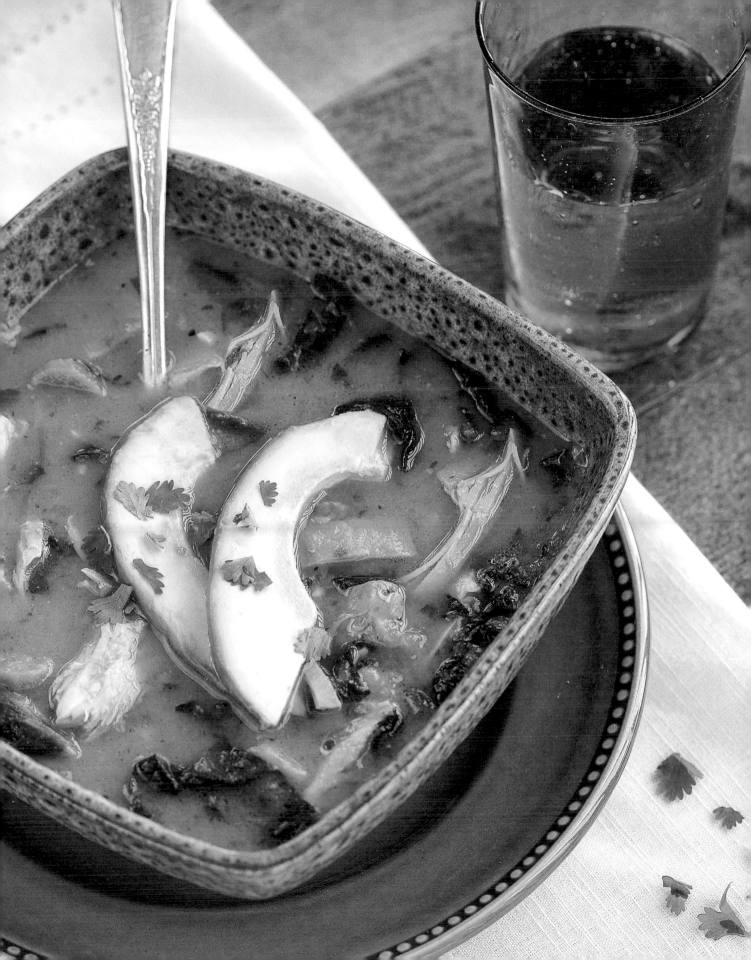

roasted butternut squash soup with sausage

prep time: *30 minutes*   cooking time: *30 minutes*   yield: *6 servings*

Roasted vegetables and robust browned sausage radiate an incomparable depth of flavor throughout every spoonful of this soup, turning it into a hearty meal that will warm you from the inside out on a cold evening. And, yes, those are grain-free breadsticks! You can find the recipe for them on page 240.

ingredients

- 3-4 pounds butternut squash, peeled and seeded
- 2 large carrots, peeled
- 1 small yellow onion, peeled and quartered
- 3 cloves garlic, peeled
- 1 tablespoon extra-virgin olive oil
- ¾ teaspoon sea salt, divided
- ½ teaspoon cracked black pepper, divided
- ½ pound mild Italian sausage, casings removed, crumbled
- 4 cups vegetable or Chicken Broth (page 316), divided
- ½ teaspoon cinnamon
- ½ teaspoon ground ginger
- ¼ teaspoon allspice
- 1 bay leaf
- Garnish: toasted hazelnut pieces and fresh sage leaves

method

1. Preheat the oven to 400°F.
2. Cut the squash, carrots, and onion into 1-inch chunks.
3. Toss the vegetable chunks and garlic in the olive oil and spread out on a baking sheet. Sprinkle with ¼ teaspoon salt and ⅛ teaspoon pepper.
4. Place the vegetables in the oven and roast for 20 minutes, stirring once.
5. Cook the sausage in a stockpot over medium heat until cooked through, about 5 minutes.
6. Remove the vegetables from the oven and place them in a blender.
7. Add half of the broth and purée until smooth.
8. Add the purée and the remainder of the broth to the pot with the sausage, stirring to combine.
9. Season with the cinnamon, ginger, allspice, bay leaf, and the remaining salt and pepper. Bring to a boil then reduce the heat to low and simmer for 10 minutes.
10. Serve hot, garnished with fresh sage and toasted hazelnut pieces.

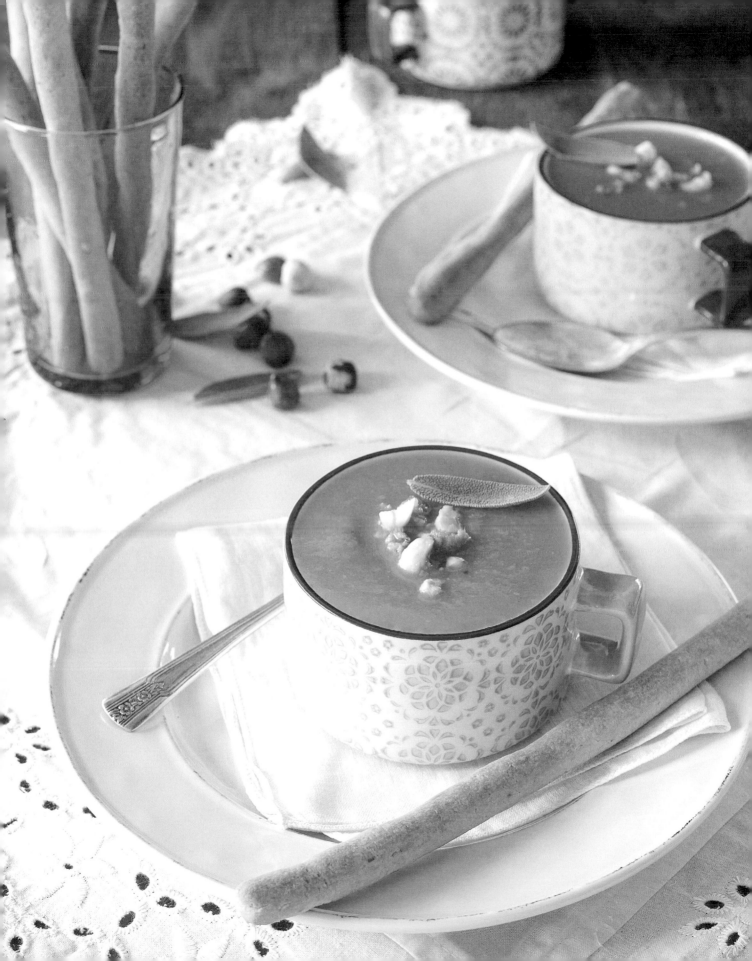

slow-cooker beef chuck chili

prep time: 15 minutes   cooking time: 6 hours   yield: 8 servings

Besides greatly cutting down on dairy, one of the biggest modifications I made when switching from the Specific Carbohydrate Diet to a more Paleo-style diet was eliminating all legumes. Even when soaked and cooked properly, beans always did a number on my digestion. So this chili is made the classic way—all meat, no fillers. I prefer to make chili with dried spices from my pantry, so I can make it practically whenever I want to.

ingredients

- 2 teaspoons coconut oil
- 2½ pounds beef chuck, cut into ½-inch cubes
- 2 red bell peppers, seeded and diced
- 1 small yellow onion, chopped
- 1 28-ounce box or jar chopped tomatoes
- 1½ cups beef broth
- 2 tablespoons tomato paste
- 2 cloves garlic, minced
- 1 bay leaf
- 2½ tablespoons chili powder
- 3 teaspoons sea salt
- 2 teaspoons cumin
- ½ teaspoon paprika
- ½ teaspoon curry powder
- ½ teaspoon cinnamon
- ¼ teaspoon black pepper
- ¼ teaspoon cayenne pepper
- ¼ teaspoon red pepper flakes
- 1 ounce unsweetened chocolate*
- Garnishes: chopped fresh cilantro, red onion

method

1. Place the oil in a large skillet over medium-high heat. Add the meat and brown on all sides, about 10 minutes.
2. Drain half of the fat, and then pour the remaining fat and meat into a slow cooker.
3. Add the remaining ingredients, except the chocolate, and cook for 6 hours on low.
4. Stir in the chocolate at the very end and adjust the salt to taste.
5. Serve garnished with cilantro and red onion, if desired.

tidbits:

Beef chuck, commonly used for stews or ground beef, tenderizes beautifully as it cooks slowly in the acidity of the tomatoes.

*Omit unsweetened chocolate for SCD.

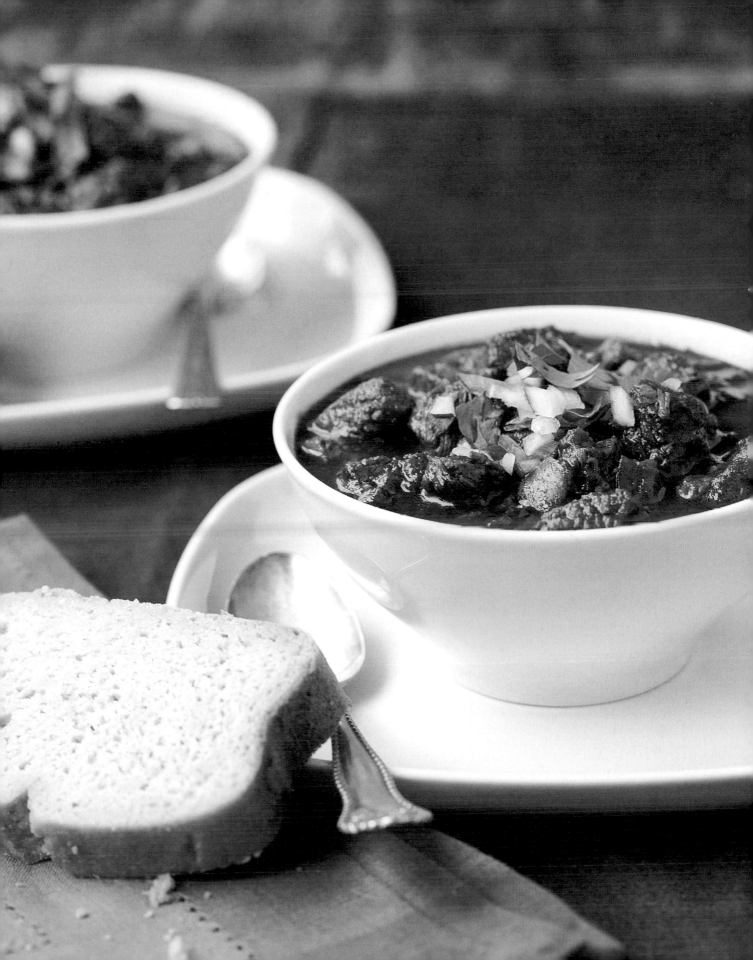

thai coconut soup
(tom kha gai)

prep time: 15 minutes   cooking time: 20 minutes   yield: 6 servings

I rate a Thai restaurant based on its tom kha gai. If it doesn't meet my expectations, I know it's not worth ordering anything else on the menu. This soup is my favorite way to start out a Thai meal, but it can also serve as a substantial and soul-warming lunch. A traditional soup in Thai cuisine, this dish combines the flavors of coconut, lime, lemongrass, and ginger, and moderate heat from Thai chilies. If you can't find the ingredients fresh in your grocery store or local Asian market, they can all be conveniently found dried in jars lining the Asian food aisles at most supermarkets.

ingredients

- 2 teaspoons coconut oil
- 8 whole Thai bird's eye chilies
- 2 13.5-ounce cans full-fat coconut milk
- ½ cup Chicken Broth (page 316)
- 2-inch piece galangal, or fresh ginger, thinly sliced
- 1 stalk lemongrass, sliced diagonally into 3-4 pieces and crushed with the butt of a knife
- 8 kaffir lime leaves, dried or fresh
- 4 tablespoons fish sauce
- 1 pound boneless chicken thighs, trimmed of all fat and thinly sliced
- 1 cup sliced white button mushrooms
- ½ yellow onion, thinly sliced
- 2 tablespoons fresh lime juice
- 8 cherry tomatoes, halved
- Garnishes: chopped fresh cilantro and scallions

method

1. Place the coconut oil in a stockpot over medium heat to melt. Add the chilies and stir for 1 to 2 minutes, until fragrant.

2. Pour in the coconut milk and bring to a boil.

3. Add the chicken broth, galangal, lemongrass, kaffir leaves, fish sauce, and chicken and simmer for 10 minutes, until the chicken is cooked through.

4. Add the mushrooms, onion, lime juice, and cherry tomatoes and simmer for 5 minutes more.

5. Remove the lemongrass, galangal, and kaffir leaves.

6. Serve garnished with fresh cilantro and scallions.

tidbits:

Kaffir lime leaves will yield the most authentic flavor, but if you can't find them you can substitute 2 teaspoons finely grated lime zest plus 3 small bay leaves.

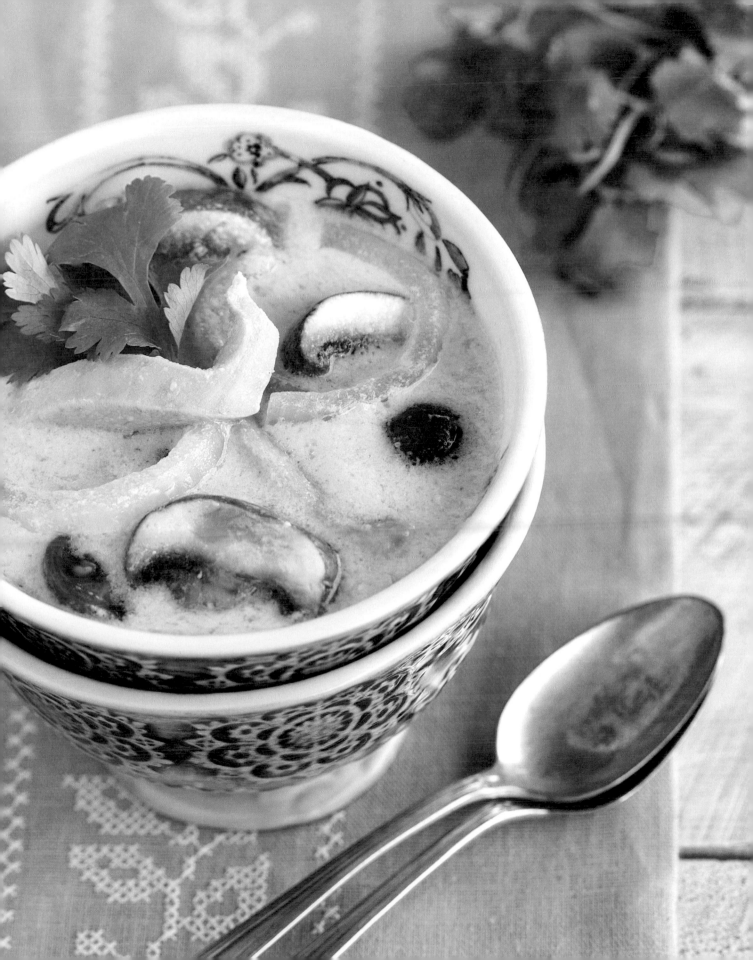

starter salads

*Being a Californian means starting your meals with a small salad usually overflowing with
ambrosial fruits, avocados, and crunchy nuts. Here are four charming starter salads to add some
color and flavor to your dinner rotation.*

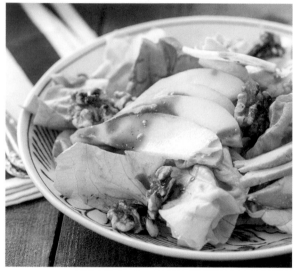

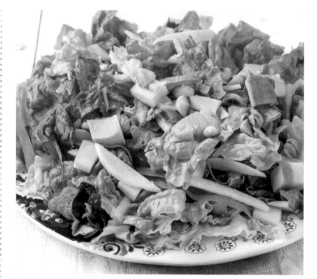

bibb lettuce with d'anjou pears, shaved fennel, avocado, and toasted walnuts

Prep time: 10 minutes   yield: 4 servings

ingredients

- 1 head Bibb lettuce, washed and torn
- 1 d'anjou pear, sliced
- 1 avocado, diced
- 1 fennel bulb, stems and leaves removed, then thinly sliced
- 2 tablespoons chopped toasted walnuts
- ¼ cup Basil-Thyme Vinaigrette (page 320)

method

Combine all salad ingredients in a bowl. Drizzle with dressing and toss to coat.

summer island salad with thai "peanut" vinaigrette

Prep time: 15 minutes   yield: 4 servings

ingredients

- 1 head red-leaf lettuce, washed and shredded
- ½ cup sliced jicama*
- ½ cup shredded carrots
- 1 avocado, diced
- 1 mango, diced
- ¼ cup macadamia nuts, toasted and chopped
- 3 tablespoons Thai 'Peanut' Vinaigrette (page 318)

Omit for SCD.

method

Combine salad ingredients and dressing in a bowl and toss. Top with toasted macadamia nuts.

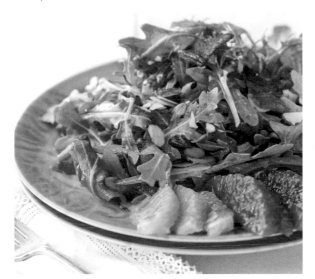

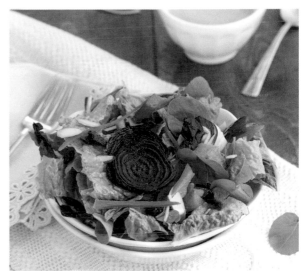

arugula, citrus, and bacon salad

Prep time: 10 minutes   yield: 4 servings

ingredients

- 1 large orange
- 1 small grapefruit
- 6 cups arugula
- 4 slices cooked bacon, chopped
- 2 tablespoons slivered almonds
- Salt and pepper

DRESSING

- 1 tablespoons apple cider vinegar
- 1 teaspoon Dijon mustard
- ¼ cup extra-virgin olive oil

method

Segment the orange and grapefruit, discarding the membranes. Combine the citrus pieces in a bowl with the arugula, bacon, almonds, and a pinch of salt and pepper. Place the vinegar and mustard in a small bowl and whisk. Add the olive oil in a slow, steady stream, whisking constantly until smooth. Drizzle over salad and toss to coat.

winter salad with roasted beets and butternut squash with champagne vinaigrette

prep time: 20 minutes

cooking time: 25 minutes   yield: 4 servings

ingredients

- ½ cup peeled and cubed butternut squash
- ½ cup peeled and sliced red beets
- 1 tablespoon extra-virgin olive oil
- Salt and pepper
- 2 cups washed and torn romaine lettuce
- 1 cup trimmed watercress
- 2 cups torn radicchio
- 1 carrot, shredded
- 2 tablespoons toasted almonds
- 2 tablespoons dried, unsweetened cranberries

DRESSING

- 2 tablespoons champagne vinegar
- 1 teaspoon Dijon mustard
- ½ teaspoon fresh lemon juice
- ¼ cup extra-virgin olive oil

method

Toss the squash and beets in olive oil and season with salt and pepper. Roast at 400°F for 15 minutes, until tender. Remove from the oven and let cool.

Toss together the butternut squash, beets, lettuces, carrot, almonds, and cranberries in a bowl. In another small bowl, whisk together the vinegar, mustard, lemon juice, and olive oil. Drizzle over the salad and toss to coat.

Danielle Walker

curried chicken salad

prep time: 30 minutes   chilling time: 60 minutes
cooking time: 15 minutes   yield: 4 servings

My great-grandmother used to make a version of this salad for family outings to the county fair. According to my grandma, she would wrap it up in pretty bowls and always bring real china and napkins instead of plastic picnic wear. She tells me we would have gotten along well. So it's no wonder that I obsessively collect small dishes and other various props for photographing my creations!

ingredients

- 2 pounds skinless, boneless chicken breasts
- 2 teaspoons coconut oil, melted
- Salt and pepper
- ½ cup Mayonnaise (page 308)
- ½ cup grapes, halved
- ½ cup cashew halves, toasted
- ¼ cup finely chopped celery
- ¼ cup finely chopped red onion
- ¼ cup finely shredded carrots
- ½ teaspoon sea salt
- Curry Spice Mix (recipe follows)
- 1 tablespoon chopped fresh mint leaves

CURRY SPICE MIX
(or substitute 2 tablespoons curry powder)

- 2 teaspoons cumin
- 2 teaspoons coriander
- 1½ teaspoons turmeric
- 1½ teaspoons ground ginger
- 1 teaspoon ground mustard
- ½ teaspoon cardamom
- ½ teaspoon ground fenugreek
- ¼ teaspoon cayenne pepper

method

1. Preheat the oven to 350°F.
2. Place the chicken on a baking sheet, drizzle with the coconut oil, and sprinkle with a pinch of salt and pepper.
3. Bake for 15 to 17 minutes, until cooked all the way through.
4. Remove the chicken from the oven and cut it into cubes. Chill in the refrigerator for 30 minutes.
5. Combine the Mayonnaise, grapes, cashews, celery, red onion, carrots, salt, and Curry Spice Mix in a bowl.
6. Add the chicken and toss to coat. Chill in the refrigerator for at least 30 minutes, or up to 24 hours, before serving.
7. Sprinkle with fresh chopped mint right before serving.

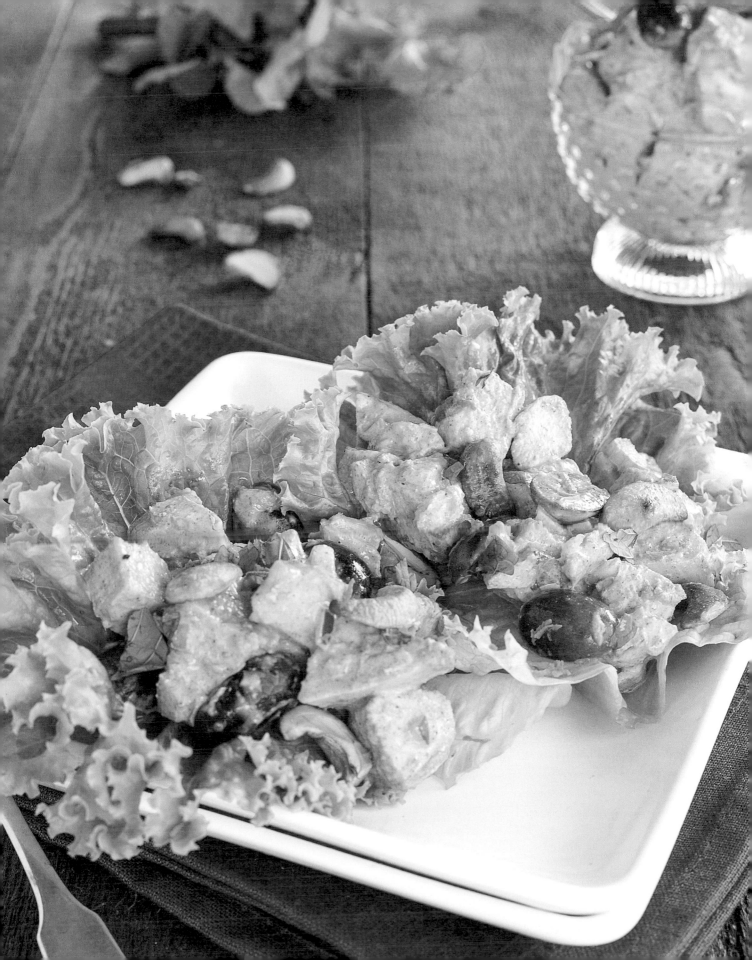

green papaya salad

prep time: 20 minutes   cooking time: 5 minutes

chilling time: 60 minutes   yield: 6 servings

Green papaya salads have always been one of my favorite appetizers at Thai restaurants, but when we lived in Kona, Hawaii for a short period, I realized that they were actually really easy to make at home. Green papayas are pretty abundant at the farmers' markets there, so we were able to enjoy this salad anytime a craving hit. If you're not in a tropical area, you can find these fruits at Asian markets, or substitute unripe mangos or even jicama. The dressing complements any relatively crunchy, julienned fruit or vegetable.

ingredients

- **4 ounces green beans (about ½ cup)**
- **½ pound green papaya**
- **1 cup shredded carrots**
- **¼ cup diced tomatoes**
- **2 tablespoons fish sauce**
- **2 tablespoons chopped fresh cilantro**
- **2 tablespoons honey**
- **1 tablespoon fresh lime juice**
- **¾ teaspoon minced garlic**
- **¼ teaspoon cayenne pepper**
- **1 tablespoon cashew pieces, toasted in a skillet for 5 minutes**
- **1 green onion, finely sliced**

method

1. Boil a large pot of water and blanch the green beans for 5 minutes, until bright green and tender.

2. Peel the papaya and remove the seeds. Slice it into thin noodles using a julienne slicer or a sharp knife.

3. Combine the papaya noodles, green beans, carrots, and tomatoes in a bowl.

4. In a separate bowl, whisk together the fish sauce, cilantro, honey, lime juice, garlic, and cayenne pepper. Pour over the vegetables and toss to coat.

5. Refrigerate for 1 hour. Serve with toasted cashew pieces and sliced green onion.

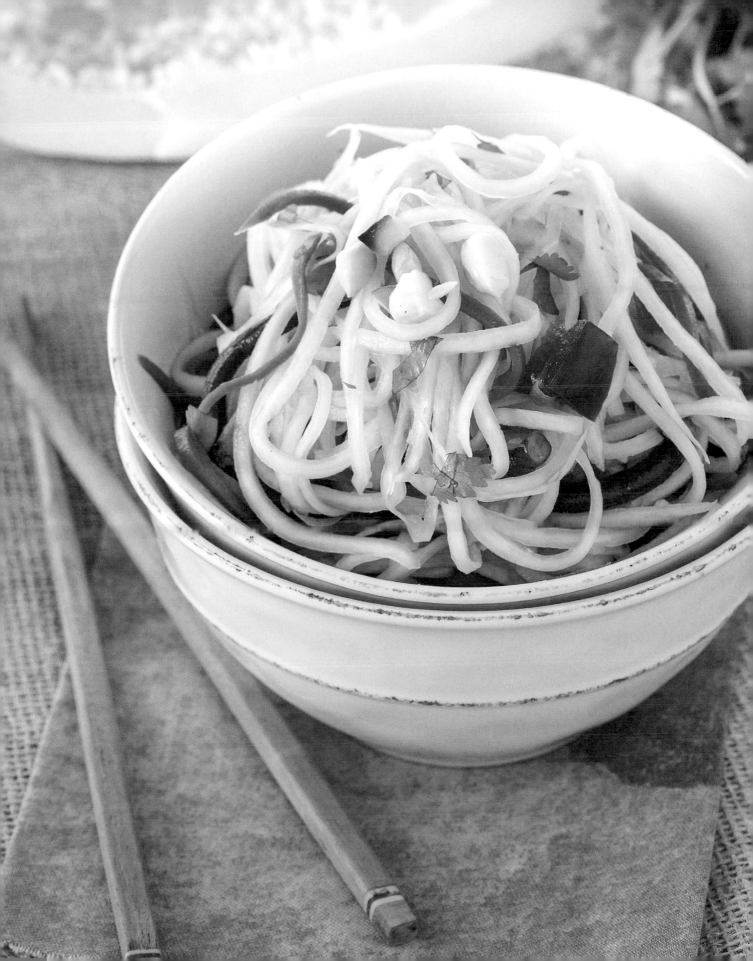

asian mango slaw

prep time: 10 minutes   chilling time: 30 minutes   yield: 4 servings

This vibrant Thai-inspired slaw has just the right balance of sweet and salty. Serve it as a side salad with Asian dishes or top it with grilled prawns for a meal in itself.

ingredients

- 1 cup broccoli-slaw mix
- ½ cup seeded and julienned red bell peppers
- ½ cup peeled and julienned carrots
- 2 teaspoons chopped fresh basil
- 1 mango, peeled and julienned
- ¼ cup Thai 'Peanut' Vinaigrette (page 318)
- Garnish: sliced almonds

method

1. Place all the ingredients together in a bowl and stir to combine. Cover and refrigerate for 30 minutes before serving.

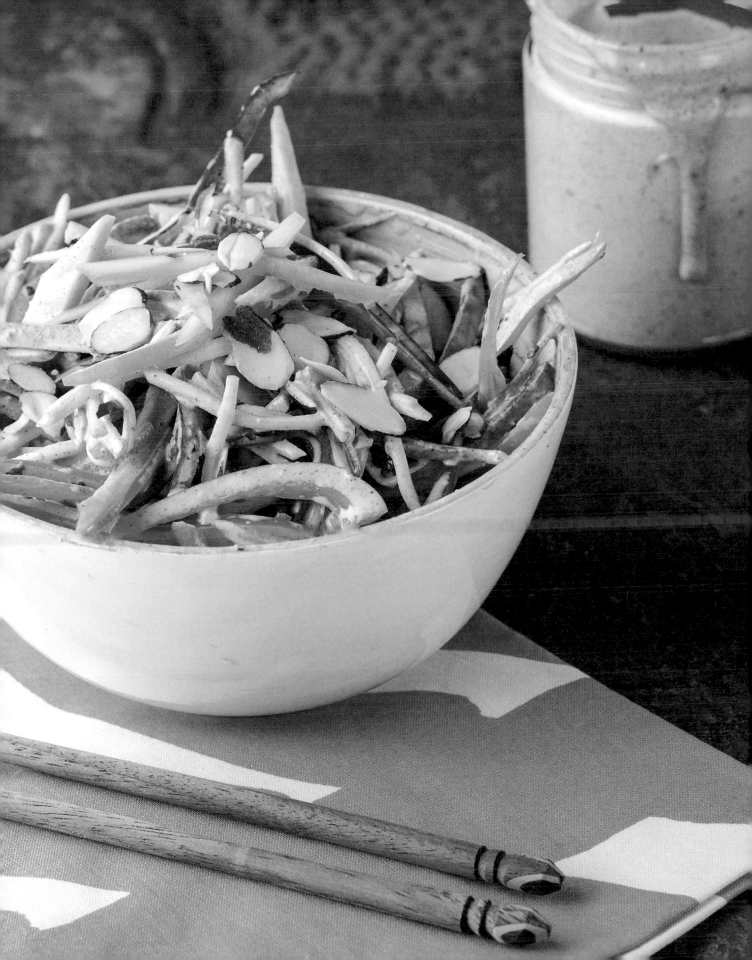

warm spinach salad
with bacon and mushrooms

prep time: 10 minutes   cooking time: 35 minutes   yield: 4 servings

Caramelized onions, salty bacon, sautéed mushrooms, and chicken served atop a bed of baby spinach with Basil–Thyme Vinaigrette.

ingredients

- 4 slices bacon
- 1 medium yellow onion, thinly sliced
- ¼ teaspoon sea salt
- 1 pound chicken breasts, cubed
- 4 ounces Portobello mushrooms, sliced
- 8 ounces baby spinach
- 2 tablespoons Basil-Thyme Vinaigrette (page 320)

method

1. Place the bacon in a skillet over medium heat and cook for 5 minutes, until slightly crisp. Set the bacon aside and drain half of the fat from the pan.

2. Add the onion and salt to the skillet and cook over medium-low heat for 20 minutes, stirring occasionally.

3. Increase the heat to medium-high, and then add the chicken and mushrooms and continue to cook for 8 minutes, until the chicken is cooked through.

4. Roughly chop the bacon, then return it to the pan just long enough to reheat it. Remove the skillet from the heat.

5. Place the spinach in a bowl, toss with the vinaigrette, and then spoon the hot toppings over the spinach.

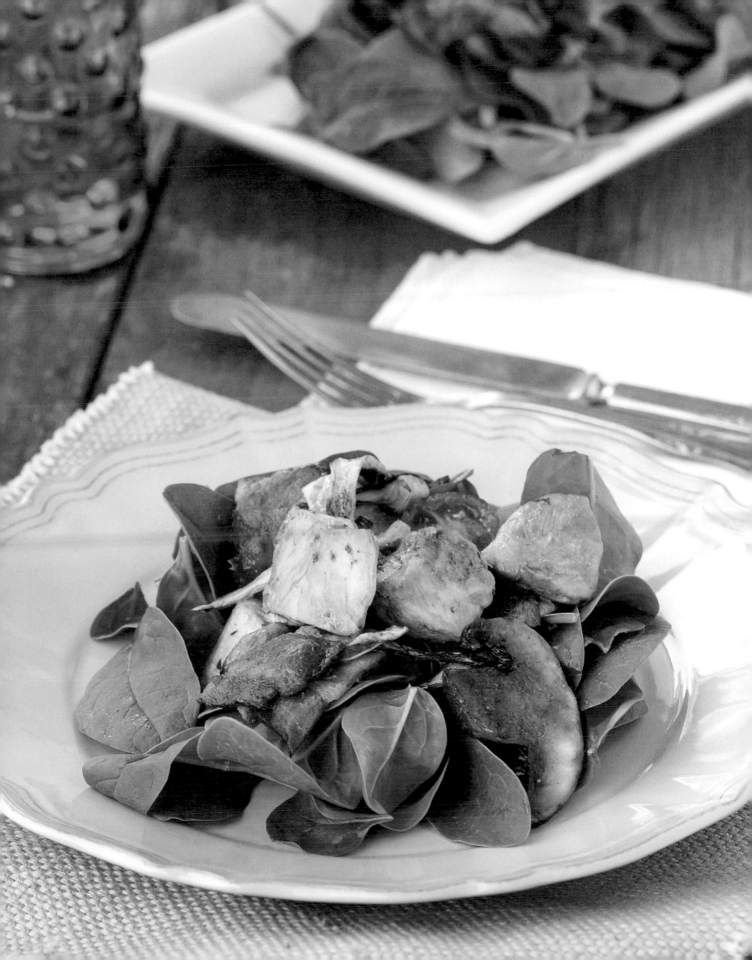

roasted-garlic mashed faux-tatoes

prep time: 15-20 minutes   cooking time: 25 minutes   yield: 4 servings

While the flavor of licorice is a characteristic of raw fennel, roasting the bulbs brings out a subtler, savory taste. In this dish roasted fennel and garlic are puréed with celeriac, or celery root, to mimic the texture of mashed potatoes, but with a third of the carbohydrates. This is a great alternative for those who don't like cauliflower, which is the most frequent substitute for mashed potatoes.

ingredients

- 4 fennel bulbs, stalks and leaves removed
- 2 cloves garlic
- 2 tablespoons extra-virgin olive oil
- ¾ teaspoon sea salt, divided
- ¼ teaspoon freshly cracked black pepper, divided
- 3 celeriac, peeled and cubed (about 4 cups)
- 3 tablespoons ghee
- ½ cup unsweetened almond milk

method

1. Preheat the oven to 425°F.

2. Cut the fennel into quarters and place it in an oven-safe dish with the garlic. Drizzle olive oil over it and sprinkle with ¼ teaspoon of the salt and ⅛ teaspoon of pepper. Cover and place in the oven and roast for 25 minutes.

3. Bring a large stockpot of water to a boil and boil the celeriac until soft, about 12 minutes. Drain and add to a food processor.

4. Add the roasted garlic and fennel mixture, ghee, almond milk, ½ teaspoon salt, and remaining pepper to the food processor and process until smooth.

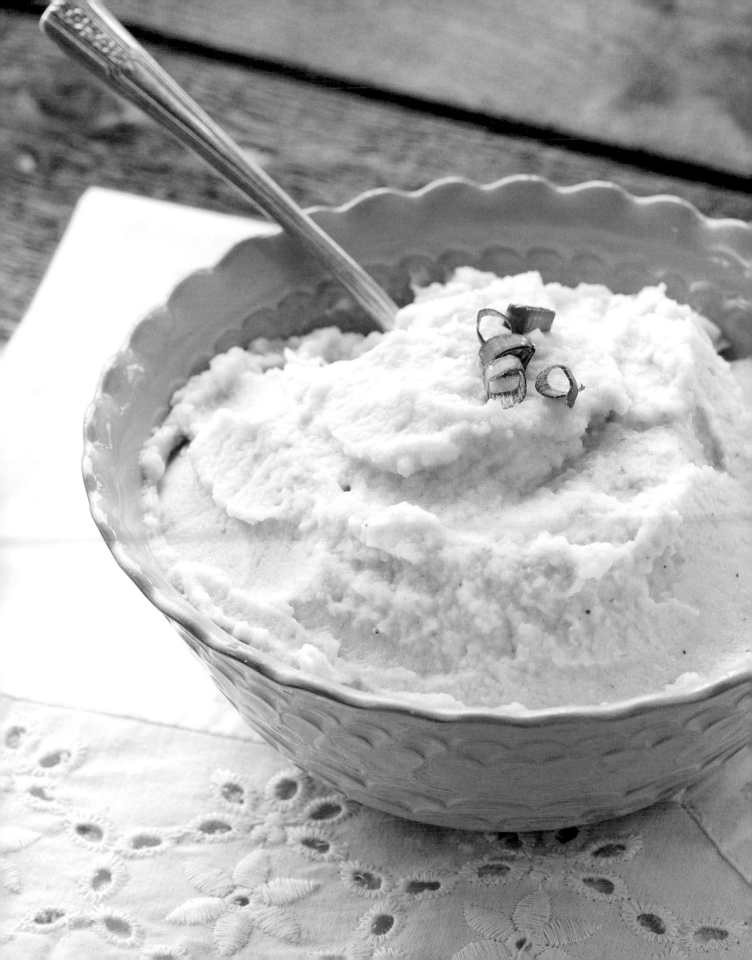

ginger-garlic broccoli

prep time: 5 minutes   cooking time: 16 minutes   yield: 4 to 6 servings

This Chinese–takeout–inspired side dish is a snap to make and so scrumptious that even your kids will ask for seconds.

ingredients

- 1 tablespoon coconut oil
- 1 tablespoon dark sesame oil
- 1 tablespoon minced garlic
- 1 tablespoon minced ginger
- 2 pounds broccoli, trimmed into florets
- ½ teaspoon sea salt
- 2 tablespoons coconut aminos
- ¼ cup water

method

1. Place the oils in a skillet or wok, heat over medium-high heat, and then add the garlic and ginger. Sauté until fragrant, but not browned.

2. Add the broccoli and salt and stir-fry for 10 minutes.

3. Add the coconut aminos and water and bring to a boil.

4. Reduce the heat, then cover and simmer for 3 to 5 minutes, until the broccoli is just tender and bright green.

tidbits:
Dark sesame oil is the same as toasted sesame oil or Chinese sesame oil.

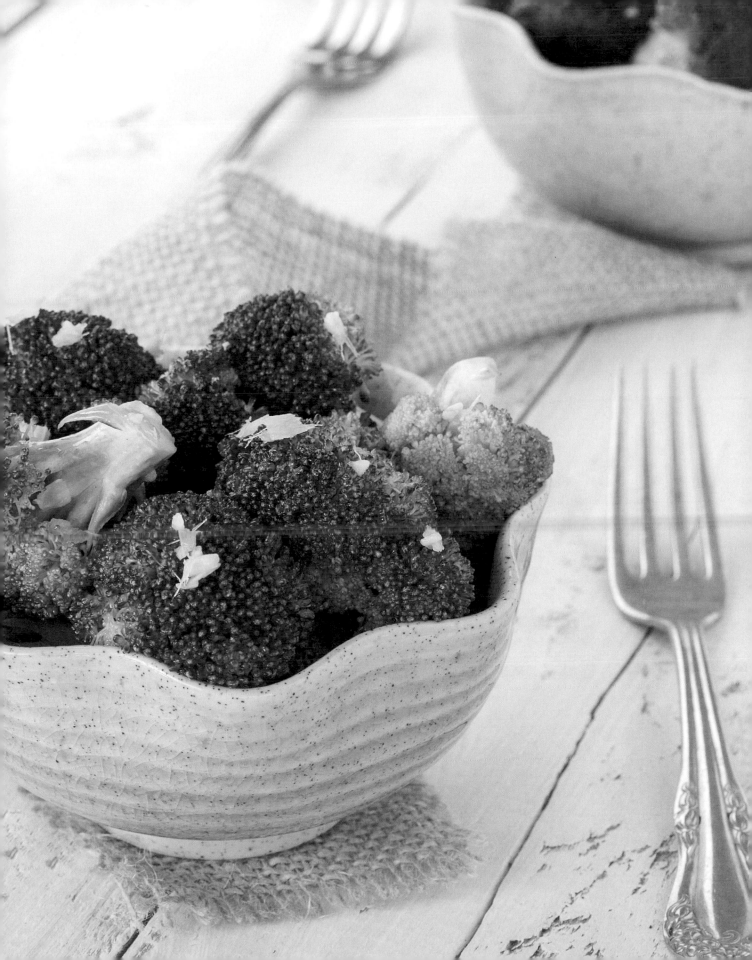

grilled artichokes with rémoulade

prep time: 20 minutes   cooking time: 30 minutes   yield: 4 servings

Artichokes are most often served steamed, but grilling gives them a smoky kick, which is perfectly paired with this pungent rémoulade for dipping.

ingredients

- 4 artichokes
- 1 lemon, halved
- 2 tablespoons extra-virgin olive oil
- Salt and pepper

REMOULADE

- 2 tablespoons Mayonnaise (page 308)
- 1 teaspoon Dijon mustard
- 1 clove garlic, crushed
- 1 teaspoon anchovy paste
- 1 tablespoon fresh lemon juice
- 1 teaspoon chopped capers
- ⅛ teaspoon cayenne pepper
- ¼ teaspoon apple cider vinegar
- 1 tablespoon chopped fresh parsley

method

1. Fill a large pot a quarter of the way with water and bring to a boil.

2. Trim the stems two inches from the base of the artichokes and cut them in half. Cut off and discard the top pointy ½-inch of each half and use a strong metal spoon to scrape away the fuzzy chokes and the small inner artichoke leaves. To prevent the cut portions from browning, immediately rub with lemon piece.

3. Squeeze the juice from the lemon into the pot. Add the halves and the artichokes to the pot. The water should reach about halfway up the artichokes, not submerge them. Reduce the heat to medium and cook, covered, for 20 minutes.

4. Meanwhile, make the rémoulade. Place all the ingredients in a bowl and whisk to combine. Season with salt and pepper to taste.

5. Heat a grill to medium-high heat. Drain the water from the pot and place the artichokes on a cutting board. Drizzle the flat sides with olive oil and sprinkle with salt and pepper.

6. Grill the artichokes cut side down for 10 minutes. Serve with rémoulade on the side.

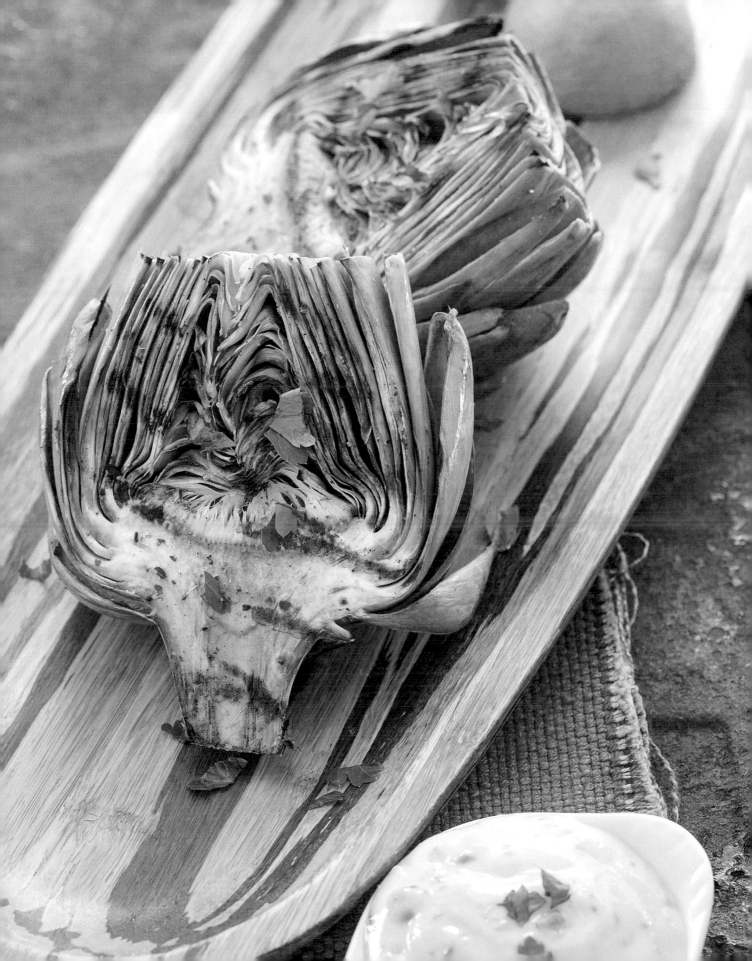

stir-fried baby bok choy

prep time: 5 minutes   cooking time: 8 minutes   yield: 4 servings

Baby bok choy has a sweeter, more delicate flavor than the adult variety and tenderizes nicely when stir-fried in this piquant sauce of sesame, ginger, and garlic.

ingredients

- 2 teaspoons coconut oil
- 1 teaspoon sesame oil
- 2 teaspoons minced garlic
- 1 teaspoon grated ginger
- 1 pound baby bok choy
- 1 tablespoon fish sauce

method

1. Place all the oil in a large skillet or wok and heat over medium-high heat.

2. Add the garlic and ginger and sauté until fragrant but not browned, about 1 minute.

3. Trim the large white stalks from the bok choy, leaving about a ½-inch at the bottom.

4. Add the bok choy to the skillet and cook, stirring occasionally, for 3 minutes.

5. Add the fish sauce, then cover and steam the bok choy for 2 to 3 minutes, until the leaves are wilted and the stalks are semisoft.

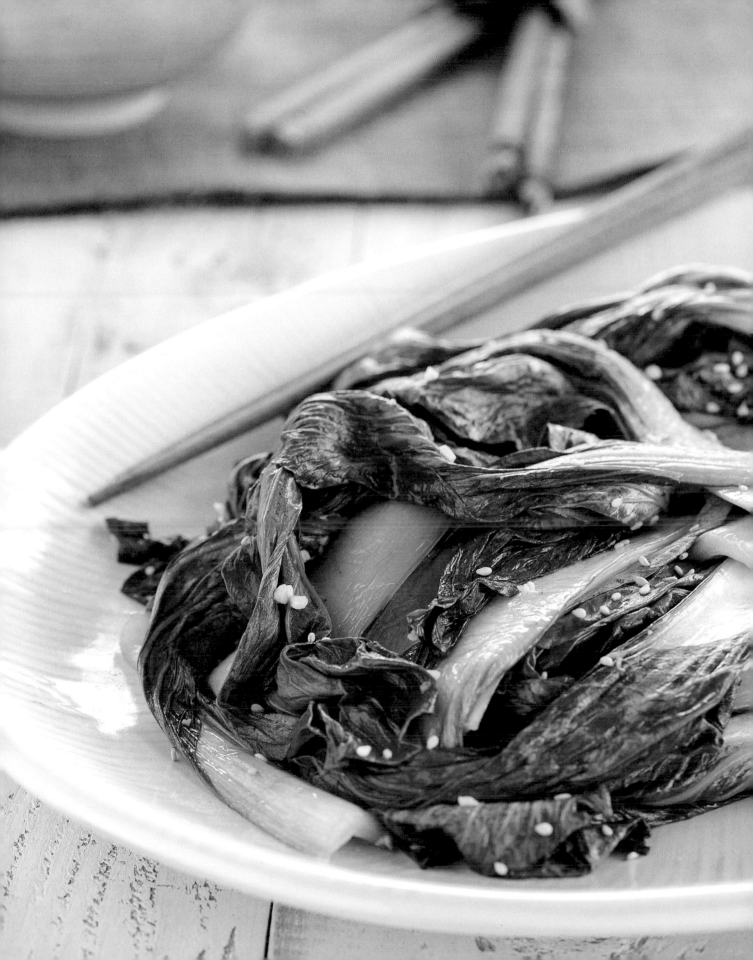

basic cauli-rice

prep time: 15 minutes   *cooking time:* 17 minutes   *yield:* 4 servings

Cauliflower is the chameleon of vegetables—it can easily replace many of the starchy vegetables in the dishes you used to adore so you don't have to miss them. With my love for Asian food, the elimination of rice left a big, black hole on my plate and nothing to soak up the velvety, spice-laden sauces. "Riced" cauliflower is a magnificent grain-free substitute and can be served with anything from Thai to Indian cuisines.

ingredients

- 1 head cauliflower, trimmed and cut into florets
- 2 teaspoons extra-virgin olive oil
- 1 teaspoon sesame oil
- ½ cup finely diced yellow onion
- 1 clove garlic, finely minced
- ½ cup water

method

1. Place the cauliflower florets in a food processor fitted with a grating attachment and process, until grated into "rice grains." Alternatively, grate the cauliflower with a cheese grater.

2. Heat the oil in a large skillet or wok over medium-high heat. Add the onion and garlic and sauté for 5 minutes.

3. Add the riced cauliflower and continue cooking for 5 to 7 minutes, until the onions are translucent.

4. Add the water, then cover and steam for 5 minutes, until the cauliflower is cooked and the water has been absorbed.

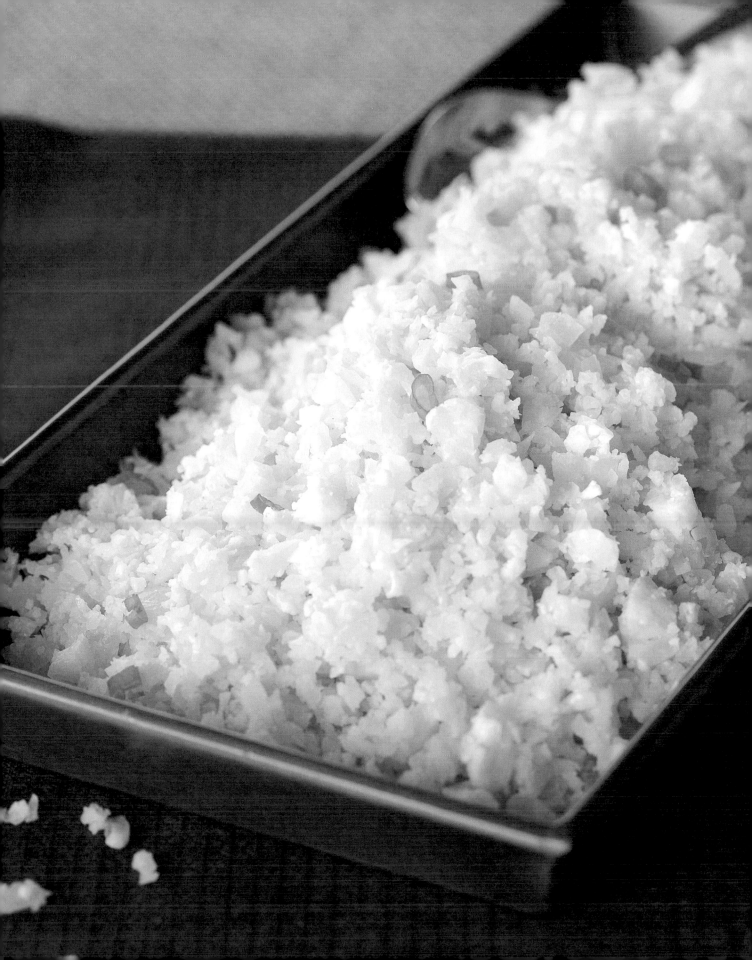

shaved brussels sprouts with bacon, leeks, and pomegranate seeds

prep time: 15 minutes   cooking time: 8 minutes   yield: 6 servings

Shaving Brussels sprouts makes them tender and lends a great texture to a dish. I like to combine them with bacon, leeks, and pomegranate seeds for a savory side dish that surprises with its pop of tang.

ingredients

- 2 pounds Brussels sprouts
- 5 slices bacon, chopped
- 1 leek, sliced, white part only
- 1 clove garlic, minced
- ⅔ cup Chicken Broth (page 316)
- ¾ teaspoon sea salt
- Pinch cracked black pepper
- 2 tablespoons pomegranate seeds

method

1. Shred the Brussels sprouts using the grater attachment on a food processor or a mandoline.
2. Cook the bacon in a large skillet or stockpot set over medium-high heat until crisp.
3. Remove the bacon from the pan, and set aside, leaving the grease in the pan.
4. Add the Brussels sprouts, leek, and garlic to the pan and sauté for 5 minutes.
5. Add the chicken broth, salt, and pepper. Cover and steam for 5 minutes, until the Brussels sprouts are bright green and tender. Return the bacon to the pan.
6. Garnish with pomegranate seeds and serve warm.

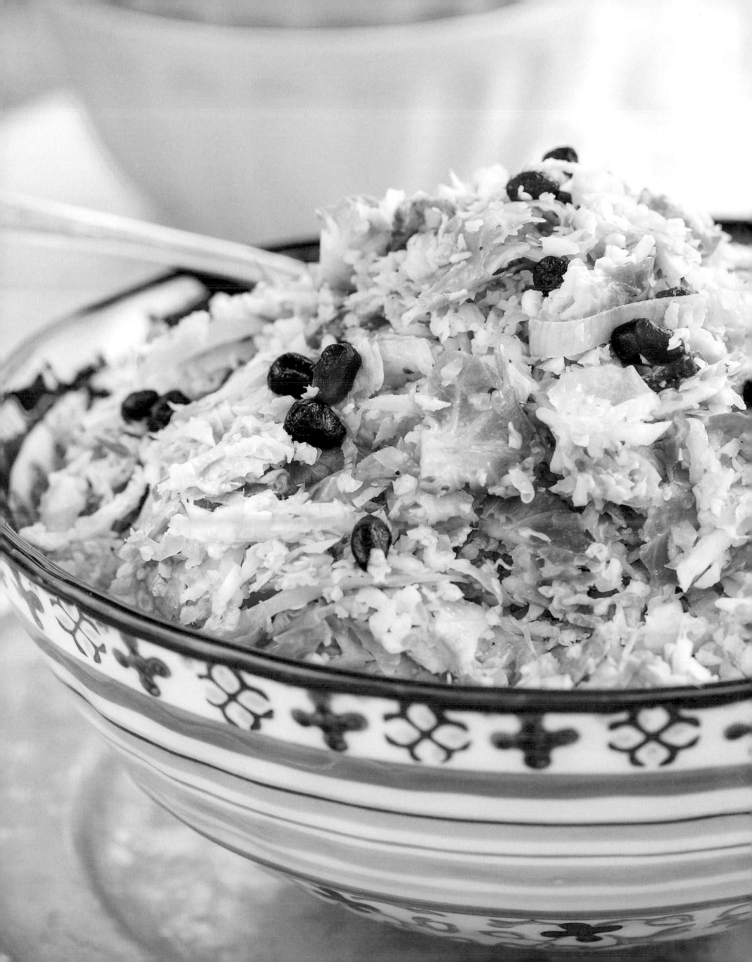

mashed cauliflower

prep time: 15 minutes   cooking time: 15 minutes   yield: 4 servings

An exceptional mashed potato substitute when you're looking to cut down on starches, mashed cauliflower will complement all of your favorite comfort-food dishes without leaving you feeling heavy—or guilty—afterward. When roasted, garlic becomes smooth and buttery. I love to add it to my mash for extra flavor and richness.

ingredients

- 5 cloves garlic, unpeeled
- 1 tablespoon extra-virgin olive oil
- 1 head cauliflower, trimmed into florets
- ¼ cup almond milk, warmed
- 3 tablespoons ghee or preferred butter substitute
- 1½ teaspoons sea salt
- Dash cracked black pepper

method

1. Preheat the oven to 425°F.
2. Place the garlic cloves in a small, heatproof dish and drizzle with the olive oil. Cover and roast in the oven for 15 minutes.
3. Meanwhile, put the cauliflower in a saucepan with ½-inch of water. Cover, and steam for 10 minutes. Drain the water completely and place the cauliflower in a food processor.
4. Squeeze the papery garlic skins to release the cloves. Add the garlic to the food processor along with the almond milk, ghee, salt, and pepper. Process until smooth and fluffy.

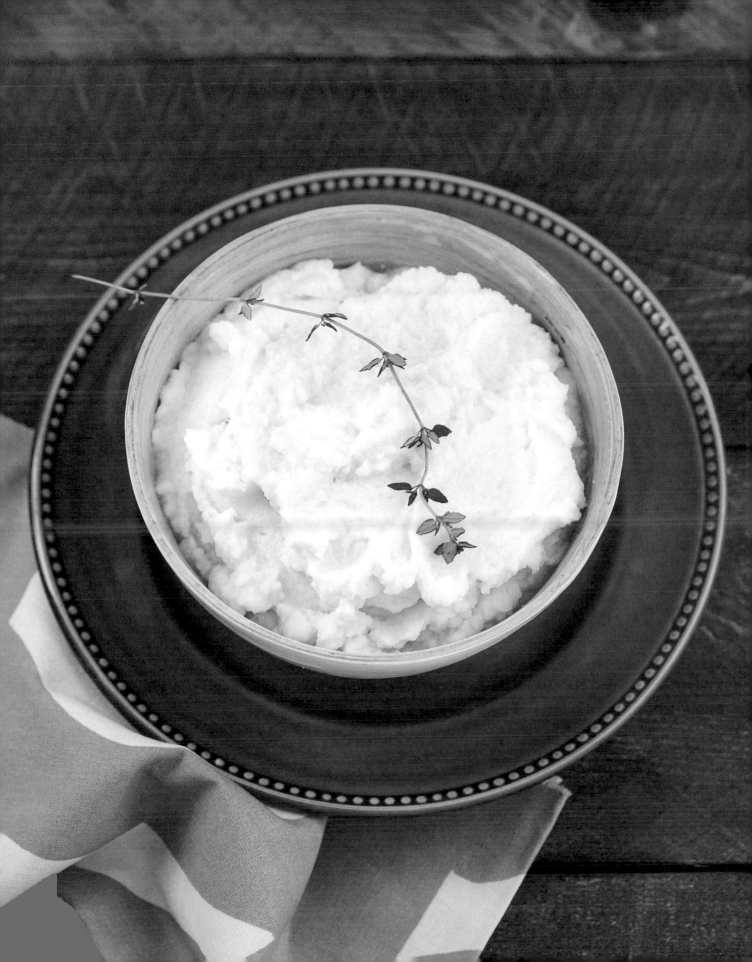

grilled lemon-garlic zucchini

prep time: 20 minutes   cooking time: 6 minutes   yield: 4 servings

Marinated in lemon, garlic, and parsley before grilling, this zucchini dish pairs nicely with any barbecued meat as-is or can be chilled and tossed with Marinated Artichoke Hearts (page 76) for a refreshing summer salad.

ingredients

- 1 tablespoon extra-virgin olive oil
- 2 teaspoons chopped flat-leaf parsley
- ½ teaspoon fresh lemon juice
- ¼ teaspoon sea salt
- Dash garlic salt
- Dash freshly ground black pepper
- 1 pound zucchini, edges trimmed and thinly sliced

method

1. Place all the ingredients, except the zucchini, in a small bowl and whisk to combine.

2. Place the zucchini in a shallow dish, pour the marinade over, and let sit for 15 minutes.

3. Meanwhile, preheat a grill to medium heat.

4. Grill the zucchini for 3 minutes on each side, until tender and bright green.

slow cooker sesame-orange chicken

prep time: 10 minutes   cooking time: 4 hours 20 minutes   yield: 6 servings

This classic Chinese dish is a favorite among many when ordering take-out, but the fried batter and sugary sauce can be overwhelming. I use tender chunks of chicken thighs and cook them slowly in a slow cooker with a tangy and sweet sauce to give you a meal with the flavor of the original, but without the negative health consequences. Serve over Basic Cauli-Rice (page 118) and create your own fortune!

ingredients

- 2 pounds boneless, skinless chicken thighs
- ⅓ cup coconut aminos
- ⅓ cup honey
- 2 tablespoons orange juice
- 2 tablespoons tomato paste
- 1 tablespoon toasted sesame oil
- 2 teaspoons minced garlic
- ½ teaspoon ground ginger
- ¾ teaspoon sea salt
- ½ teaspoon red pepper flakes
- ¼ teaspoon cracked black pepper
- Garnish: sesame seeds

method

1. Trim any visible fat from the chicken, then place it in a single layer in the bottom of a slow cooker.

2. Place the remaining ingredients, except sesame seeds, in a bowl, whisk together, and pour over the chicken.

3. Turn the chicken once to ensure even coating.

4. Cook the chicken on low for 4 hours.

5. Remove the chicken from the sauce and cut it into cubes.

6. Spoon any fat off the top of the sauce, then transfer the sauce to a small pan.

7. Simmer the sauce over medium heat for 20 minutes, until it has reduced by half and is thick and shiny.

8. Toss the chicken in the sauce and serve with a sprinkle of sesame seeds.

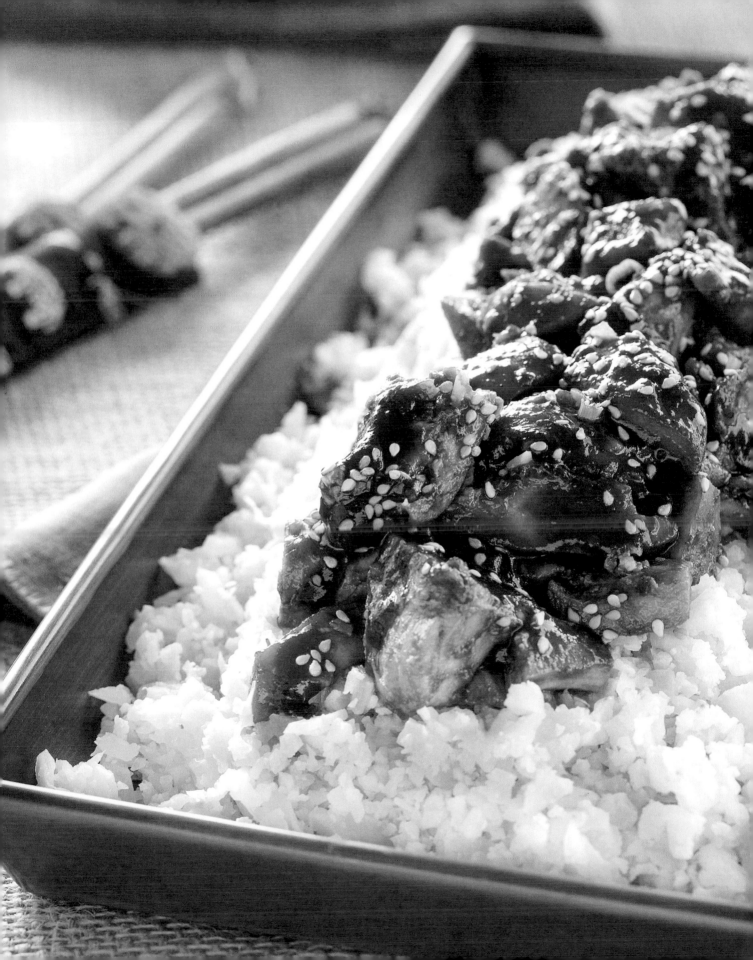

braised chicken
in artichoke-mushroom sauce

prep time: 15 minutes   cooking time: 60 minutes   yield: 4 to 6 servings

My mom has made us a version of this dish for as long as I can remember, and it was the first thing she made me when I got out of the hospital after the birth of my son. Even though I could only grab bites between bouncing and rocking, it was sweet to enjoy a familiar meal after eating hospital food for days while living on little to no sleep! My mom's recipe calls for quite a few ingredients that I am now unable to eat, but I've adjusted it so that I can enjoy it once again.

ingredients

- 6 tablespoons bacon fat, ghee, or unsalted butter, divided
- 2 pounds chicken leg quarters
- 2 pounds chicken drumsticks
- 1 teaspoons sea salt, plus more for finishing
- ¼ teaspoon cracked black pepper
- ½ teaspoon paprika, plus more for finishing
- ½ pound sliced cremini mushrooms, stems removed
- ¾ cup Chicken Broth (page 316)
- 1½ tablespoons apple cider vinegar
- 1 teaspoon honey
- 1 tablespoon coconut flour
- 2 cups Marinated Artichoke Hearts (page 76 or from a jar)

method

1. Preheat the oven to 375°F.

2. Place 4 tablespoons bacon fat in a large Dutch oven or stockpot and heat over medium-high heat.

3. Rinse and dry all the chicken, then sprinkle with the salt, pepper, and paprika.

4. Add the chicken to the pot and cook for 8 minutes, turning every 2 minutes to brown evenly on all sides.

5. Remove the chicken and set aside.

6. Add the remaining 2 tablespoons bacon fat to the pot, then add the mushrooms, and sauté for 5 minutes.

7. Stir in the Broth, vinegar, honey and coconut flour and simmer for 10 minutes.

8. Return the chicken to the pot, and then scatter the artichoke hearts around it.

9. Spoon a bit of the sauce over top of the chicken and artichokes, cover, place in the oven, and bake for 40 minutes.

10. Remove from the oven and finish with a pinch of salt and paprika.

tidbits:

Chicken leg quarters contain the thigh, drumstick and a portion of the back. Asher enjoys eating the drumsticks by themselves, so I use a combination of both. Feel free to substitute chicken breasts or thighs as well.

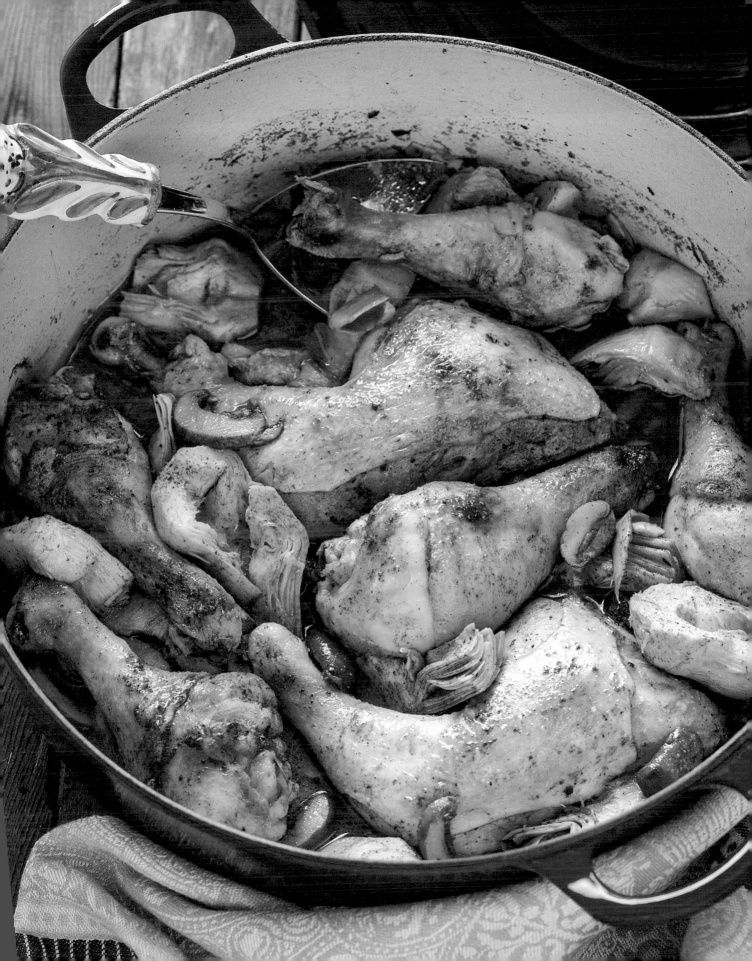

"fettuccine" alfredo with blackened chicken

prep time: 40 minutes   cooking time: 30 minutes   yield: 4 servings

My dad has always favored creamy Alfredo sauce over red sauce, so I created this dish with him in mind. I add prosciutto to the sauce to make it rich and flavorful and serve it with a Cajun spiced grilled chicken breast on the side.

ingredients

- 1 cup raw cashews
- 1½ pounds boneless, skinless chicken breasts
- 1 tablespoon Cajun Spice Rub, recipe to follow
- 4 large zucchini, about 2 pounds
- 1¼ teaspoons sea salt, divided
- 1 tablespoon extra-virgin olive oil
- ½ pound asparagus, trimmed and cut into 1-inch pieces
- 1 leek, white part only, thinly sliced
- ½ cup chopped cremini mushrooms
- 2 ounces prosciutto, chopped
- 2 cups water
- 1 tablespoon fresh lemon juice
- 1 clove garlic, minced
- ¼ teaspoon white pepper
- ⅛ teaspoon nutmeg
- Garnish: toasted pine nuts

CAJUN SPICE RUB

- 2 teaspoons extra-virgin olive oil
- 1 teaspoon coarse sea salt
- ¾ teaspoon paprika
- ½ teaspoon fresh cracked pepper
- ¼ teaspoon chili powder
- ¼ teaspoon cayenne pepper
- ¼ teaspoon cumin
- ¼ teaspoon onion powder
- ¼ teaspoon dried thyme
- ¼ teaspoon dried oregano
- 1 garlic clove, crushed

method

1. Place the cashews in a bowl of water that's been heated to a boil and soak for 30 minutes.

2. Meanwhile, rub the chicken all over with the Cajun Spice Rub and heat a grill to medium-high. Grill the chicken on both sides until it is no longer pink in the center, about 10 to 15 minutes. Remove the chicken and slice it into thin strips.

3. Peel the zucchini and slice off the ends. Using a spiral slicer or julienne peeler, turn the zucchini into long noodles, discarding the seeded portion. Bring a large pot of water to a boil. Add the zucchini noodles and boil for 3 to 5 minutes. Use tongs to remove the noodles, placing them on a baking sheet lined with paper towels. Sprinkle with ¼ teaspoon of the salt. Set aside to "sweat" until the sauce is done.

4. Place the asparagus in the zucchini water and return to a boil. Blanch for 2 to 3 minutes, until slightly tender and bright green. Drain the asparagus and wipe the pan dry.

5. Return the pan to the heat. Add the olive oil, asparagus, leek, mushrooms, and prosciutto. Sauté for 5 minutes over medium-high heat. Reduce the heat to low.

6. Drain the cashews and place in a blender with the 2 cups water. Add the lemon juice, garlic, white pepper, nutmeg, and remaining teaspoon salt. Blend on high until smooth.

7. Add the sauce to the prosciutto mixture and simmer for 7 to 10 minutes.

8. Place the noodles and chicken in a large bowl, add the sauce, and toss to combine. Garnish with toasted pine nuts.

tidbits:

Zucchini holds a lot of moisture, which is released when it's cooked. To achieve a tender noodle that does not water down the sauce, the noodles are first blanched in hot water and left to sweat their liquid out while the remainder of the dish is prepared.

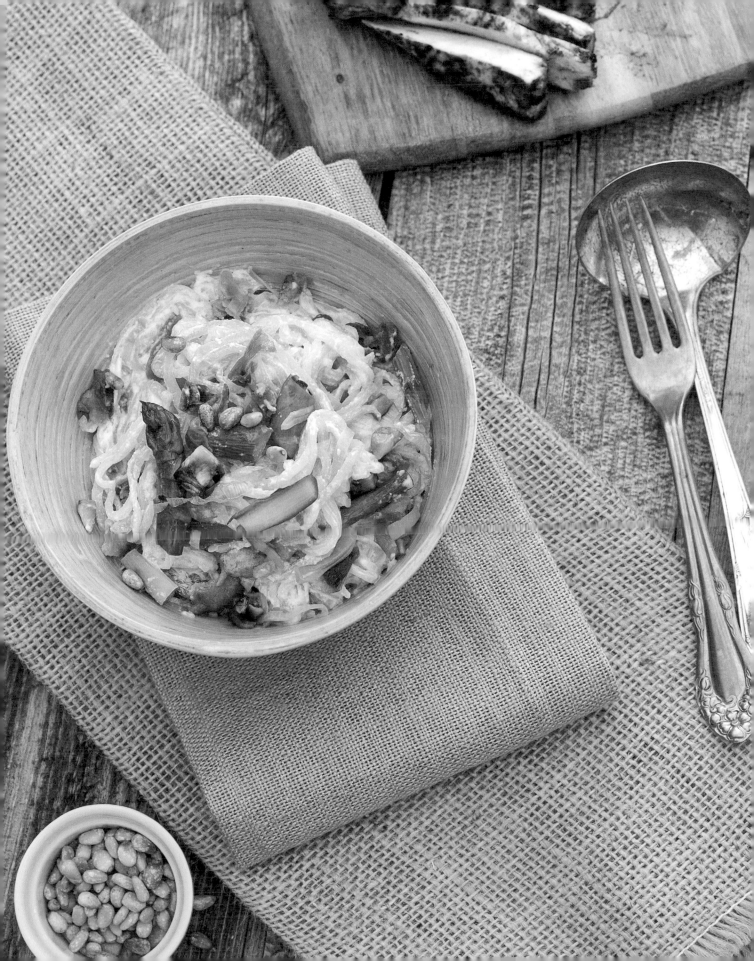

chicken cobb salad

prep time: 15 minutes + 30 minutes marinating time

cooking time: 14 minutes   yield: 4 to 6 servings

Even my husband is happy to eat this salad as a meal because it's so hearty. The Dijon and basil lend complexity to the dressing, and the artichoke hearts provide the extra layer of flavor that blue cheese does in the traditional version.

ingredients

- 2 tablespoons extra-virgin olive oil
- 2 tablespoons Dijon mustard
- 1 clove garlic, crushed
- ¼ teaspoon sea salt
- pinch cracked black pepper
- 2 boneless, skinless chicken breasts
- 2 cups baby romaine or spring mix
- 2 cups shredded romaine hearts
- ¼ cup Basil-Thyme Vinaigrette (page 320)
- 1 cup chopped plain artichoke hearts
- 1 cup chopped baby tomatoes
- 4 hard-boiled eggs, chopped
- 6 slices cooked bacon, chopped
- 1 avocado, diced

method

1. Place the oil, mustard, garlic, salt, and pepper in a bowl and whisk to combine.

2. Place the chicken in a shallow dish, pour the marinade over it, and marinate for 30 minutes.

3. Heat a grill to medium and grill the chicken until the thickest part reaches 170°F on a meat thermometer. Remove the chicken from the heat, dice, and set aside to cool.

4. Place all the lettuce in a bowl, add the vinaigrette, and toss. Arrange the remaining ingredients with the chicken on top or toss everything together to serve.

tidbits:

To make perfect hard-boiled eggs, place the eggs in a pot of cold water. Bring the water to a boil, then cover and remove the pot from the heat. Allow the eggs to cook in the hot water for 20 minutes.

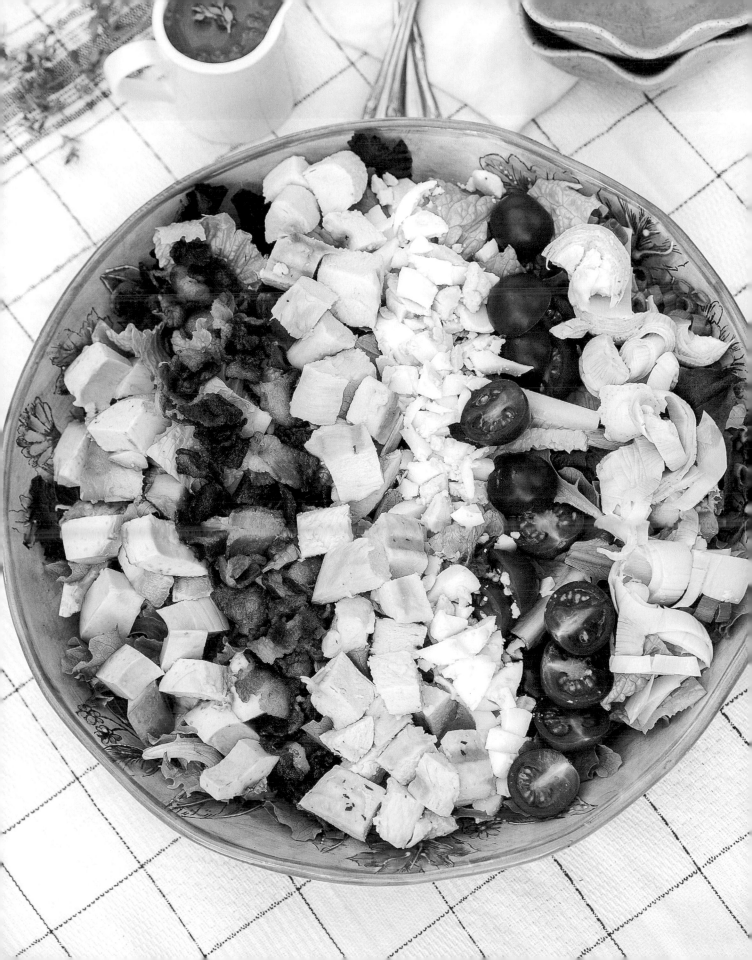

slow cooker chicken tacos

prep time: 15 minutes   cooking time: 6 hours   yield: 6 to 8 servings

This chicken melts in your mouth and smells incredible when you walk in the house after a long day at work or running kids to and from activities. Serve in butter lettuce cups with all of your favorite taco fixings or wrapped in my Crepes (see recipe on page 302).

ingredients

- 1 pound boneless chicken thighs, trimmed of fat
- 1 pound boneless chicken breasts
- 3 cups diced tomatoes in juices, from a jar or fresh
- 1 small yellow onion, diced
- 4 cloves garlic, minced
- 2 serrano chilies, seeded and chopped
- 2 tablespoons chopped cilantro
- 1 tablespoon cumin
- 1 tablespoon chili powder
- 2½ teaspoons coriander
- 2 teaspoons sea salt
- ½ teaspoon cayenne pepper
- ½ teaspoon black pepper
- Topping suggestions: avocado, jalapenos, Pico de Gallo (page 332), cilantro

method

1. Place all the ingredients in a slow cooker and cook on low for 5 hours.
2. Remove the chicken, shred with two forks, then return to sauce for an additional hour.

tidbits:

If you're short on time, use a jar of your favorite salsa instead of the tomatoes, onions, and chilies.

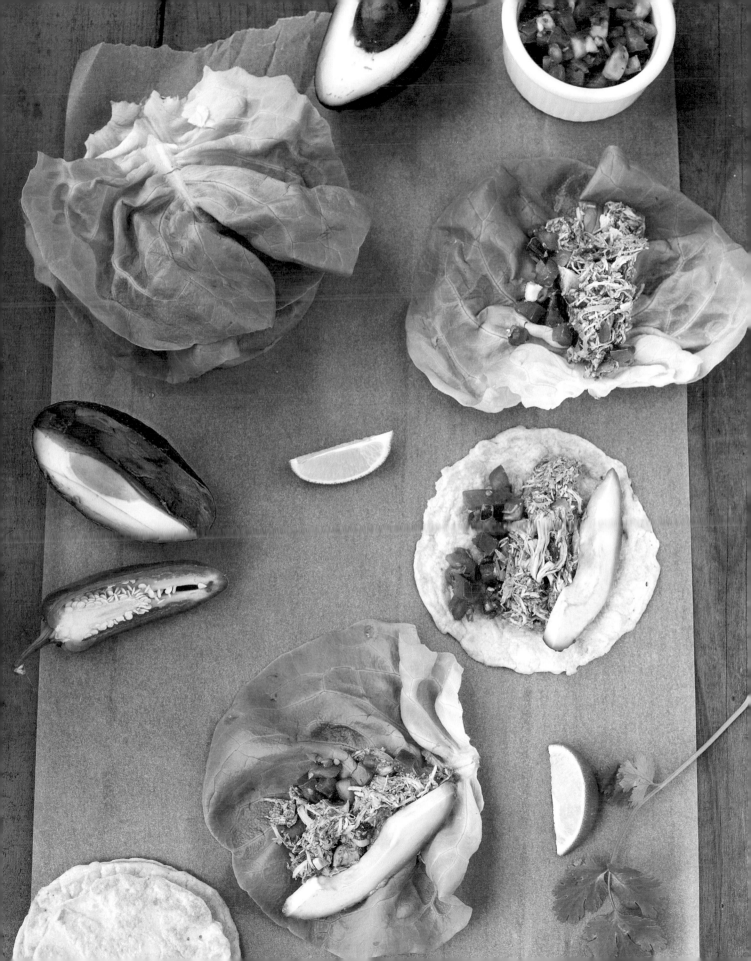

pulled barbecue chicken sandwiches with coleslaw

prep time: 10 minutes   *cooking time:* 4 hours   *yield:* 6 servings

While we often use lettuce wraps in grain-free cuisine, sometimes it is just too flimsy and won't soak up the juicy sauces that accompany the slow-cooked meat, like with this pulled barbecue chicken. Although there are a lot of ingredients, you will probably have most of them in your pantry, and all you have to do is throw them all in the pot and forget about it—cooking doesn't get better than this if you ask me!

ingredients

- Hamburger Buns (page 242)

CHICKEN

- 1 pound boneless, skinless chicken breasts
- 1½ pounds boneless, skinless chicken thighs
- ¾ cup diced yellow onion
- ½ cup + 2 tablespoons white vinegar
- ½ cup honey
- ¼ cup tomato paste
- 2 tablespoons coconut aminos
- 1½ tablespoons all-natural liquid smoke
- 2 teaspoons minced garlic
- 2 teaspoons fish sauce
- 1½ teaspoons chili powder
- 1½ teaspoons sea salt
- 1 teaspoon paprika
- 1 teaspoon Dijon mustard
- ¾ teaspoon cayenne pepper
- ½ teaspoon allspice
- ¼ teaspoon cracked black pepper

COLESLAW

- 1 cup shredded green cabbage
- 1 cup shredded red cabbage
- ½ cup shredded carrots
- ¼ cup Mayonnaise (page 308)
- 1 tablespoon finely chopped red onion
- 1 tablespoon apple cider vinegar
- 1 teaspoon Dijon mustard
- ½ teaspoon honey
- ¼ teaspoon sea salt
- Dash cracked black pepper

method

1. Place all the chicken ingredients in a slow cooker and cook on high for 3 hours. Remove the chicken, shred with two forks, then return to the pot and continue cooking for 1 hour.

2. Meanwhile, make the coleslaw. Place all the coleslaw ingredients in a bowl and stir to combine. Refrigerate for at least 30 minutes before serving.

3. Serve the chicken on grain-free Hamburger Buns with the coleslaw on top or alongside.

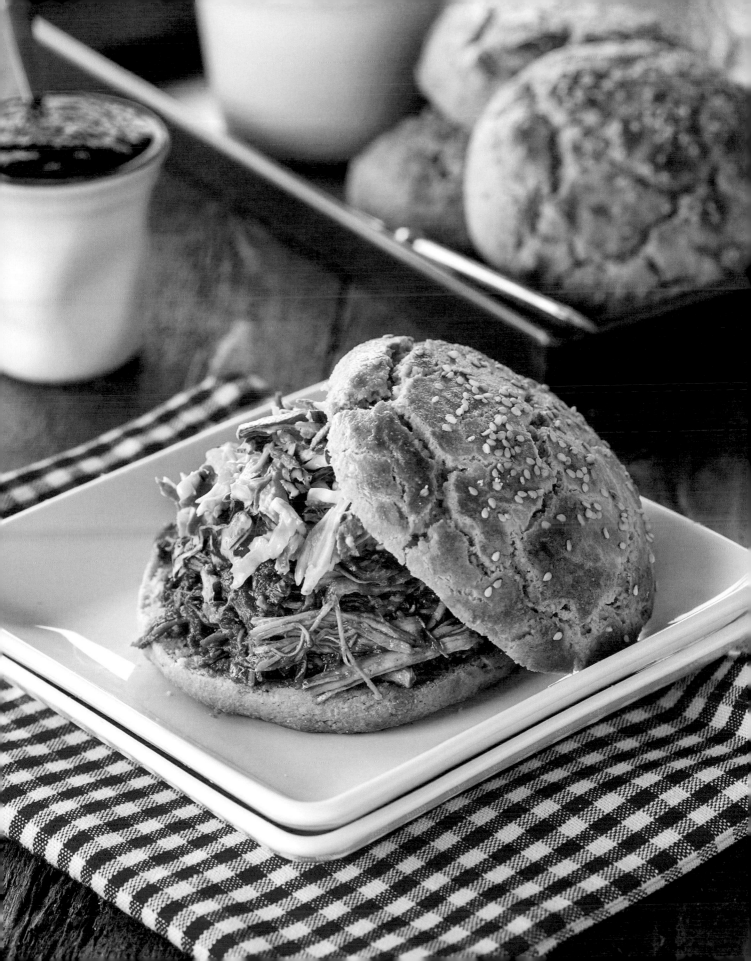

citrus-cumin chicken

prep time: 15 minutes + 2 hours for marinating

cooking time: 15 minutes   yield: 6 servings

This easy marinade is tangy and sweet with just a hint of spice. Feel free to choose your own cuts of chicken, but I prefer a combination to appeal to everyone's preference.

ingredients

- ¼ cup extra-virgin olive oil
- ¼ cup orange juice
- 2 tablespoons fresh lime juice
- 1 tablespoon minced garlic
- 1 tablespoon coconut aminos
- 1 tablespoon cumin
- 2 teaspoon apple cider vinegar
- 1 teaspoon minced ginger
- 4 pounds chicken pieces, bone-in and skin-on (a combination of drumsticks, thighs, and breasts)
- ½ teaspoon sea salt
- ¼ teaspoon cracked black pepper

method

1. Place the oil, orange juice, lime juice, garlic, coconut aminos, cumin, vinegar, and ginger in a nonreactive baking dish large enough to hold all the chicken and whisk to combine. Add the chicken pieces and turn to coat. Let marinate for at least 30 minutes, or up to a couple of hours in the refrigerator.

2. Preheat a grill to medium heat. Remove the chicken from the baking dish and let excess marinade drip back into the dish. Place the chicken on the hot grill without overcrowding. Season with salt and pepper. Grill until fully cooked through, turning occasionally, about 15 minutes total.

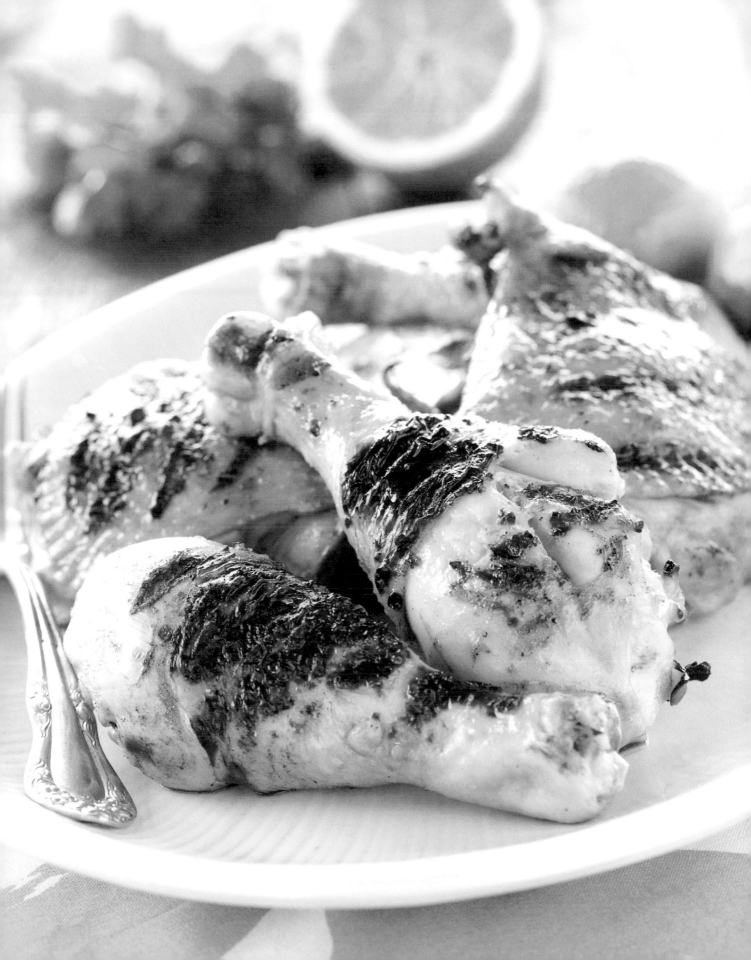

club sandwich wraps

prep time: 15 minutes   yield: 4 servings

Sandwiches are an easy lunch option and don't have to disappear from your life just because you're grain-free. This club sandwich uses sturdy iceberg lettuce to wrap the contents inside in a tight package for a finger-friendly meal.

ingredients

- 8 large iceberg lettuce leaves
- ½ cup Pesto Mayo (page 308)
- 8 slices crispy cooked bacon
- 8 ounces sliced roasted turkey or thinly sliced chicken breast
- 4 slices vine-ripened tomato
- 1 avocado, sliced
- Dill pickles

method

1. Layer 2 pieces of lettuce on top of each other and spread with Pesto Mayo.

2. Add 2 pieces of bacon, a quarter of the turkey, 1 tomato slice, and a quarter of the avocado.

3. Gently pull the lettuce around the fillings and secure with a toothpick.

4. Use a serrated knife to cut the sandwich diagonally.

5. Repeat with remaining ingredients.

tidbits:
To give your sandwich a spicy or smoky kick, try the Roasted Red Pepper or Chipotle Mayo (page 308).

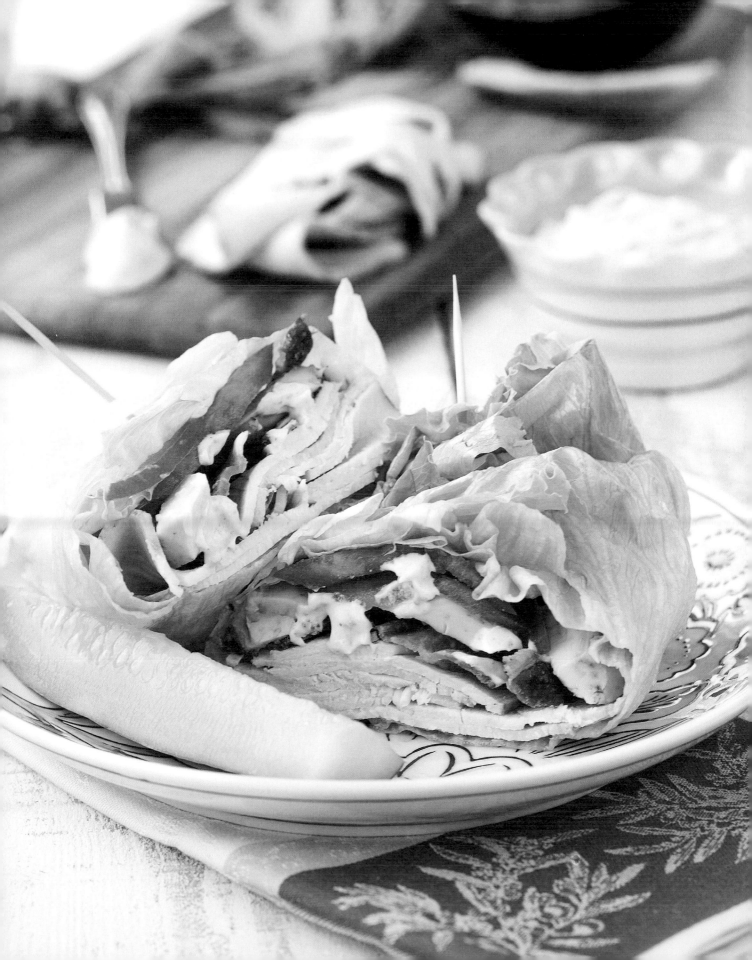

lemon herb-roasted chicken and vegetables

prep time: 30 minutes   cooking time: 55 minutes   yield: 4 to 6 servings

Roasted chicken is a basic dish that every home cook should master. It can be the centerpiece for a quiet family gathering or an elegant dinner party. It also provides superb leftovers for soups or sandwiches. Use the bones and giblets to make stock so you don't waste a single bit of the bird.

ingredients

- 1 4- to 5-pound roasting chicken
- 1 bunch sage
- 4 sprigs rosemary
- 1 lemon, halved
- 6 cloves garlic, peeled and crushed
- Salt and pepper
- 4 tablespoons extra-virgin olive oil or melted ghee, divided
- ¾ teaspoon Dijon mustard
- ½ teaspoon lemon juice
- 1 tablespoon chopped fresh sage
- 1 teaspoon chopped fresh rosemary
- 1 clove garlic, minced
- 1 teaspoon fresh thyme leaves
- 1 teaspoon sea salt
- ¼ teaspoon cracked black pepper
- 5 large carrots, peeled and cut into 2-inch pieces
- 3 cups peeled and cubed butternut squash
- ½ yellow onion, sliced

method

1. Remove the giblets from the chicken cavity. Reserve for another use or discard. Rinse the chicken and pat very dry with paper towels. Leave at room temperature for 1 hour.

2. Preheat the oven to 425°F.

3. Stuff the cavity with the bunch of sage, rosemary sprigs, lemon halves, and garlic cloves. Generously sprinkle salt and pepper inside the cavity. Tie the legs together with kitchen string and tuck the wing tips under the body of the chicken.

4. Place 2 tablespoons of the oil and the mustard, lemon juice, chopped sage, chopped rosemary, minced garlic, thyme leaves, teaspoon salt, and ¼ teaspoon cracked pepper in a bowl and stir well. Rub all over the bird and underneath the skin.

5. Add the remaining oil to a bowl with the carrots, squash, and onion and toss. Spread the vegetables around the bottom of a roasting pan and place the chicken on top, breast side up.

6. Place the chicken in the oven and roast for 15 minutes. Reduce the heat to 350° and roast for 40 more minutes, or until the juices run clear when you cut between a leg and thigh and an internal thermometer reads 180°. Remove the chicken to a platter and cover for about 20 minutes. Slice the chicken and serve it with the vegetables.

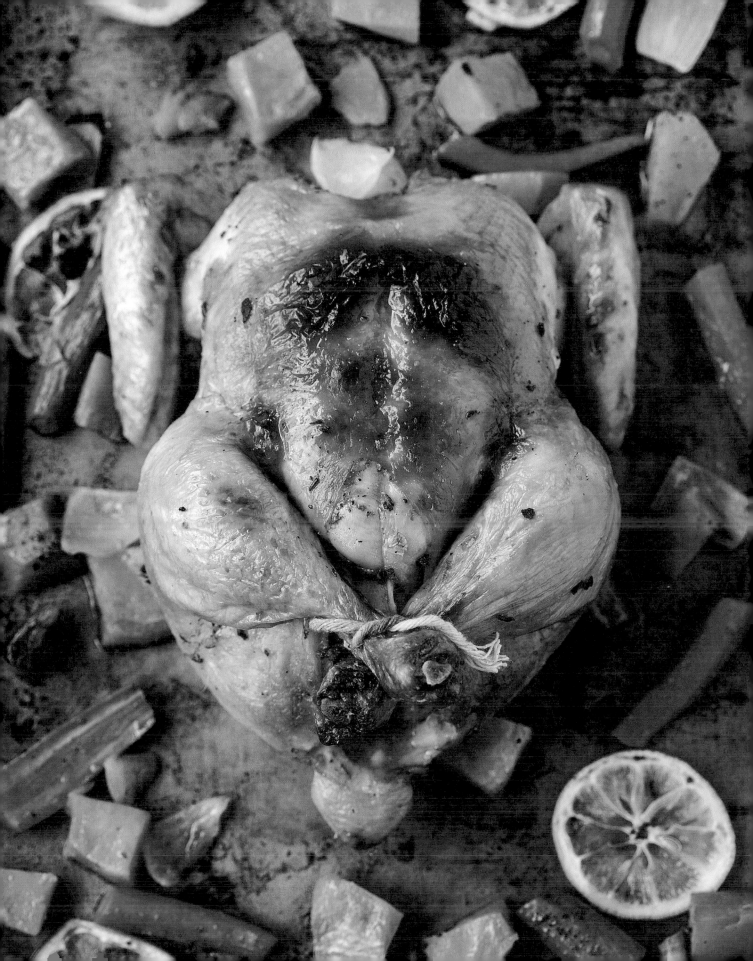

thai pad see ew

prep time: 30 minutes   *cooking time:* 15 minutes   *yield:* 4 to 6 servings

Pad See Ew is a Thai dish featuring wide, flat rice noodles in a light brown sauce with broccolini, carrots, and a scrambled egg. It's sort of like Chinese fried rice, but with noodles. I use a vegetable peeler to make very thin ribbon noodles from carrots and then sauté them with the other ingredients until they are soft and flavorful.

ingredients

- 10 medium carrots (about 1 pound), peeled
- 1 pound boneless, skinless chicken breasts
- 2 tablespoons coconut oil
- 6 cloves garlic, minced
- 3 cups broccolini, stalks trimmed to 1-inch long
- ⅓ cup coconut aminos
- 2 eggs

method

1. Lay the peeled carrots on a cutting board and use a vegetable peeler to create very thin but wide ribbons. Peel down to the core of the carrot, then flip over and continue peeling.

2. Slice the chicken very thinly on a diagonal. Place the oil in a deep sauté pan or wok over medium heat to warm. Add the garlic and chicken and stir-fry them for 5 minutes, until the chicken is white on the outside.

3. Add the broccolini and coconut aminos and cook for 5 more minutes, until the broccolini has softened a bit. Add the carrot noodles and stir-fry for another 5 minutes.

4. Push the stir-fry aside in the pan, then crack the eggs into the pan and stir vigorously to scramble them. Let them cook until firm, then mix everything together. Serve immediately.

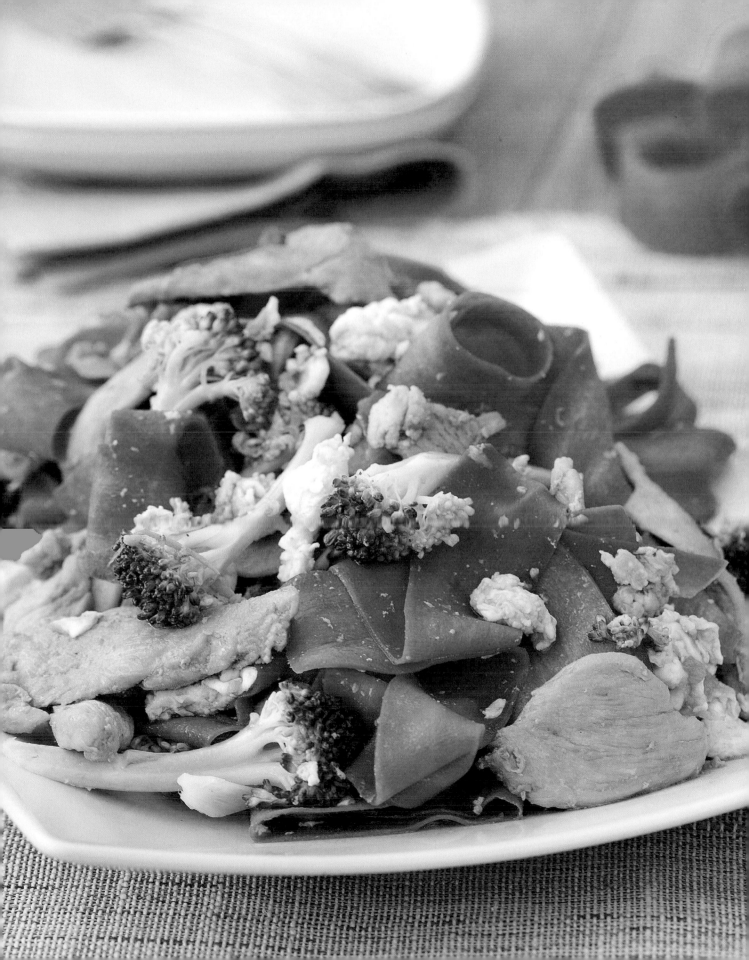

petrale sole
with lemon-caper sauce

prep time: 15 minutes cooking time: 15 minutes yield: 4 servings

Petrale sole, a mild and delicate white fish with a buttery flavor, is complemented by a tangy and salty lemon–caper sauce and served with a side of wilted spinach.

ingredients

- 1 tablespoon coconut oil
- 4 6-ounce sole fillets
- ½ teaspoon sea salt
- ⅓ teaspoon cracked black pepper
- 12 ounces baby spinach
- ½ cup Chicken Broth (page 316)
- 2 tablespoons fresh lemon juice
- 2 tablespoons chopped fresh parsley
- 1 tablespoon capers, drained

method

1. Place the oil in a skillet over medium-high heat and swirl to coat the bottom.

2. Sprinkle the fish with the salt and pepper. Place in the skillet and cook for 3 minutes on each side, or until slightly flaky in the center. Remove the fish from the pan and keep warm.

3. Place the spinach in the same skillet and sauté for 5 minutes, until wilted. Remove the spinach from the pan and keep warm with the fish.

4. Place the broth, lemon juice, parsley, and capers in the same skillet and bring to a boil. Spoon the sauce over the fish and spinach to serve.

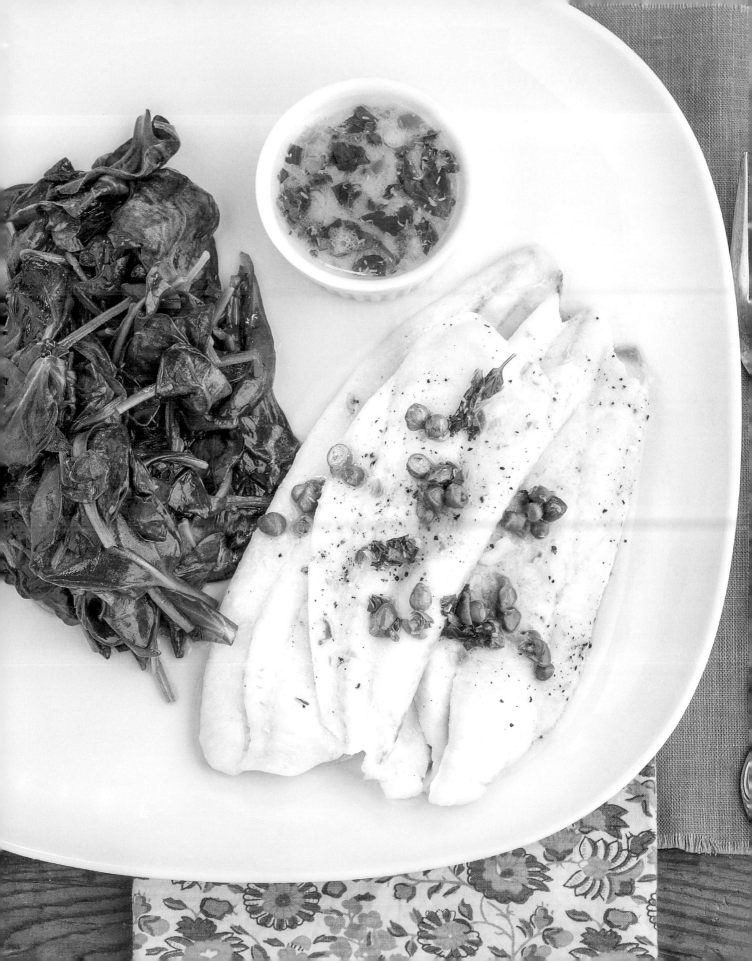

macadamia-coconut crusted ono with mango coulis

prep time: 15 minutes + 1 hour marinating time cooking time: 15 minutes yield: 4 servings

We were living in Kona, Hawaii when I started writing this book, so the flavors and cuisines of Hawaii have had a noticeable impact on my recipes. Among my favorites is this one. Luckily you don't have to live on a tropical island to enjoy it, as the ingredients are pretty widely available around the world.

ingredients

- 4 6-ounce skinless ono fillets
- 1 cup coconut milk
- 1 teaspoon fresh lemon juice
- ½ cup dry-roasted macadamia nuts
- ¼ cup shredded unsweetened coconut
- ½ teaspoon finely minced lemon zest
- 1 tablespoon chopped parsley
- ½ teaspoon sea salt
- 1 tablespoon coconut oil, melted
- 1 large mango, peeled and seeded
- 2 teaspoons pineapple juice
- 1 teaspoon fresh lime juice
- Coconut-Lime Rice (page 126), optional

method

1. Place the fish in a shallow dish.

2. Pour the coconut milk and lemon juice into a small bowl and stir to combine. Pour the mixture over the fish and place the fish in the refrigerator to marinate for 1 hour.

3. Preheat the oven to 400°F.

4. Place the macadamia nuts in a food processor. Pulse 8 to 10 times, until the nuts are finely chopped but haven't turned into nutbutter.

5. Add the coconut, lemon zest, parsley, and salt to the food processor and pulse twice to incorporate. Empty the mixture into a shallow dish.

6. Remove the fish from the marinade and pat dry. Press each fillet into the macadamia mixture, coating it on all sides.

7. Grease the bottom of a baking dish with 1 teaspoon of the coconut oil. Place the fish in the dish and drizzle with the remaining coconut oil. Bake for 15 minutes, until the fish is cooked through.

8. Place the mango, pineapple juice, and lime juice in a blender and purée. Drizzle on a plate and top with fish. Serve with Coconut-Lime Rice if you like.

tidbits:

Halibut, mahi-mahi, or any other firm white fish will also work beautifully in this recipe.

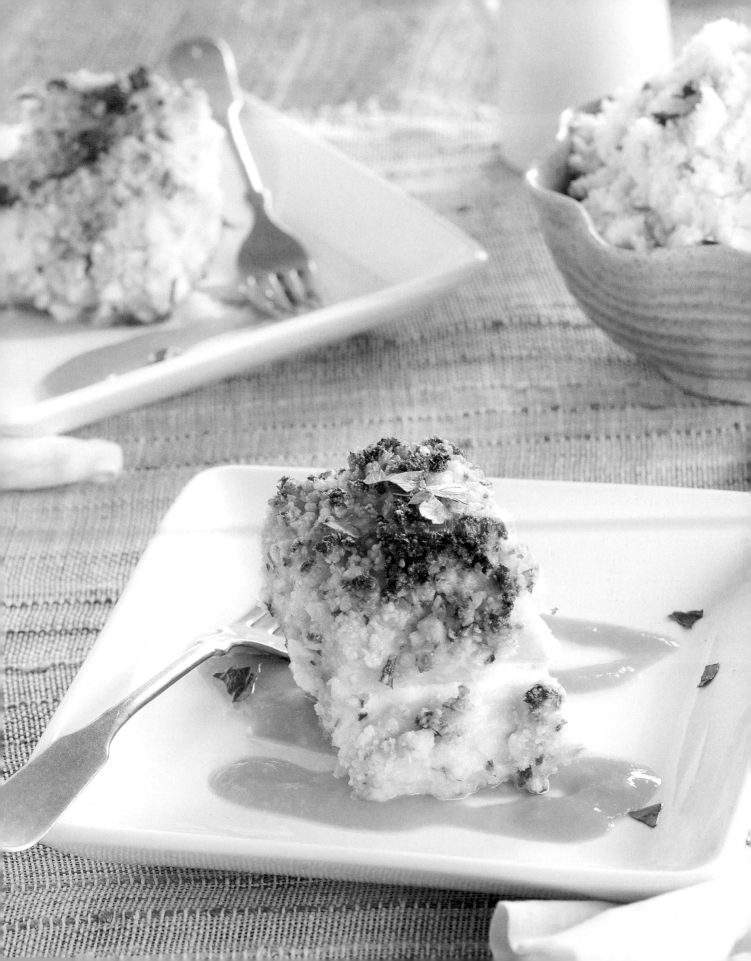

seafood, chorizo, and chicken paella

prep time: 25 minutes   cooking time: 50 minutes   yield: 4 servings

Paella is a traditional Spanish dish made with short-grain rice, saffron, and good-quality olive oil. Cauliflower's versatility shines again, as it is used in this dish as a low-carb replacement for the rice. Simmered until tender in an aromatic saffron broth, it is virtually undetectable as an impostor.

ingredients

- 1 head cauliflower (about 4 cups chopped)
- 1½ cups Chicken Broth (page 316)
- 1 cup clam juice
- 2 tablespoons extra-virgin olive oil, divided
- 2 boneless, skinless chicken thighs, cubed
- 6 ounces chorizo sausage, casings removed, crumbled
- 1 medium yellow onion, chopped
- 2 cloves garlic, minced
- 2 Roma tomatoes, chopped
- 2 teaspoons sea salt
- ¼ teaspoon cracked black pepper
- ¼ teaspoon smoked paprika
- 1 teaspoon saffron threads
- 6 littleneck clams, scrubbed clean
- 6 mussels, scrubbed clean
- ½ pound jumbo shrimp, peeled and deveined
- ¼ cup chopped fresh parsley
- Lemon wedges

method

1. Place the cauliflower in a blender or food processor and process until it resembles grains of rice. Discard any large portions that did not break down.

2. Place the chicken broth and clam juice in a saucepan set over medium heat. Keep warm until ready to use.

3. Place 1 tablespoon of the olive oil in a large skillet and heat over medium-high heat. Brown the chicken and sausage in the skillet on all sides, about 5 minutes.

4. Add the remaining tablespoon of oil and the onion, garlic, tomatoes, salt, pepper, paprika, and saffron. Sauté for 7 more minutes, until the onions have softened.

5. Pour ¾ cup of the broth mixture into the skillet, stirring to scrape up the browned bits from the bottom of the skillet. Stir in the riced cauliflower and simmer for 15 minutes.

6. Meanwhile, add the clams and mussels to the remaining broth and bring to a boil. Cover and cook for 6 to 7 minutes, until the shells have opened up. Remove the mussels and clams with a slotted spoon and set aside. Add the shrimp to the pan and cook for 2 to 3 minutes, until pink. Set aside with the mussels and clams.

7. When the cauliflower is tender and most of the juices have evaporated, nestle the shrimp, clams, and mussels into the paella. Cook for 10 minutes until warmed through, then remove from the heat. Let stand for 10 minutes before serving.

8. Sprinkle the parsley over the top and serve each dish with a lemon wedge. Paella is best with a squeeze of fresh lemon right before eating.

tidbits:

Never cooked shellfish before? Don't fret—it's really simple. If you don't like seafood, feel free to make this paella your own by adding more chicken or sausage or replacing the meat with vegetables. If seafood is omitted, substitute additional chicken broth for the clam juice.

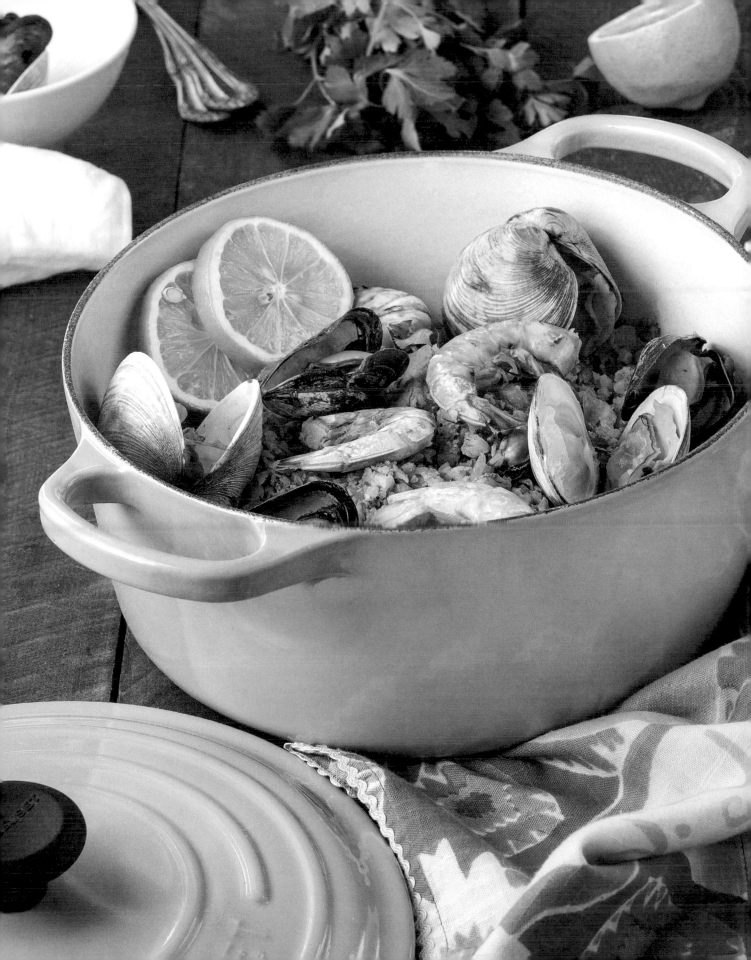

pan-seared salmon in red curry sauce

prep time: 10 minutes   cooking time: 12 minutes   yield: 4 servings

Salmon is first coated in a sweet-and-spicy paste then quickly pan-seared to create a crusty glaze. It is then poached in a savory Thai red curry sauce to ensure even cooking and an impeccably moist and flaky entrée.

ingredients

- 1 tablespoon coconut oil, melted, divided
- 1½ teaspoon red curry paste, divided
- 1½ teaspoons coconut crystals or honey, divided
- 4 6-ounce salmon fillets with skin
- ½ cup coconut milk
- 1 teaspoon fish sauce
- ½ teaspoon fresh lime juice
- ½ teaspoon grated fresh ginger
- ½ teaspoon minced garlic

method

1. Place 2 teaspoons of the oil, 1 teaspoon of the curry paste, and 1 teaspoon of the coconut crystals in a small bowl and stir well. Rub the paste onto the top and sides of each salmon fillet.

2. Place the remaining teaspoon of oil in a large skillet and heat over medium-high heat.

3. Add the salmon, skin side up, and pan-sear for 3 minutes. Carefully flip the fillets over.

4. Add the rest of the ingredients and the remaining ½ teaspoon curry paste to the skillet. Poach the salmon in the liquid for 5 to 7 minutes, until the center of each fillet just cracks and flakes.

5. Remove the fillets and keep warm on a plate covered with foil.

6. Simmer the sauce for 3 to 5 minutes, until it has reduced by half.

7. Serve the fillets topped with the red curry sauce.

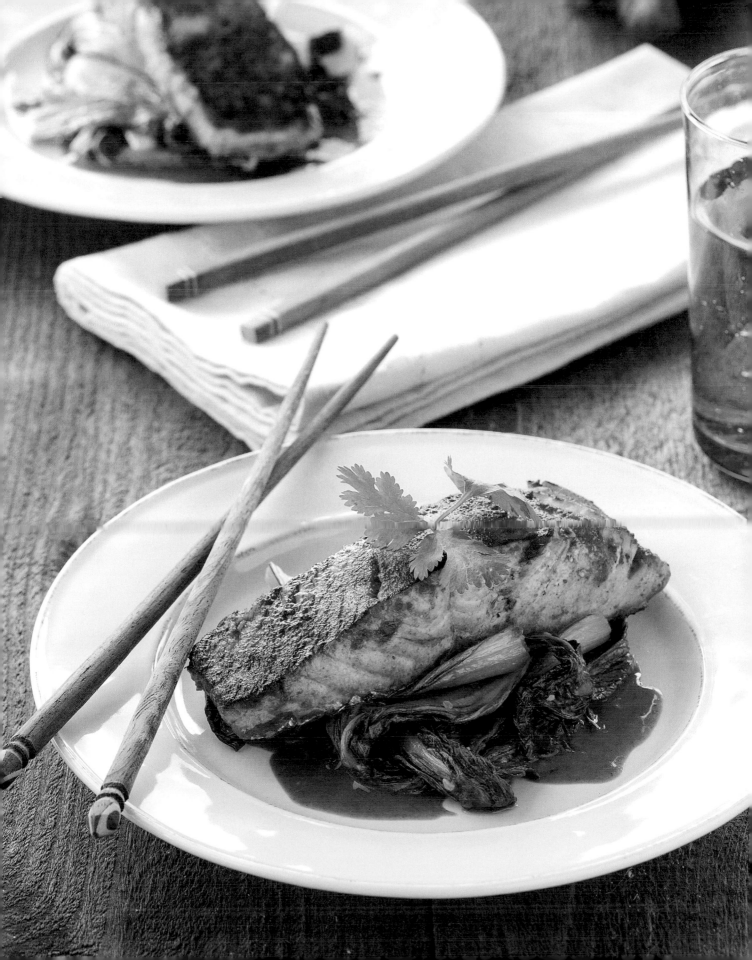

lemon-basil sea bass
en papillote

prep time: 15 minutes   *cooking time:* 10-12 minutes   *yield:* 4 servings

With this French technique of baking a white fish en papillote, or wrapped in parchment, the paper traps moisture, gently steaming the fish in its own juices, infused with whatever seasonings you've tucked inside. The best part of this method? Minimal cleanup!

ingredients

- 3 zucchini, julienne-sliced into noodles
- ¼ cup chopped fresh basil
- 4 6-ounce sea bass fillets (or any firm white fish)
- 2 Roma tomatoes, sliced into 12 slices
- 2 lemons, sliced into 12 slices
- 2 cloves garlic, minced
- 3 tablespoons extra-virgin olive oil
- Salt and pepper
- 4 sheets parchment paper (each about 12 inches long)

method

1. Preheat the oven to 375°F.

2. Place 1 sheet of parchment paper on a rimmed plate and pile ¼ of the zucchini noodles on one half of the paper. Sprinkle with basil.

3. Place 1 fish fillet on top, then layer with 3 slices of tomato and 3 slices of lemon.

4. Sprinkle ¼ teaspoon garlic on top, drizzle with 2 teaspoons olive oil, and generously sprinkle with salt and pepper.

5. Fold the other half of the paper over the fish, then pinch and roll the sides toward the contents to form a tightly sealed pouch.

6. Repeat with the remaining fish, then arrange the 4 pouches on a rimmed baking sheet.

7. Bake for 10 to 12 minutes, until the pouches have puffed up and the fish is slightly firm to the touch.

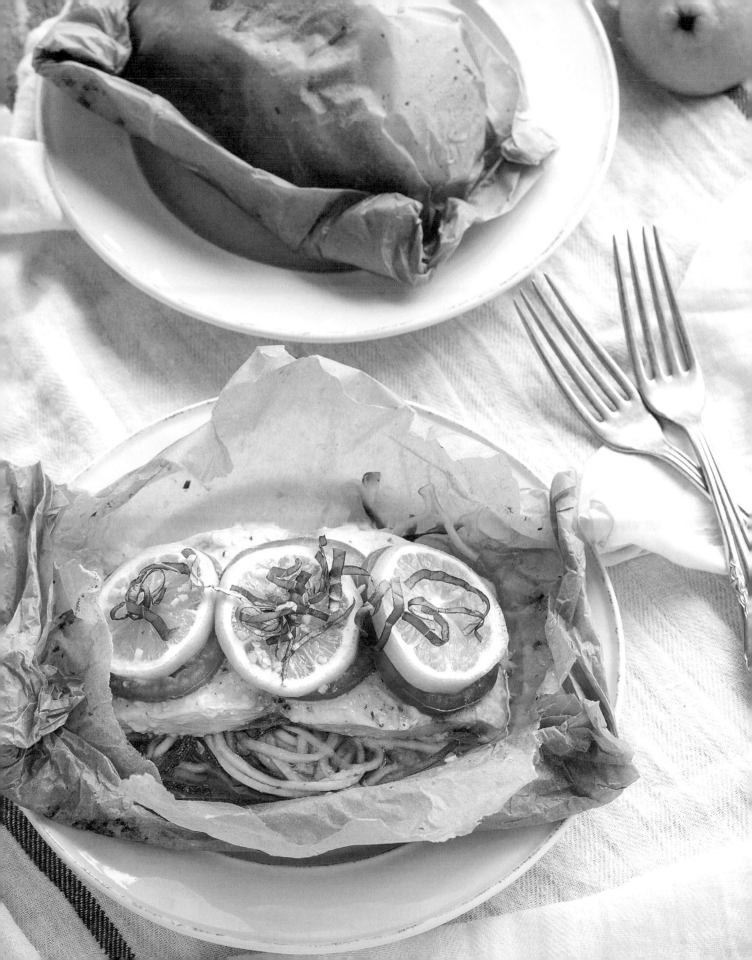

prawn and pumpkin yellow curry

prep time: 15 minutes   cooking time: 25 minutes   yield: 4 servings

Making homemade curry paste is very simple and yields a much more authentic and pungent result than store-bought versions. This yellow curry can be used with more than just prawns as it also tastes incredible with chicken or a vegetable medley.

ingredients

- 1 shallot, peeled
- 3 cloves garlic, peeled
- 1 1-inch piece ginger, peeled and cut in half
- 1½ teaspoons cumin
- 1 teaspoon coriander
- ¾ teaspoon turmeric
- ¼ teaspoon fennel seeds
- ⅛ teaspoon nutmeg
- ¼ teaspoon dried Thai chilies, ground
- 3 tablespoons fish sauce
- 1 13.5-ounce can coconut milk
- 2 kaffir lime leaves
- 1 tablespoon coconut crystals*
- 1 tablespoon tomato paste
- 1 tablespoon coconut butter
- 3 cups mixed stir-fry vegetables
- 1 cup diced pumpkin, seeds removed
- 1 pound prawns, peeled and deveined

For SCD, substitute honey for the coconut crystals.

method

1. Place the shallot, garlic, ginger, cumin, coriander, turmeric, fennel, nutmeg, chilies, and fish sauce in a food processor and pulse until finely chopped and a paste has formed.

2. Scrape the paste into a saucepan. Whisk in the coconut milk, kaffir lime leaves, coconut crystals, tomato paste, and coconut butter. Cook over medium-high heat until it comes to a low boil.

3. Reduce the heat to medium-low and add the vegetables, pumpkin, and prawns. Simmer for 10 to 12 minutes, until the vegetables are cooked and slightly softened and the prawns have turned pink and are firm to the touch.

4. Remove from the heat and let the sauce sit for 10 minutes to thicken.

tidbits:

- *The flavor will be slightly different, but you can substitute cayenne pepper if Thai chilies are not available.*
- *For each kaffir lime leaf, you may substitute ½ a small bay leaf plus ¼ teaspoon lime zest.*

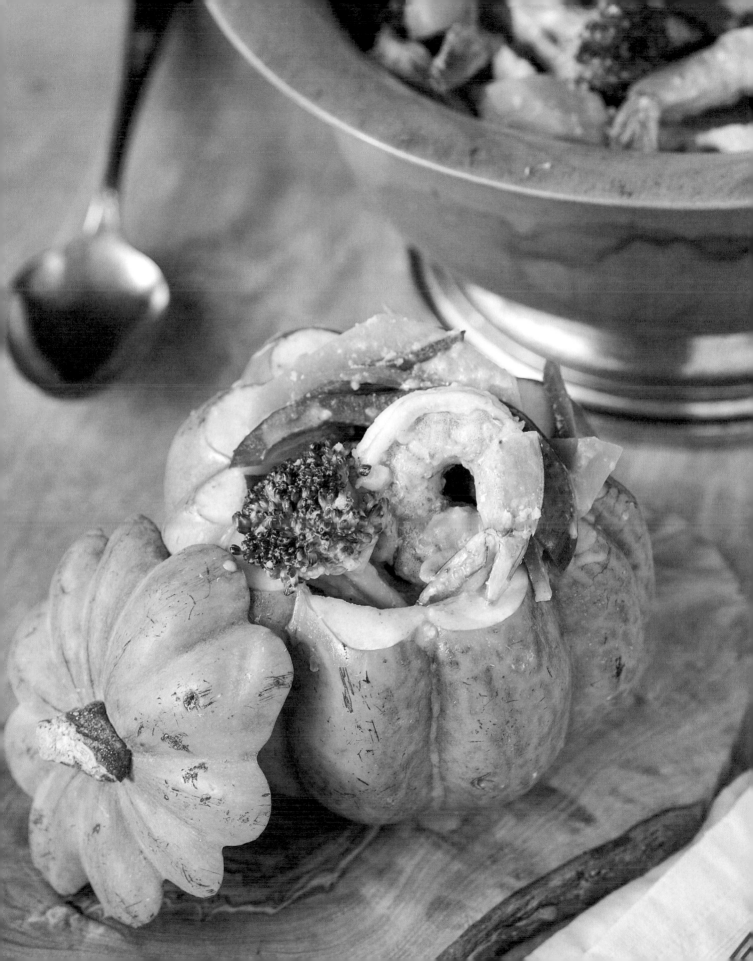

honey-lime salmon tostadas

prep time: 15 minutes + 30 minutes marinating time

cooking time: 10-12 minutes   yield: 4 servings

Marinated in a blend of honey, lime juice, and spices, this salmon obtains a sweet- and- spicy crust when it's pan-seared. The salmon can also be served over a bed of lettuce, but if you are feeling the urge to bite into something crispy, these almond flour tostada shells uniquely complement the bold flavors of the salmon and sauces.

ingredients

SALMON

- 2 tablespoons fresh lime juice
- 2 teaspoons honey
- 1 teaspoon cumin
- ½ teaspoon sea salt
- ½ teaspoon chili powder
- ¼ teaspoon cracked black pepper
- 1 pound salmon fillet with skin
- 1 tablespoon coconut oil

SHELLS

- 2½ cups blanched almond flour
- 1 teaspoon sea salt
- 2 tablespoons extra-virgin olive oil
- 2 large eggs
- ½ teaspoon baking soda
- 2 teaspoons chopped cilantro
- 1 teaspoon fresh lime juice

TOPPINGS

- Roasted-Tomatillo Salsa (page 333)
- Avocado Sour Cream (recipe follows)
- Shredded carrots
- Shredded red cabbage

method

1. Place all the ingredients for the salmon, except the salmon and the oil, in a shallow dish and stir to combine. Add the salmon and turn a couple of times to coat thoroughly. Cover and let marinate for 30 minutes.

2. Preheat the oven to 350°F.

3. To make the tostadas, place all the shell ingredients in the bowl and mix until a dough forms.

4. Divide the dough into 8 even balls, rolling them between your hands until smooth.

5. Place the balls of dough on a piece of parchment paper cut to the size of a baking sheet. Place another piece of parchment paper on top, then use a rolling pin to roll each ball out into a circle ⅛-inch thick. Remove the top sheet.

6. Carefully transfer the parchment paper to the baking sheet, and bake for 18 minutes, flipping halfway through.

7. Heat the tablespoon of oil in a skillet over medium heat. Pan-fry the salmon for 3 to 4 minutes on each side, until it is evenly browned and slightly flaky on top.

8. Remove the skin and slice the salmon into 8 pieces.

9. Serve on top of the tostada shells with desired toppings.

avocado sour cream:

Soak ½ cup raw cashews in water for 4 hours. Drain, then purée with 1 avocado, 2 tablespoons fresh lime juice, ½ seeded jalapeño pepper, ½ teaspoon sea salt, and ⅛ teaspoon cayenne pepper. Chill for 30 minutes.

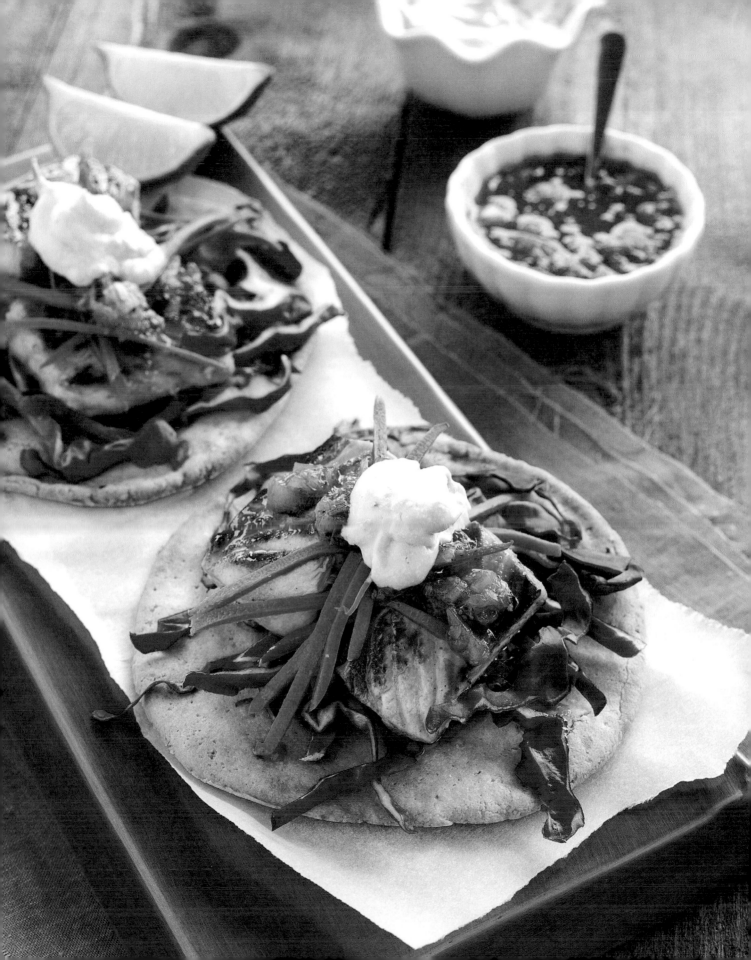

sausage and butternut squash stuffed tomatoes

prep time: 30 minutes   cooking time: 60 minutes   yield: 4 servings

Tomatoes are a plump and juicy vessel for a savory blend of sausage, sautéed vegetables, and aromatic herbs. While the vibrant and uniquely shaped heirloom tomato presents strikingly in this recipe, these stuffed tomatoes can be made all year round using a beefsteak or another large variety.

ingredients

- 4 large tomatoes
- 1 tablespoon extra-virgin olive oil
- ½ pound mild Italian sausage, casings removed and crumbled
- 1 cup peeled and finely diced butternut squash
- ½ cup diced yellow onion
- 4 ounces mushrooms, chopped
- 2 cloves garlic, minced
- 1 tablespoon chopped fresh basil
- 1 teaspoon chopped fresh rosemary
- ½ teaspoon sea salt
- ¼ teaspoon cracked black pepper
- ¼ cup almond meal

method

1. Preheat the oven to 350°F.

2. Core the tomatoes, leaving the bottoms intact. Using a small spoon, gently scrape out the seeds and half of the flesh, carefully leaving the skin intact.

3. Drain the tomatoes, cut side down, on paper towels while preparing the filling.

4. Heat the oil in a skillet over medium heat and brown the Italian sausage, about 5 minutes.

5. Add the squash, onion, mushrooms, garlic, basil, rosemary, salt, and pepper and sauté until the vegetables are soft, about 15 minutes. Remove from the heat and stir in the almond meal.

6. Spoon the filling into the tomatoes, packing it down slightly.

7. Place the stuffed tomatoes in a lightly greased baking dish, and bake until tomatoes are cooked through and the filling is golden brown on top, about 40 minutes.

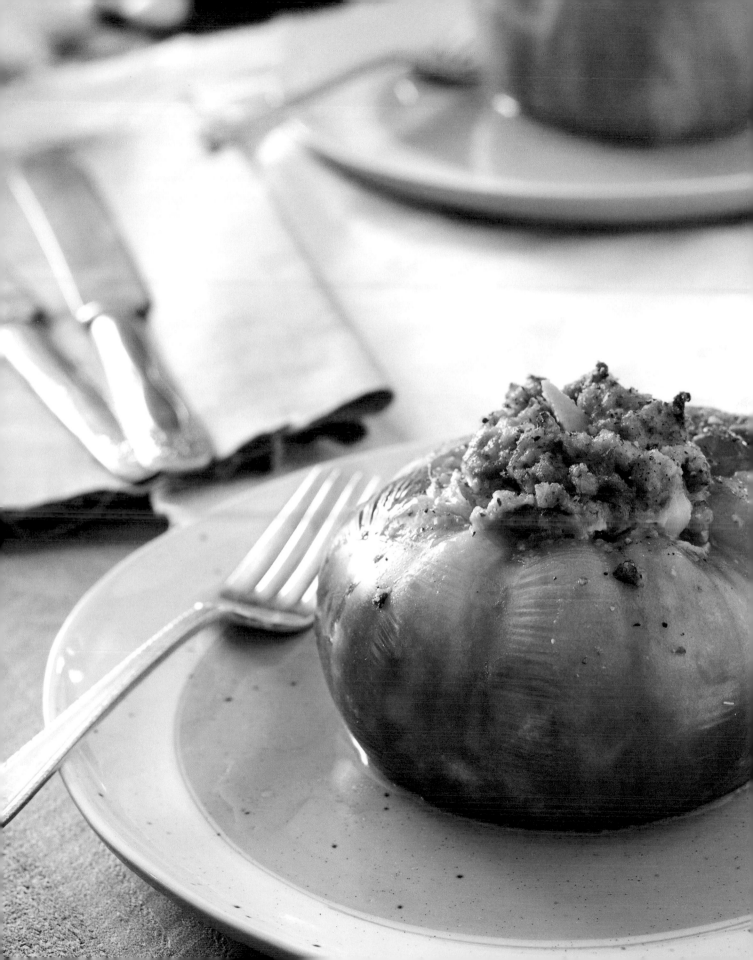

greek gyro pasta with lamb meatballs

prep time: 20 minutes + 30 minutes marinating time

cooking time: 25 minutes   yield: 4 servings

Juicy marinated lamb meatballs are served over zucchini pasta with a cool cucumber tzatziki sauce, which makes this dish taste like a traditional gyro wrap even though it looks like spaghetti and meatballs!

ingredients

MEATBALLS

- 1½ pounds ground lamb
- 1½ tablespoons fresh lemon juice
- 1½ tablespoons extra-virgin olive oil
- 3 cloves garlic, minced
- 1½ teaspoons chopped fresh rosemary
- 1½ teaspoons chopped fresh oregano
- 1 teaspoon sea salt
- ¼ teaspoon cracked black pepper

TZATZIKI SAUCE

- ¾ cup Coconut Milk Yogurt (page 46 or store-bought)
- 1 small cucumber, peeled, seeded, and finely chopped
- 1 tablespoon fresh lemon juice
- 1 teaspoon chopped fresh dill
- 1 teaspoon chopped fresh mint
- 1 clove garlic, minced
- ½ teaspoon balsamic vinegar
- ¼ teaspoon sea salt

PASTA

- 4 large zucchini
- 1 tablespoon fresh lemon juice
- 1 tablespoon extra-virgin olive oil
- 1½ teaspoons chopped fresh oregano
- ½ teaspoon sea salt
- 1 cup cherry tomatoes, halved
- ½ red onion, thinly sliced

method

1. Place all the meatball ingredients in a bowl and mix well. Let marinate at room temperature for 30 minutes.

2. Meanwhile, make the sauce. Place all the sauce ingredients in a bowl and whisk to combine. Cover and refrigerate while the meatballs are cooking.

3. Preheat the oven to 375°F.

4. Form the meat into 2-inch balls and place them on a rimmed baking sheet.

5. Bake until no longer pink in the center, 20 to 25 minutes.

6. Meanwhile, make the pasta. Peel the squash and make noodles using a spiral slicer or julienne peeler. Place the noodles in a bowl and toss with the lemon juice, olive oil, oregano, and salt. Allow the noodles to marinate while the meatballs cook.

7. Remove the meatballs from the oven and let them cool for 5 minutes. Mix the tomatoes and onion into the pasta.

8. Serve the meatballs atop the marinated zucchini pasta with a dollop of tzatziki sauce.

tidbits:

You can purée ½ cup soaked cashews plus ¼ cup almond milk in the blender to substitute for yogurt in the tzatziki sauce.

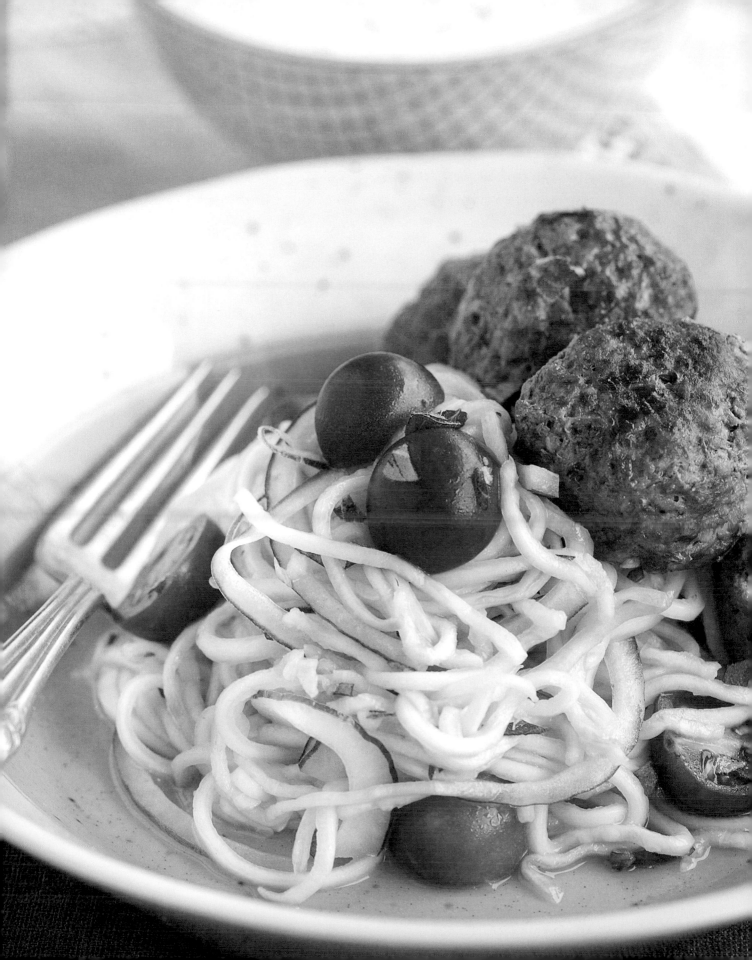

spinach sausage lasagna

prep time: 30 minutes   cooking time: 60 minutes   yield: 6 to 8 servings

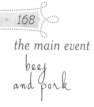

This recipe has been up on my blog for quite some time now and has received nothing but rave reviews. The most common version of grain-free lasagna uses thinly sliced zucchini as the noodle substitute, but here I use a coconut-flour-based crepe. Zucchini lasagna is decent, but this recipe much more mimics the flavors and textures of the Italian dish we all know and love. It's a process to prepare, but you will know it was worth it in the end when you take your first steaming bite.

ingredients

- ½ pound uncooked Italian sausage
- 2 cups Marinara Sauce (page 306)
- 2 cups baby spinach
- 1¼ cups Basic Nut Cheese (page 304)
- ¼ teaspoon sea salt
- ⅛ teaspoon pepper
- 1 tablespoon chopped fresh parsley
- 1 tablespoon chopped fresh basil
- 10 Crepes (page 302), cut into 2-inch-wide strips, scraps reserved

method

1. Preheat the oven to 375°F.

2. Remove the casings and crumble the sausage into a skillet. Brown over medium-high heat for 5 to 6 minutes, until cooked through. Remove the sausage and leave the juices in the pan. Combine sausage with the Marinara Sauce in a bowl.

3. Place the spinach in the same skillet and sauté over medium heat until wilted, about 5 minutes.

4. Place the Nut Cheese, salt, pepper, parsley, and basil in a bowl and mix.

5. Spoon 2 tablespoons of the sauce into the bottom of an 8-by-11-inch baking dish.

6. Layer Crepe strips on top of it, overlapping them ever so slightly so the fillings don't seep through the cracks. If there are gaps around the edges of the dish, fill them in with the reserved Crepe scraps.

7. Next, gently spread ⅓ of the cheese mixture over the surface. Sprinkle ½ of the spinach over it, then top with ⅓ of the meat sauce.

8. Repeat in this order: Noodles, cheese, spinach, and meat sauce. Finish by sprinkling the remaining ¼ cup of nut cheese over the top.

9. Bake uncovered for 20 to 30 minutes, until the corners are bubbling. Let sit for 10 to 15 minutes before serving.

> tidbits:
> *Making traditional lasagna is already a bit labor-intensive even without the additional steps of making homemade lasagna "noodles." You can easily make the crepes and the marinara the night before. You can also purchase store-bought marinara to save time—just make sure to get a really good one!*

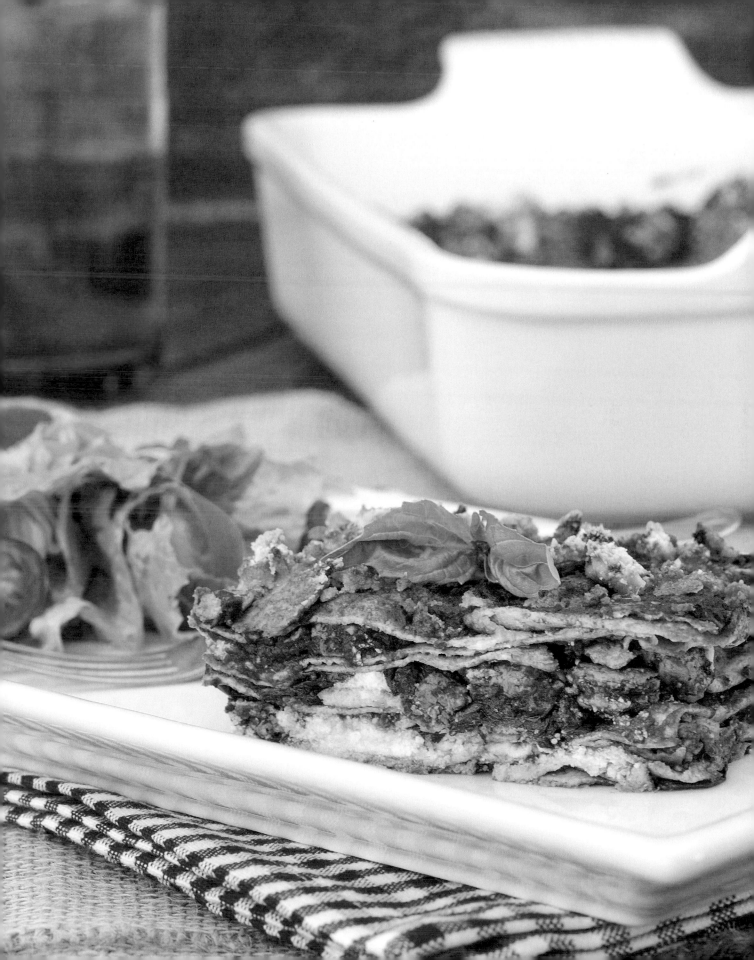

slow cooker pot roast

prep time: 20 minutes   cooking time: 10 hours   yield: 6 to 8 servings

A chuck roast is one of the less expensive types of roasts, but you would never know it after it has cooked in a tomato broth all day long. The meat shreds easily and melts in your mouth. Bonus: This is made in a slow cooker, so you can start it in the morning and have dinner ready by 6 p.m.!

ingredients

- 1 boneless beef chuck roast, 3-4 pounds, tied with kitchen twine
- 2 teaspoons sea salt, plus more to taste
- ½ teaspoon black pepper, plus more to taste
- 2 tablespoons coconut oil
- 1 yellow onion, halved
- 6 medium carrots, peeled and cubed
- 3 stalks celery, chopped
- 1 cup chopped leeks, green and white parts
- 4 cloves garlic, crushed
- 1 26-ounce jar or box chopped tomatoes
- 1 cup Chicken Broth (page 316)
- ¾ cup Burgundy wine
- 3 branches fresh thyme
- 2 sprigs fresh rosemary

method

1. Pat the beef dry with a paper towel and season with the salt and pepper. Place the oil in a Dutch oven and heat over medium heat. Add the roast and brown on all sides, about 10 minutes.

2. Place the onion, carrots, celery, leeks, and garlic in a slow cooker. Place the roast on top of the vegetables, then add the tomatoes and their juices, the Chicken Broth, and wine. Tie the thyme and rosemary together with kitchen twine and add to the pot. Cook on low for 8 hours, basting the meat twice to keep it moist on top.

3. Transfer the roast to a cutting board and remove the twine. Slice the meat against the grain or shred with two forks.

4. Discard the thyme and rosemary and skim off the top layer of fat from the sauce. Transfer half the sauce, all the onion, and half of the other vegetables to a blender and purée until smooth.

5. Pour the gravy back into the pot and return the meat to the pot. Continue cooking on low for another 1 to 2 hours.

6. Adjust salt and pepper as needed. Serve hot with extra gravy on the side.

tidbits:

While most pot roast recipes use white flour to thicken the sauce, I like to purée the cooked vegetables to create a thick and satisfying gravy to serve with the roast.

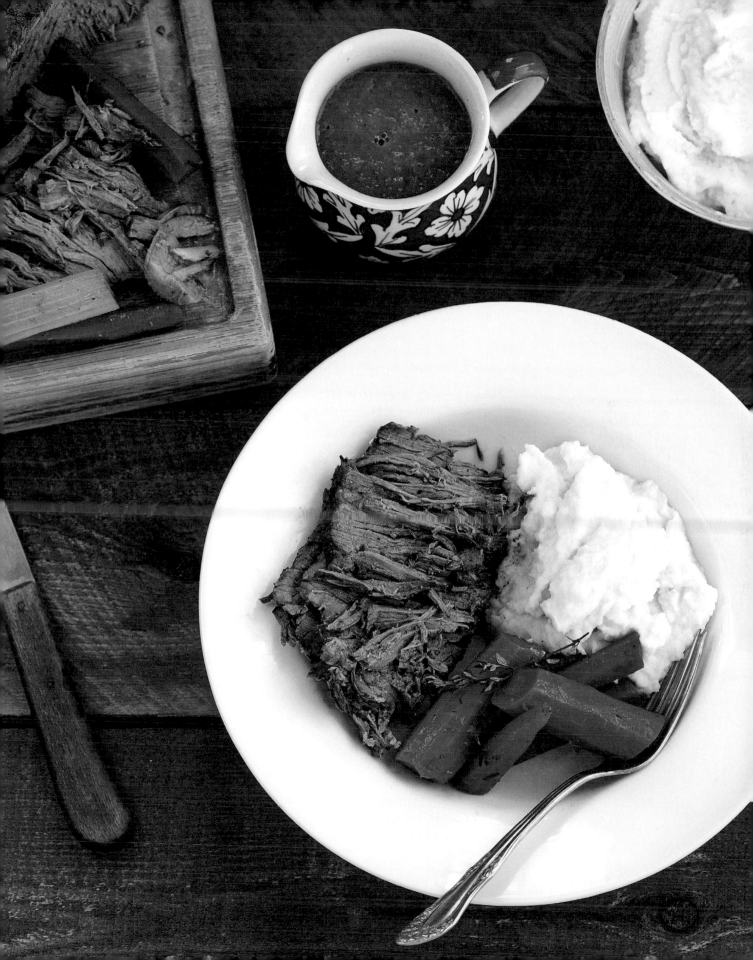

granny sarella's spaghetti sauce

prep time: 20 minutes   cooking time: 3 hours 15 minutes   yield: 6 servings

This is my great-grandmother's sauce recipe that has been passed down and perfected over many generations, with a few Paleo modifications. There are two secret ingredients: cinnamon and pork chops. The pork chops, which I admit are a totally bizarre ingredient for spaghetti sauce, simmer with the sauce and makes it stand head and shoulders above the myriad of store-bought sauces and even other homemade versions. The story goes that the men in Granny Sarella's family used to fight over who got to eat the chops after they were pulled out of the sauce—so don't discard them!

ingredients

- ¼ cup extra-virgin olive oil, divided
- 1 pound ground beef
- 1 pound pork chops, bone in
- ½ cup chopped onion
- 2 cloves garlic, minced
- 1 cup water
- 1 26.5-ounce box or jar tomato puree
- 2 tablespoons tomato paste
- 1 tablespoon honey
- 1 tablespoon dried oregano
- 1½ teaspoons sea salt
- 1 teaspoon fresh basil, chopped
- ¼ teaspoon black pepper
- 10 sprigs fresh parsley, chopped (or ¼ cup dried)
- ¼ teaspoon cinnamon

method

1. Place 2 tablespoons of the olive oil in a large stockpot over medium-high heat. Add the beef and pork chops and brown.

2. Remove the meat and drain the grease from the pot. Add the remaining olive oil and the onion and garlic. Sauté for 5 minutes, until fragrant and softened.

3. Return the meat to the pot. Add 1 cup water, tomato puree, tomato paste, honey, oregano, salt, basil, and pepper. Simmer, uncovered, for 3 hours on medium low. Stir in the parsley and cinnamon during the last 20 minutes of cooking.

4. Remove the pork chops before serving.

tidbits:

- *The sauce is pictured served over zucchini noodles. You can find the method for preparing them on my blog at www.againstallgrain.com/zucchini-noodles*
- *It is also wonderful served over spaghetti squash.*

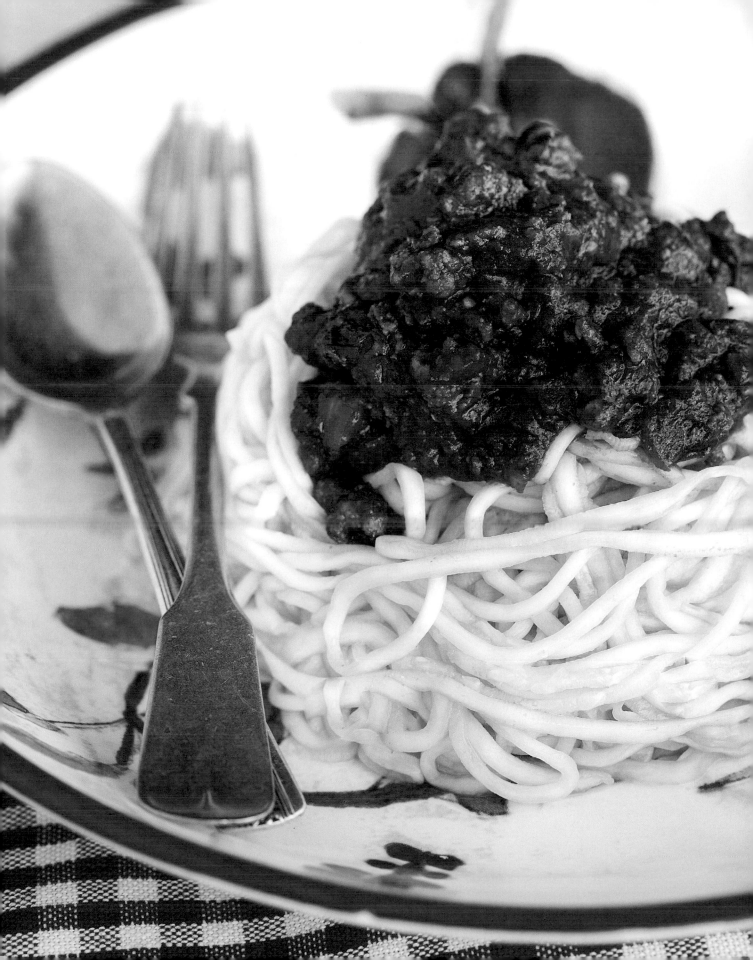

curried short ribs

prep time: 15 minutes   cooking time: 8 hours   yield: 4 servings

English-cut short ribs are slowly braised in fragrant curry to yield succulent meat that you will savor with every melt-in-your-mouth bite. Don't be alarmed that you'll need four pounds for four people—the bones and the fat make them heavy but they shrink in size as the fat slowly cooks down. My husband exclaimed that these ribs were the best dinner I ever set on the table. Pretty good for only ten ingredients and virtually no time in the kitchen!

ingredients

- 2 tablespoons coconut oil
- 4 pounds bone-in beef short ribs, cut into 3-inch pieces
- Salt and pepper
- 1 13.5-ounce can coconut milk
- 1/3 cup tomato paste
- 1/3 cup red curry paste
- 4 cloves garlic, minced
- 2 tablespoons fish sauce
- 2 teaspoons fresh lime juice
- 1 teaspoon ground ginger
- 1/2 yellow onion, sliced
- 1 pound carrots, peeled

method

1. Place the oil in a large pot over medium-high heat. Season both sides of the short ribs with salt and pepper. Place in the pot and sear on all sides, about 6 minutes.

2. Place the coconut milk, tomato paste, curry paste, garlic, fish sauce, lime juice, and ginger in a bowl and whisk to combine. Add the sauce and onions to a slow cooker. Place the short ribs on top, spooning some sauce over the meat.

3. Cook for 8 hours on low, basting and stirring once halfway through.

4. Skim off and discard all of the fat that has accumulated at the top of the pot.

5. Add the carrots and continue cooking for 1 hour more.

tidbits:

- *English style short ribs are beef ribs that are cut parallel to the bone and typically segmented into three-inch sections. Each short rib contains beef, fat, and bone which, when slowly braised, yields a succulent and flavorful dish.*

- *While I highly recommend trying the recipe as is, grass-fed short ribs are pricy and may need to be saved for a special occasion. Chuck roasts or stew meat are great budget-friendly substitutions.*

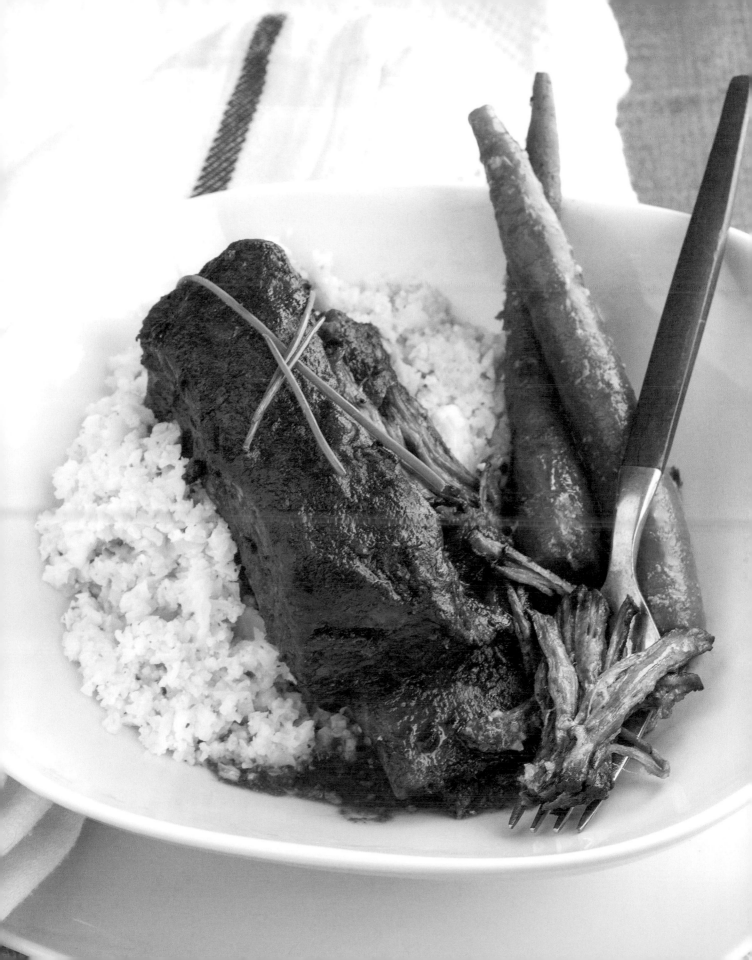

barbecue bacon burgers
with rosemary-garlic mushrooms

prep time: 20 minutes   cooking time: 15 minutes   yield: 4 servings

Barbecue sauce and bacon mixed into the beef before grilling produces an incredibly juicy burger. Mushrooms sautéed with rosemary and garlic turn up the flavor volume, but burgers are the perfect canvas for individualism, so feel free to add any or all of your favorite condiments.

ingredients

BURGERS

- 1 pound ground beef
- 4 slices cooked bacon, chopped, cooking fat reserved
- ¼ cup Smoky Barbecue Sauce (page 326)
- ½ teaspoon Dijon mustard
- ¼ teaspoon chili powder
- ¼ teaspoon sea salt
- ⅛ teaspoon paprika

MUSHROOMS

- 1 tablespoon reserved bacon fat
- 4 ounces baby bella or cremini mushrooms, sliced
- 1 teaspoon chopped fresh rosemary
- ½ teaspoon minced garlic
- ¼ teaspoon sea salt

method

1. Preheat a grill to medium-high heat.

2. To make the burgers, combine all the burger ingredients in a bowl and form into 4 patties about 1-inch thick.

3. To make the mushrooms, heat the fat in a skillet over medium heat. Add the remaining mushroom ingredients and sauté until tender, about 15 minutes.

4. Grill the burgers over direct heat for 2 minutes on each side, then move them to a lower-heat area of the grill. Continue cooking the burgers another 2-3 minutes for medium-rare burgers, 3-4 minutes for medium, or 5-6 minutes for well-done burgers. Serve with sautéed mushrooms and additional barbecue sauce.

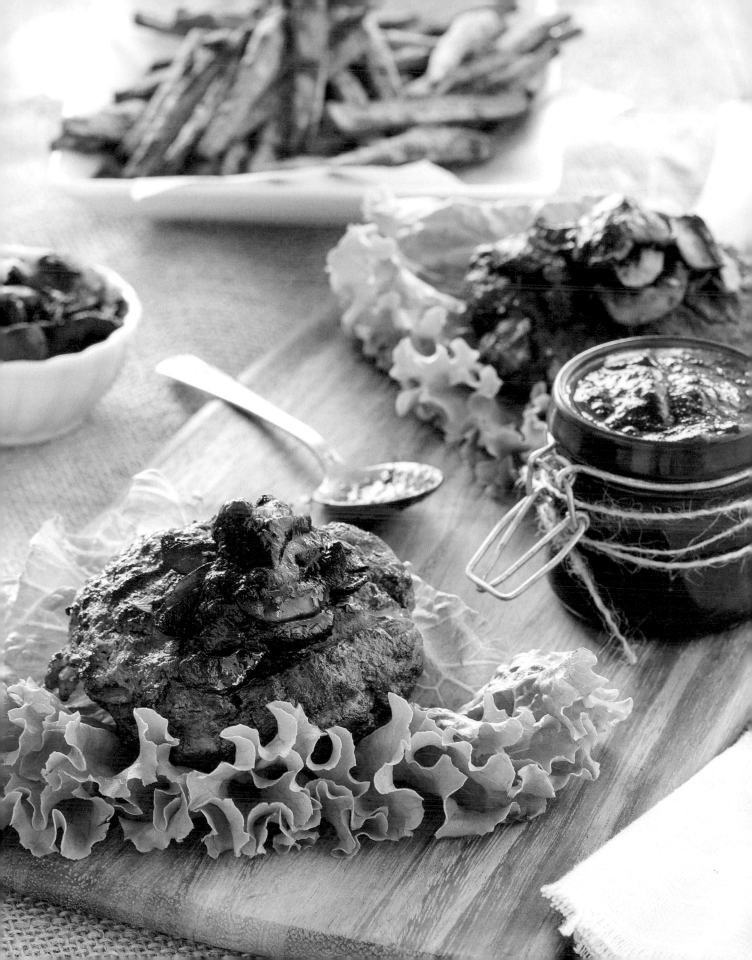

indian-spiced pork roast
with cumin-curry carrots

prep time: 15 minutes   *cooking time:* 45 minutes   *yield:* 6 to 8 servings

Garam masala is a spice mix frequently used in Indian cuisine, and just a small amount gives this roast a bold, mildly spicy flavor. You can purchase garam masala at most grocery stores, but I have also included a recipe in case you want to make your own.

ingredients

- 1 tablespoon bacon fat
- 3 pounds boneless pork top-loin center-cut roast, trimmed and tied
- 1 tablespoon garam masala
- ½ teaspoon sea salt
- 6 large carrots, peeled and cut into 2-inch pieces
- ½ teaspoon cumin
- ¼ teaspoon curry powder
- Asian Pear Chutney (page 322)

GARAM MASALA

- 2 teaspoons ground coriander
- ½ teaspoon black pepper
- ½ teaspoon cumin
- ¼ teaspoon ground cardamom
- ¼ teaspoon cinnamon

method

1. Preheat the oven to 350°F.

2. Place the bacon fat in a cast-iron skillet or other oven-safe skillet over medium-high heat.

3. Rinse the roast and pat dry. Rub the roast all over with the garam masala and salt. Place the meat in the skillet and sear on all sides, about 5 minutes.

4. Transfer the skillet to the oven. Roast for 35 minutes, or until the internal temperature reaches 150°F on a meat thermometer. Transfer the roast to a cutting board and let it rest for 10 minutes while the carrots cook.

5. Increase the oven temperature to 400°F. Place the carrots in the same skillet used for the roast. Sprinkle them with the cumin and curry powder. Place them in the oven and roast for 10 minutes, until tender.

6. Remove the strings from the roast and thinly slice. Serve with the carrots and chutney.

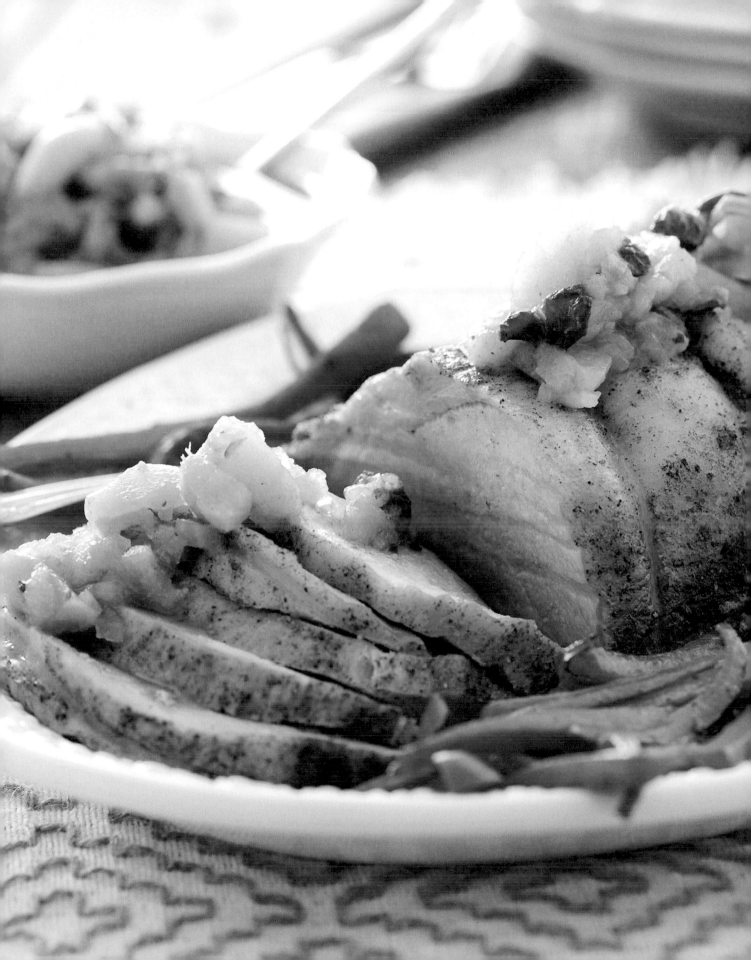

london broil with rosemary vegetables

prep time: 20 minutes + 6 hours marinating time

cooking time: 15 minutes   yield: 6 to 8 servings

Buying grass-fed meat can add up. If you're feeding a family on a tight budget, less-expensive cuts like top round or "London broil" will help you stretch your dollars—all you have to do is marinate the meat in acidic ingredients or slow cook it to make it tender. This classic recipe calls for marinating London broil in red wine and vinegar to tenderize the meat before broiling it.

ingredients

MEAT

- ¼ cup red wine
- 4 cloves garlic, finely minced
- 2 tablespoons coconut aminos
- 1 tablespoon apple cider vinegar
- 1 tablespoon whole-grain mustard
- 1 tablespoon fresh lemon juice
- 1 teaspoon chopped fresh basil
- 1 teaspoon chopped fresh thyme
- ½ teaspoon sea salt
- ¼ teaspoon cracked black pepper
- 2 pounds top round, or "London broil"

VEGETABLES

- 1 tablespoon extra-virgin olive oil
- 4 ounces baby bella mushrooms, sliced
- 1 small yellow onion, sliced
- 1 yellow bell pepper, seeded and sliced
- 1 sprig fresh rosemary
- Salt and pepper

method

1. Place all the ingredients for the meat in a shallow dish. Score both sides of the meat, diamond cut, about ⅛-inch deep. Place the meat in the refrigerator to marinate for 6 hours or overnight, turning occasionally.

2. Remove the meat from the marinade and let it sit at room temperature for 30 minutes before cooking. Lightly pat off excess marinade.

3. Position an oven rack in the top quarter of the oven. Set the oven to broil on high and cook the meat about 4 inches from the heating element for 5 to 7 minutes on each side. Let stand for 10 minutes before thinly slicing it diagonally against the grain.

4. Meanwhile, prepare the vegetables. Place the olive oil in a pan over medium heat, add the vegetables and rosemary and sauté until tender, about 15 minutes. Season with salt and pepper.

tidbits:

Butchers often label top round "London broil," but London broil actually refers to a preparation method, not a cut. Traditionally, a London broil is a tougher cut of meat that is often marinated and cooked quickly at high temperature, then sliced very thinly on the diagonal.

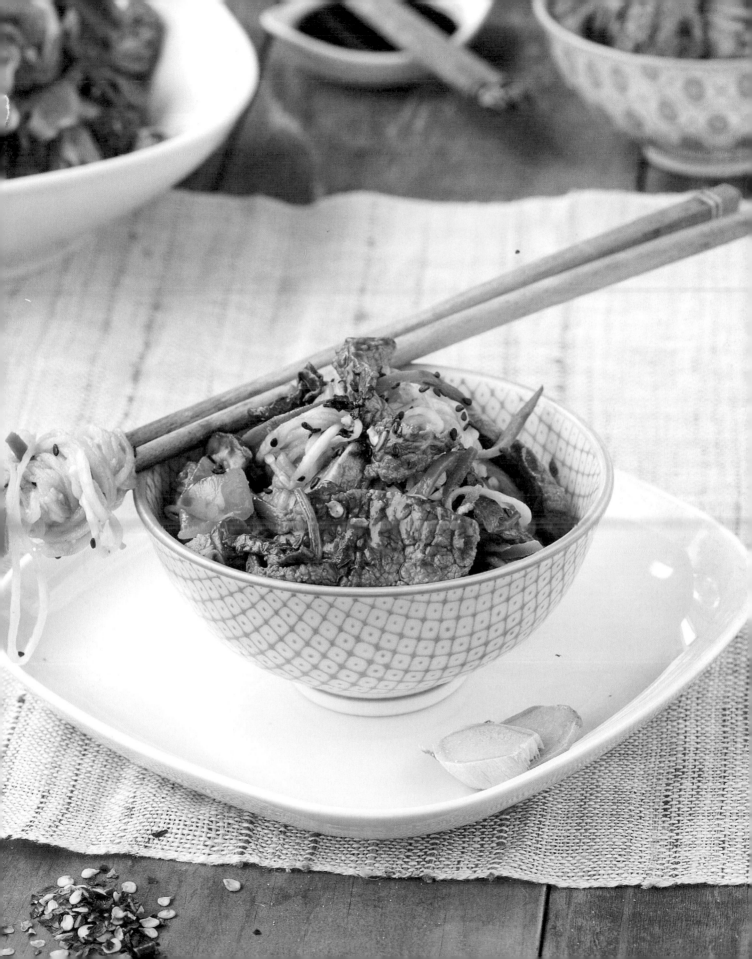

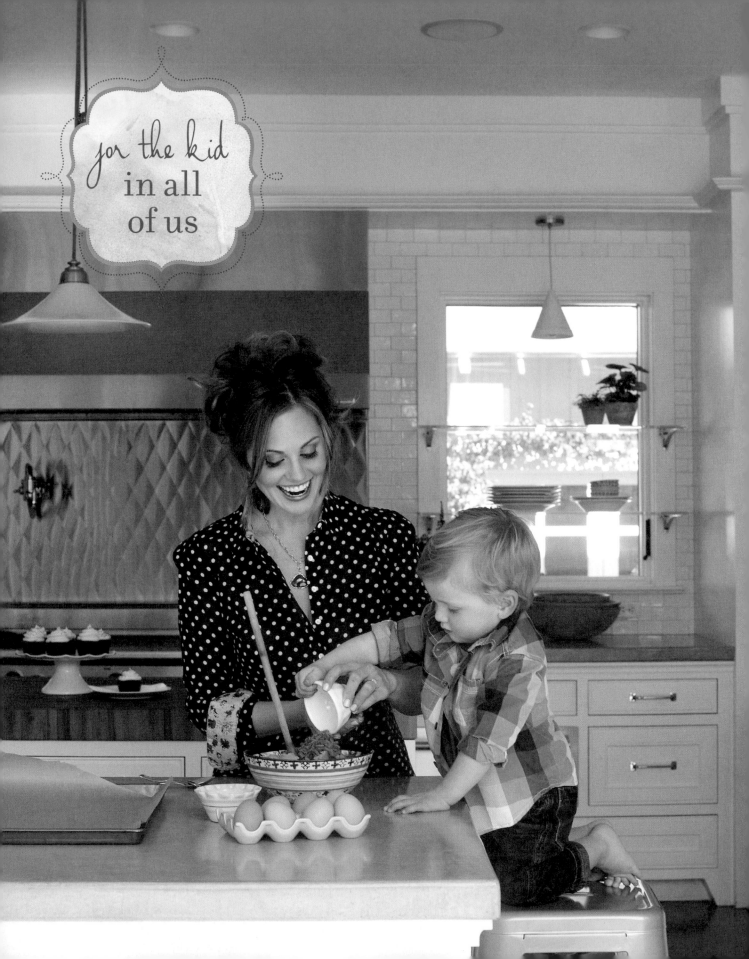

for the kid
in all
of us

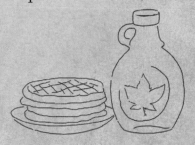

not-a-grain bars
("cereal" breakfast bars)

prep time: 50 minutes   cooking time: 12 minutes   yield: 8 bars

*for the kid
in all of us*

My blog readers helped me name these bars when I created them. The name stuck, and so has the recipe, as it has been made and enjoyed by hundreds of readers and their children. While commercial cereal bars are touted as "healthy," my version is grain-free and full of heart-healthy fats and fiber, so much better for growing bodies. When Asher hears the mixer humming, he runs into the kitchen asking to cook with me and loves to help roll out the dough. Swap the blueberry preserves for any pectin-free/refined-sugar-free jam of your choice!

ingredients

- ¾ cup blanched almond flour
- ½ cup coconut flour
- 2 teaspoons finely ground flaxseeds plus 1 tablespoon for dusting*
- ½ teaspoon baking soda
- ½ teaspoon cinnamon
- ¼ teaspoon sea salt
- ¼ cup coconut oil at room temperature
- ¼ cup honey
- 2 large eggs at room temperature
- 1 teaspoon pure vanilla extract
- ¾ cup Blueberry Preserves (page 330)

tidbits:

You can also just roll both pieces of dough into large squares rather than cutting into rectangles before baking. Spread all the fruit preserves on the bottom square, leaving a ½-inch border all the way around. Lift the parchment paper with the plain square and carefully flip it onto the other square. Seal the edges as described and bake for 12 minutes. Cut into rectangles after cooling. The jam will show with this method, but the bars will taste just as good!

method

1. Place the flours, 2 teaspoons ground flaxseeds, baking soda, cinnamon, and salt in a small bowl and stir to combine.

2. Place the coconut oil, honey, eggs, and vanilla in a large bowl and beat for 30 seconds on medium-high until creamy.

3. Slowly incorporate the dry ingredients into the wet, beating until well combined, about 45 seconds.

4. Divide the dough in half and shape into balls. Place each ball on a piece of plastic wrap and flatten into a disk. Wrap tightly and chill in the refrigerator for 20 minutes.

5. Preheat the oven to 350°F.

6. Remove 1 disk from the refrigerator and let sit at room temperature for 5 minutes to soften. Roll the dough out between 2 pieces of parchment paper until it's ¼-inch thick.

7. Using a pizza cutter, cut into rectangles about 5 inches by 2 inches.

8. Spread 1 tablespoon of the fruit preserves in the center of each rectangle, leaving a small border.

9. Repeat steps 6 and 7 with the other disk of dough.

10. Use a spatula to carefully place rectangles of plain dough on top of the rectangles with preserves. (Refrigerate the plain rectangles again to make moving them easier if necessary.)

11. Lightly wet your fingers with water and gently seal the bars by pressing the edges together. Sprinkle with additional flaxseeds.

12. Transfer the parchment paper with the bars to a baking sheet and bake for 12 minutes.

*Omit for SCD and increase coconut flour by 1 teaspoon.

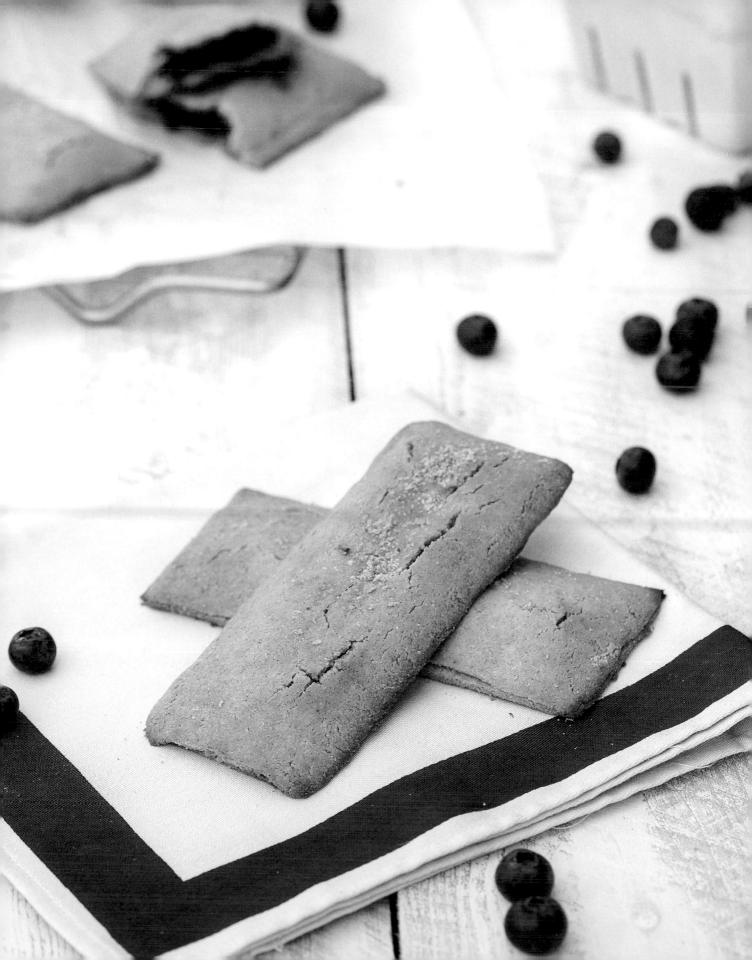

banana mouse pancakes

prep time: 8 minutes   cooking time: 10-15 minutes   yield: 12 to 14 pancakes

*for the kid
in all of us*

I vividly remember the special weekend treat my mom would make for us. I would wake up to the smell of melted chocolate and butter and come down to the kitchen to a plate full of steaming-hot chocolate chip pancakes lovingly shaped into the little, black, squeaky mouse with the big ears. Now that Asher has grown to love that character as well, I get heaps of joy out of carrying on my mom's sweet tradition with these banana pancakes.

ingredients

- 6 eggs
- 1 cup blanched almond flour
- ¾ cup sliced bananas (use overly ripe ones for more sweetness)
- ½ cup coconut milk
- ¼ cup coconut flour
- 2 teaspoons pure vanilla extract
- 2 teaspoons honey
- 1 teaspoon baking soda
- Dash of sea salt
- 1 teaspoon coconut oil or palm shortening

method

1. Place all the ingredients, except the oil, in a blender. Blend on low for 10 seconds, then on high for 30 seconds. The batter should be very smooth.

2. Let the batter sit for 5 minutes to thicken.

3. Place the oil in a shallow skillet or on a griddle over medium heat.

4. Spoon 1½ tablespoons of batter onto the hot pan for the head, then 2 teaspoons for each ear. Make sure the ears connect to the head for easier flipping.

5. Watch the pancakes closely and carefully flip them once bubbles rise to the surface, after about 1 minute.

6. Cook on the second side for just 15 to 30 seconds, then keep warm in an oven set to 200°F while you cook the remaining batter.

tidbits:

- *If the batter begins to get too thick halfway through the cooking process, add a little water to thin it out.*

- *The pancakes can burn easily if too much oil is in the pan. Use just enough oil to coat the surface.*

- *Use a thin spatula, working it under the pancake from the side, for the easiest flipping.*

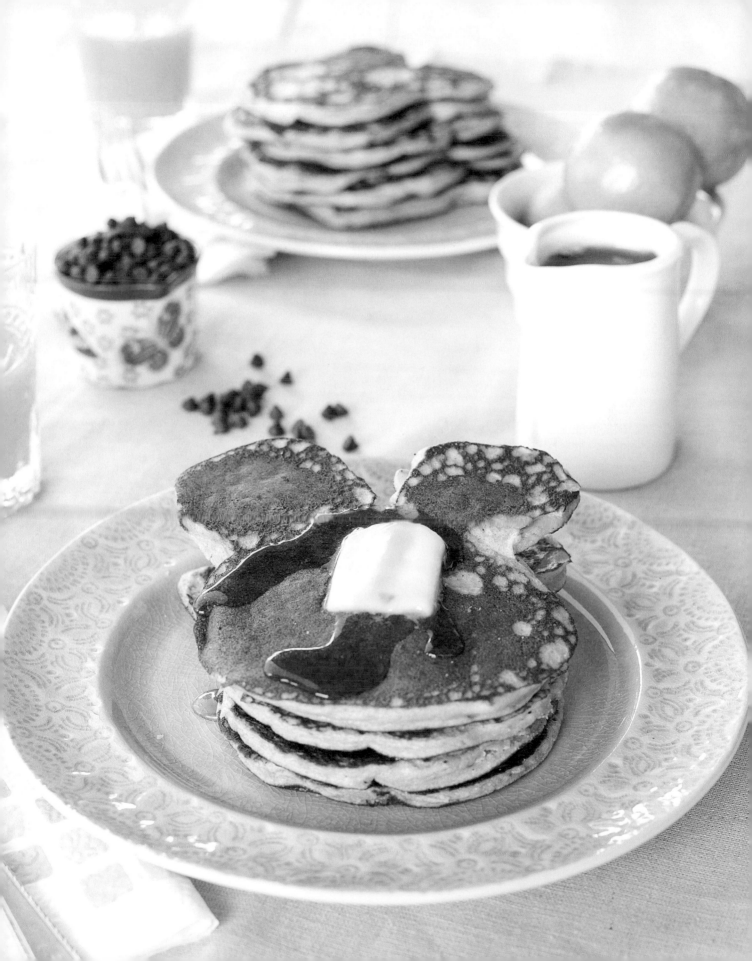

spaghetti squash boats with mini-meatballs

prep time: 15 minutes   cooking time: 50 minutes   yield: 4 servings

Sometimes cooking for children is less about trying new recipes and more about a fresh presentation of the same old same old. This is just your typical grain-free spaghetti and meatballs, but it is served in a "boat" for fun. I'm fortunate that Asher doesn't know the difference between spaghetti squash and wheat spaghetti, but his face sure lights up when I put this big, yellow boat before him. And I enjoy serving it knowing that he's getting a hefty serving of vegetables, from both the squash and the hidden leafy greens in the sauce!

ingredients

- 2 small spaghetti squash, about 1 pound each
- 2 teaspoons extra-virgin olive oil, divided
- Marinara Sauce (page 306)
- 2 cups baby spinach leaves, chopped
- 1 zucchini, very finely grated
- ½ pound mild sugar-free Italian sausage, uncooked
- ¼ teaspoon garlic salt

method

1. Preheat the oven to 400°F.

2. Cut each squash in half lengthwise and scoop out the seeds.

3. Place cut side down on a rimmed baking sheet. Rub 1 teaspoon of the olive oil on the skins, then roast for 30 to 40 minutes, until the squash is soft when you touch it and the skin has shriveled slightly.

4. Prepare the Marinara Sauce. Stir in the baby spinach and grated zucchini during the last 15 minutes of simmering.

5. Meanwhile, discard the casings from the sausage and roll the meat into 12 meatballs about the size of golf balls. Place them on a rimmed baking sheet lined with parchment paper.

6. Remove the spaghetti squash from the oven and cool cut side up on a cutting board.

7. Place the meatballs in the oven and bake for 8 minutes, turning them once to ensure even cooking.

8. Using the tines of a fork, release the "noodles" by dragging the fork lengthwise along the spaghetti squash.

9. Place the noodles in a bowl and toss with the remaining teaspoon of olive oil. Sprinkle with garlic salt.

10. Divide the noodles among the squash cavities, ladle ½ cup marinara over it, and top with 3 meatballs.

tidbits:

For more richness, toss "pasta" with ghee instead of olive oil.

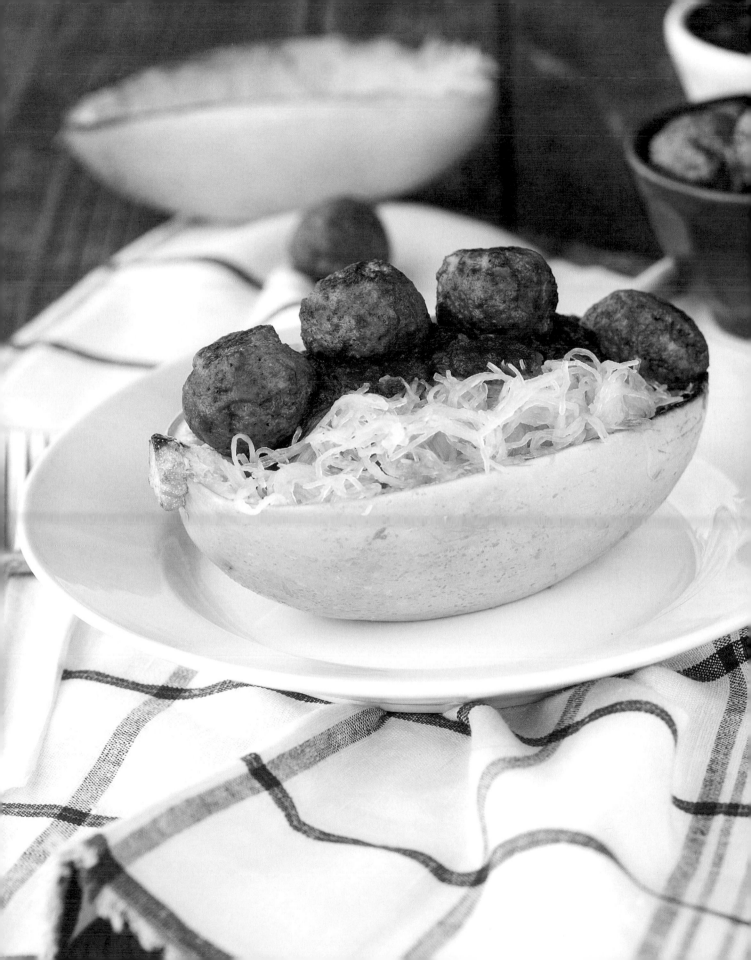

hidden-veggie muffins

prep time: 10 minutes   cooking time: 30 minutes   yield: 1 dozen muffins

*for the kid
in all of us*

Asher devours these little muffins without a clue that they are stuffed with two types of veggies. Naturally sweetened from the fruit and carrots, they taste like a real treat to little ones!

ingredients

- Coconut oil for greasing, optional
- ¾ cup pitted dates, about 4 ounces
- ¾ cup shredded zucchini
- ½ cup shredded carrots
- 3 eggs at room temperature
- ½ cup unsweetened applesauce
- 2 cups blanched almond flour
- 1½ teaspoons baking soda
- ¾ teaspoon cinnamon
- ½ teaspoon nutmeg
- ¼ teaspoon sea salt

method

1. Preheat the oven to 350°F. Line a muffin tin with baking cups or grease with coconut oil.

2. Place the dates in a bowl of warm water for 10 minutes to soften.

3. Spread the zucchini and carrots on a tray lined with a paper towel to drain some of the moisture while you prepare the batter.

4. Place the dates, eggs, and applesauce in a food processor and process for 30 seconds, until smooth.

5. Add the almond flour, baking soda, cinnamon, nutmeg, and salt and process for 15 seconds more.

6. Wrap the paper towel around the vegetables and give them a light squeeze to remove excess moisture and fold them into the batter.

7. Divide the batter evenly among the muffin cups, filling each ⅔ of the way full. Bake for 30 minutes. Cool in the pan for 10 minutes, then on a wire rack until completely cool.

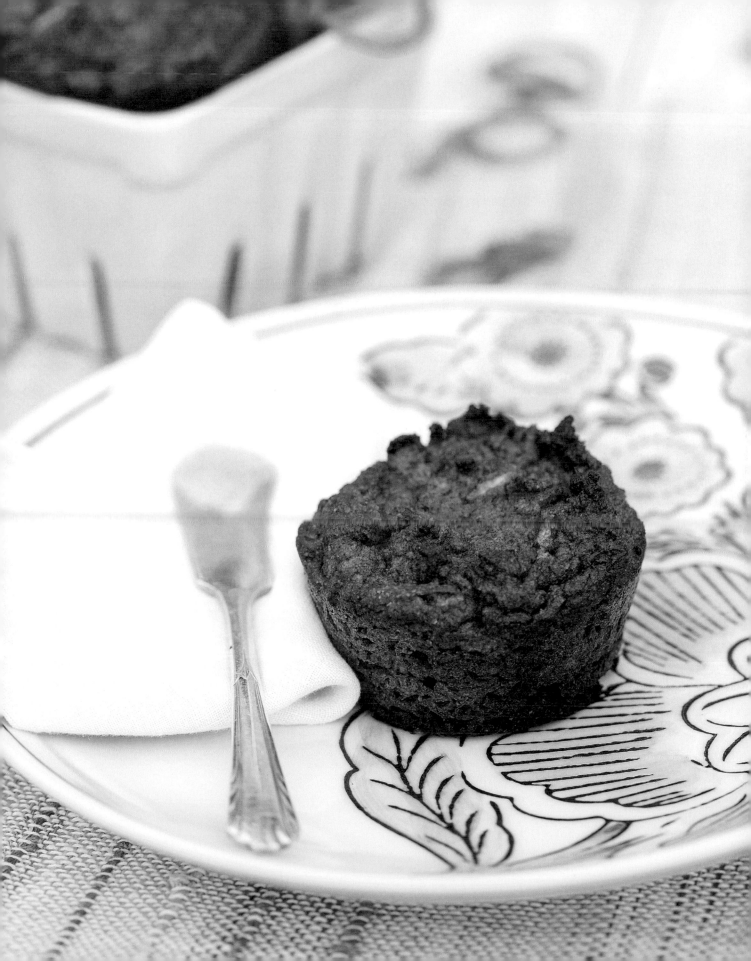

cutout cookies with frosting

prep time: 30 minutes   cooking time: 10 minutes   yield: about 1 dozen cookies

*for the kid
in all of us*

These buttery cookies are soft and chewy and the frosting pipes or spreads onto the cookies like a dream. Use this recipe all year round for your various holiday celebrations!

ingredients

DOUGH

- 2½ cups blanched almond flour
- ¼ cup honey
- 1 egg
- 2 teaspoons coconut oil
- ½ teaspoon pure vanilla extract
- ½ teaspoon baking soda
- ¼ teaspoon sea salt
- 1 teaspoon coconut flour

FROSTING

- 6 tablespoons coconut butter
- ¼ cup raw cacao butter, chopped
- ¼ cup honey
- ¼ cup cold coconut milk
- food coloring, optional

method

1. Preheat the oven to 350°F.

2. Place all the dough ingredients, except the coconut flour, in a food processor and process until a smooth ball forms, about 30 seconds.

3. Flatten the ball of dough into a ½-inch-thick disk and wrap in plastic wrap. Place in the refrigerator to chill for 20 minutes.

4. Place the dough between 2 sheets of parchment paper and roll out to ¼-inch thickness. Remove the top sheet and sprinkle the dough with the coconut flour, rubbing it in slightly with your fingertips. Dip a cookie cutter in a little flour, then cut out shapes, peeling away excess dough. Gather the excess dough into a ball and reroll it to make more cookies. If it starts to dry out or crack when rolled the second time, lightly wet hands before kneading the scraps to add a little moisture back into the dough.

5. Place the cookies on a tray lined with parchment paper and bake for 8 to 10 minutes. Cool completely on a wire rack.

6. Meanwhile, make the frosting. Place the coconut butter and cacao butter in a saucepan over low heat until melted, but not boiling. Pour into a bowl and whisk in the honey and cold coconut milk. Place in the refrigerator for 20 minutes to set.

7. Scrape the frosting into a blender or food processor and pulse a few times, until the frosting is smooth and fluffy. Divide frosting and add food coloring if desired.

8. Pipe designs or spread frosting onto cooled cookies.

tidbits:

To avoid the toxic chemicals in standard food coloring, you can find colorings made from vegetable dyes online or at some health-food stores. If you're feeling very ambitious, you can even find instructions online about how to make your own using beets, carrots, cabbage, turmeric, annatto, spinach, and ground freeze-dried fruits.

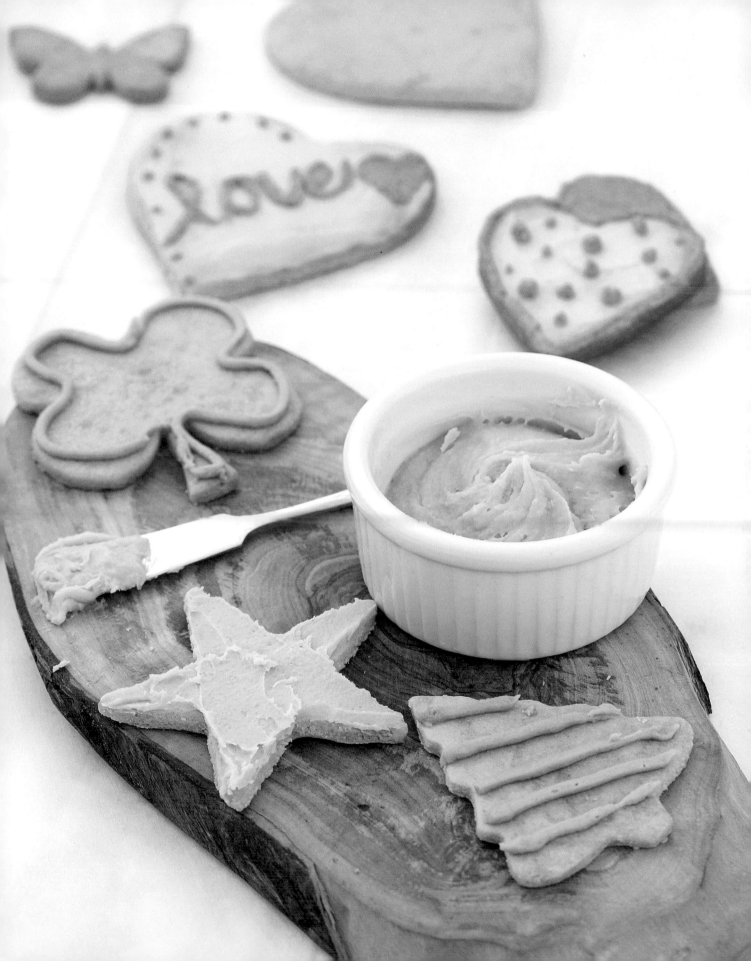

chicken-zoodle soup

prep time: 20 minutes   cooking time: 6 hours in a slow cooker, 30 minutes on the stove
yield: 8 servings

for the kid
in all of us

The classic kids' comfort food is now grain-free! Homemade broth contains healing elements essential for any little body recovering from a bug. Asher loves to slurp these "zoodles" up through his lips and picks out all the tender and flavorful chicken pieces.

ingredients

- 1 tablespoon coconut oil
- ½ cup diced yellow onion
- ½ cup chopped celery
- 1 cup sliced carrots
- 8 cups Chicken Broth (page 316)
- 2 pounds boneless chicken breasts, cubed
- 2 sprigs fresh thyme
- 8 black peppercorns
- 1 clove garlic, crushed
- 1 bay leaf
- 1 teaspoon sea salt
- 1 teaspoon parsley
- ¾ teaspoon oregano
- 2 pounds zucchini

method

1. Place the oil in a skillet over medium heat. Add the onion, celery, and carrots and sauté for 6 minutes.

2. Place the vegetables and the remaining ingredients, except the zucchini, in a slow cooker and cook for 6 hours on low. Alternatively, place in a stockpot over medium-high heat, cover, and bring to a boil. Lower the heat and simmer for 30 minutes.

3. Meanwhile, cut off the ends and peel the zucchini. Use a julienne peeler or spiral slicer to create noodles, discarding the seeded portions. Add the noodles to the slow cooker during the last 30 minutes of cooking or to the stockpot during the last 8 minutes. Stop cooking once the noodles are tender.

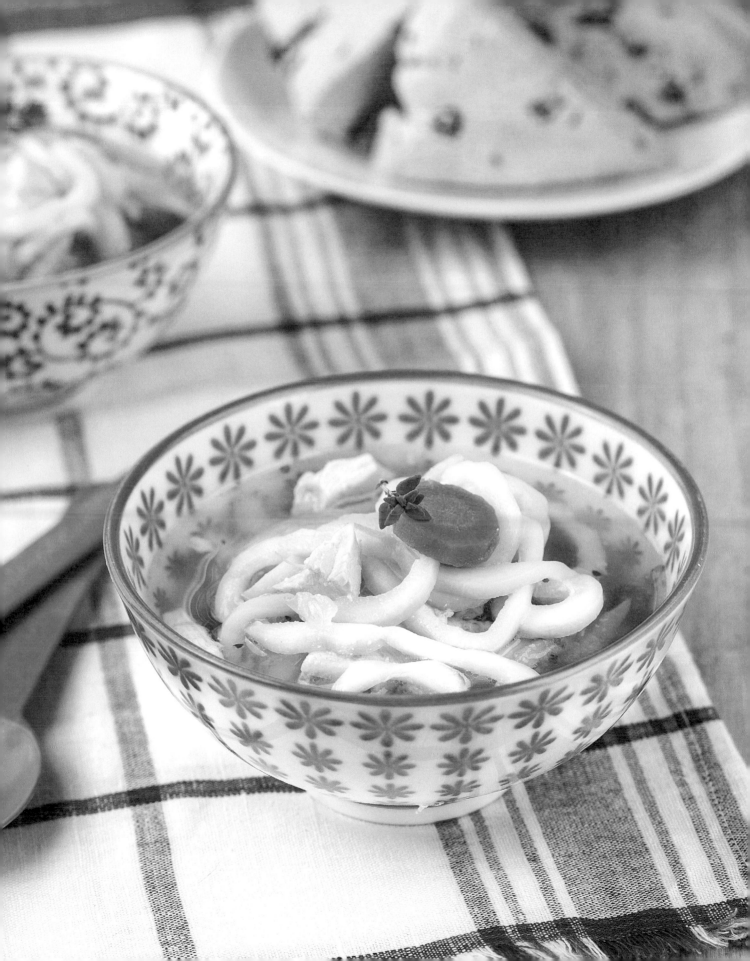

apple sandwiches

prep time: 10 minutes   yield: 6 servings

for the kid
in all of us

This is not so much an original recipe as it is simply another way to make feeding a grain-free kid fun. Kids need variety and love to eat with their hands. Asher is incredibly independent, and I have the most success with letting him take ownership in his snack choices by allowing him to choose his own toppings, like with these apple sandwiches.

ingredients

- 2 apples, cored and thinly sliced
- ¼ cup unsweetened almond or sunflower seed butter
- ¼ cup dairy-free chocolate chips
- ¼ cup Vanilla-Almond Granola (page 56)
- ¼ cup raisins

There's really no method here—just let your kids pick their fillings and sandwich them between two apple slices!

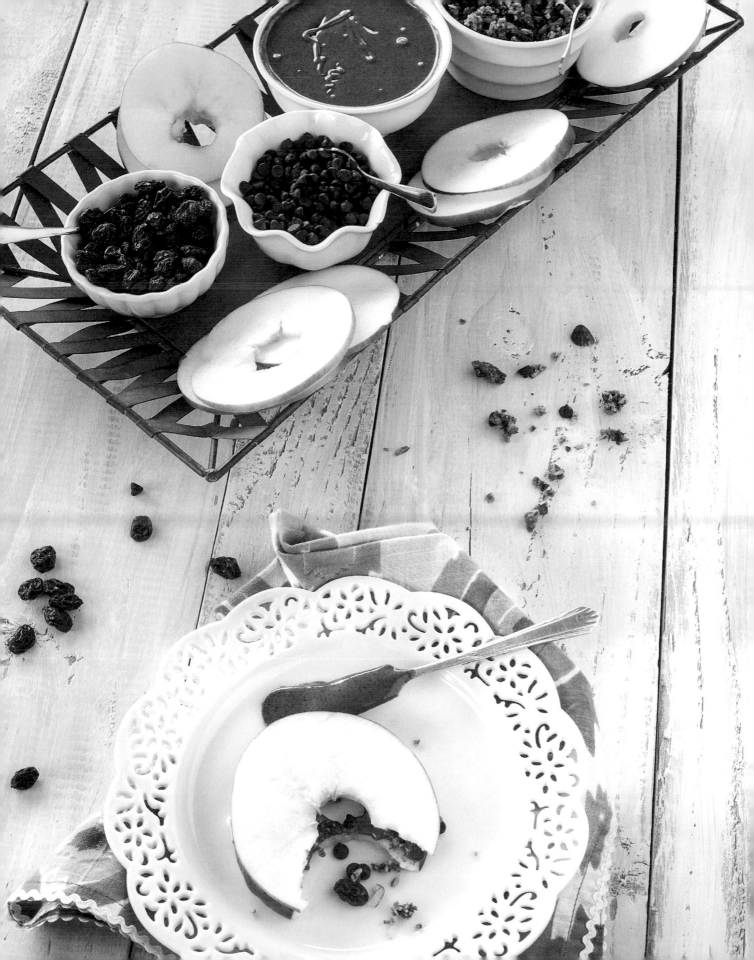

trail mix granola bars

prep time: 20 minutes   chilling time: 2 hours   cooking time: 10 minutes

yield: 1 dozen

With no baking required, this easy snack is ideal for kids' lunchboxes or after a long day of playing. Unprocessed nuts, succulent dried fruits, and honey make these chewy bars a treat for kids and adults alike.

ingredients

- ½ cup honey
- ½ cup almond butter
- 2 tablespoons coconut oil
- 1 teaspoon pure vanilla extract
- ¾ cup raw pecan halves
- ¾ cup raw cashews
- ½ cup raw almonds
- **5 large pitted dates, soaked in warm water for 15 minutes**
- ¼ cup shredded, unsweetened coconut
- ¼ cup raisins
- 2 tablespoons dried, unsweetened cranberries
- ½ cup dark chocolate pieces, optional

method

1. Line a 9-by-13-inch baking dish with parchment paper.

2. Place the honey, almond butter, oil, and vanilla in a saucepan over medium heat. Bring to a boil, then lower heat and simmer for 10 minutes.

3. Meanwhile, place the pecans, cashews, almonds, and dates in a food processor and process until the mixture resembles coarse sand. Add the coconut and pulse a few times to combine.

4. Remove the honey mixture from the stove and stir in the nut mixture. Add the raisins and cranberries, and the chocolate if desired.

5. Spoon the mixture into the baking dish, spreading it out with the back of a spoon.

6. Place a piece of parchment paper on top and use your palms to press the mixture evenly into the pan. Pack it down as tightly as possible to allow the mixture to cohere.

7. Remove the top piece of parchment and place the dish in the freezer for 2 hours.

8. Remove from the freezer and lift the mixture out of the pan using the edges of the parchment paper. Cut into 12 even rectangle-shaped bars with a sharp knife. Store in the refrigerator.

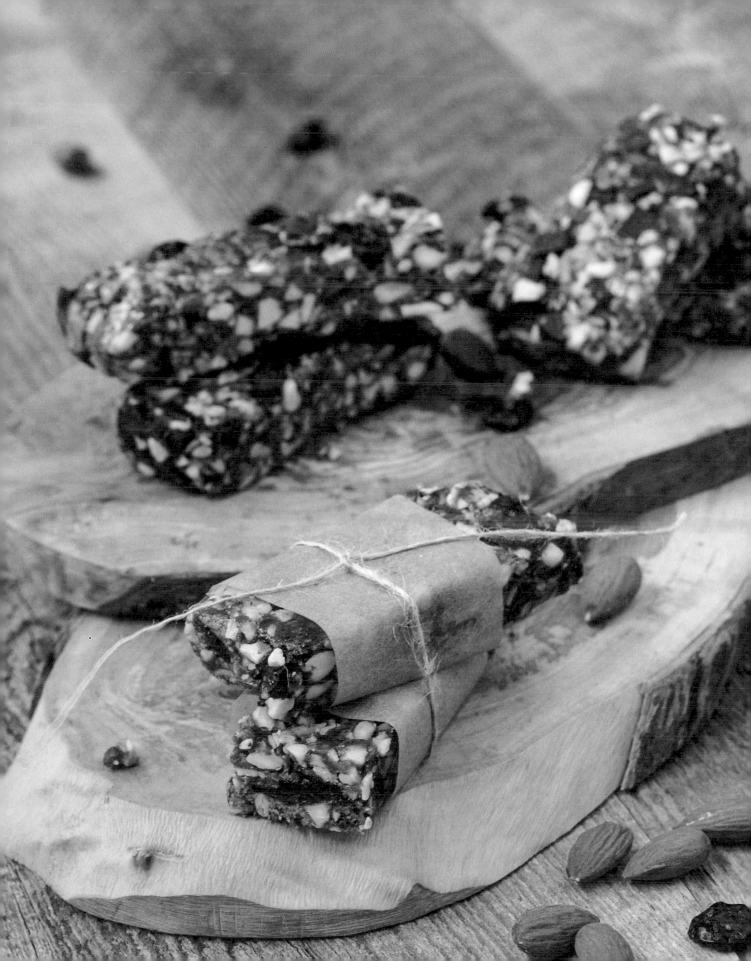

fruit roll-ups

prep time: 10 minutes   cooking time: 20 minutes
dehydrating time: 2–4 hours   yield: 4 servings

Asher loves fruit leathers, and I used to spring for the expensive organic ones at the store, but even those usually have added sugar. These fruit roll-ups can be made in the oven or dehydrator and are sweetened with applesauce, so they are a much better alternative—and are consumed just as quickly!

ingredients

- 4 cups frozen mixed fruit
- ½ cup unsweetened applesauce
- 1 teaspoon fresh lemon juice
- ¼ teaspoon lemon zest
- 1 tablespoon honey, if using tart berries

method

1. Place all the ingredients in a saucepan over medium-high heat. Bring to a boil, then lower heat and simmer for 20 minutes, until the fruit is soft and the liquid has thickened.

2. Pour the mixture into a blender or food processor. Carefully blend until smooth.

3. Line dehydrator sheets with parchment paper. Pour half of the fruit mixture through a fine-mesh sieve onto one tray and half onto the other. Use a spatula to lightly spread the mixture evenly, about ⅛-inch thick.

4. Place in the dehydrator for 3 hours at 150°F. If using an oven, bake on the lowest setting for 4 to 5 hours. Rotate trays midway through.

5. Cut the paper and fruit into 1-inch strips using scissors. Roll them up tightly and keep in an airtight container for a week.

tidbits:

Times may vary. Fruit strips are done when they are no longer sticky when you touch them lightly with your finger. If the edges get a little too brittle and dry, brush a tiny bit of water over them to rehydrate.

flavor ideas:

Mixed berries work well or create a tropical version with a mix of mango, pineapple, and peaches.

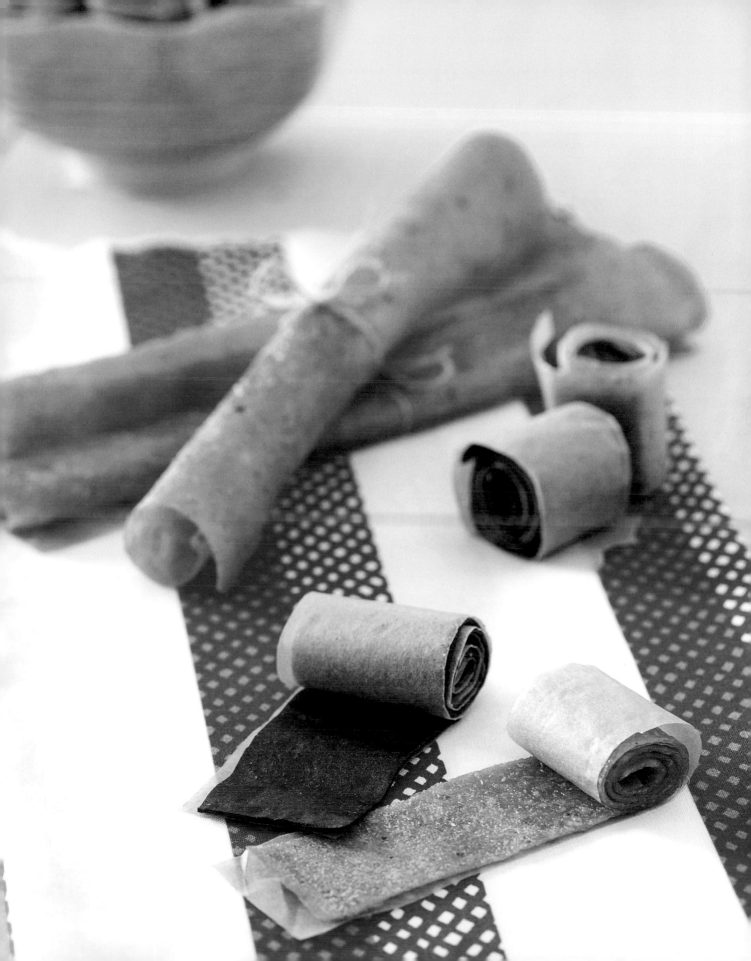

crispy chicken tenders
with honey-mustard dipping sauce

prep time: 30 minutes   cooking time: 20 to 25 minutes   yield: 4 to 6 servings

*for the kid
in all of us*

*I try to feed Asher whatever we're having for dinner, but sometimes the flavors are too mature
for his palate. For nights like those I like to have more kid-friendly options readily accessible.
The whole family actually enjoys these chicken tenders so I can also serve them without having
to make a separate meal for the adults.*

ingredients

- ¼ cup coconut flour
- ½ teaspoon coarse sea salt
- ⅛ teaspoon pepper
- ¼ teaspoon garlic salt
- ¼ teaspoon ground mustard seed
- ¼ teaspoon onion powder
- 2 eggs or ¼ cup extra-virgin olive oil
- 1 cup shredded, unsweetened coconut
- 1 pound chicken tenders
- 4 teaspoons honey
- 2 teaspoons whole-grain mustard

method

1. Preheat the oven to 375°F.

2. Place the coconut flour, salt, pepper, garlic salt, mustard seed, and onion powder in a shallow bowl and mix. Place the eggs in a separate shallow bowl and whisk. Place the shredded coconut in another shallow bowl.

3. First, dip each tender in the coconut flour mixture and lightly shake off the excess. Then, dip it into the eggs. Lastly, dip it into the coconut and press the coconut into the chicken.

4. Place the chicken strips on a baking sheet lined with parchment paper. Bake for 8 minutes, then turn the tenders over and bake another 8 minutes. Turn the oven to broil and bake for 3 to 5 more minutes, until the chicken is evenly browned.

5. Meanwhile, put the mustard and honey in a small bowl and mix.

6. Serve the chicken tenders warm with the honey-mustard sauce or sauce of your choice.

tidbits:
*Eggs help the coating stick, but
olive oil can be easily substituted
to make these egg-free.*

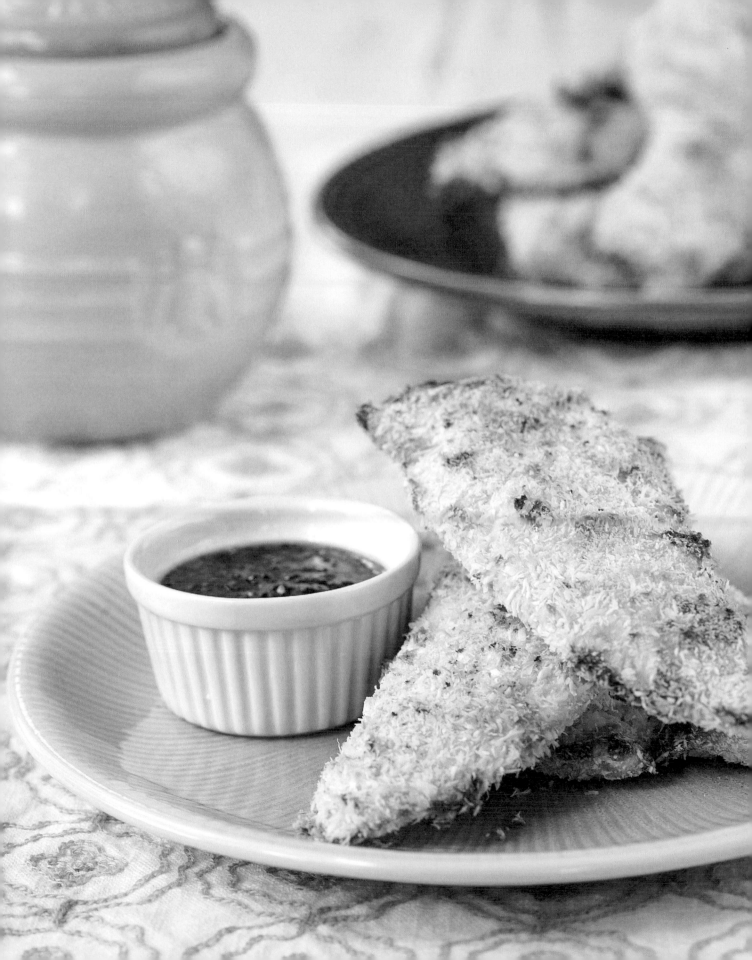

cinnamon applesauce

prep time: 20 minutes   cooking time: 6 hours   yield: 6 cups

*for the kid
in all of us*

The aromas and flavors of homemade applesauce far surpass those of store-bought, which, besides not being able to waft heavenly smells, often contain added sugars and preservatives. The scent of sweet apples and cinnamon will perfume your entire home as this sauce simmers away in the slow cooker all day.

ingredients

- 4 pounds tart apples, cored, peeled, and sliced
- 1 tablespoon fresh lemon juice
- 1 teaspoon cinnamon
- ½ teaspoon pure vanilla extract
- ½ teaspoon salt
- 1¼ cups water

method

1. Place the apples, lemon juice, cinnamon, vanilla, salt, and 1¼ cups water in a bowl and stir. Pour into a slow cooker and cook on low for 6 hours.

2. For a smooth applesauce, place in a blender in batches and purée until smooth.

tidbits:

No slow cooker? No problem, this applesauce can also be made on the stovetop. Add all of the ingredients to a saucepan, cover, and simmer for 30 minutes until soft.

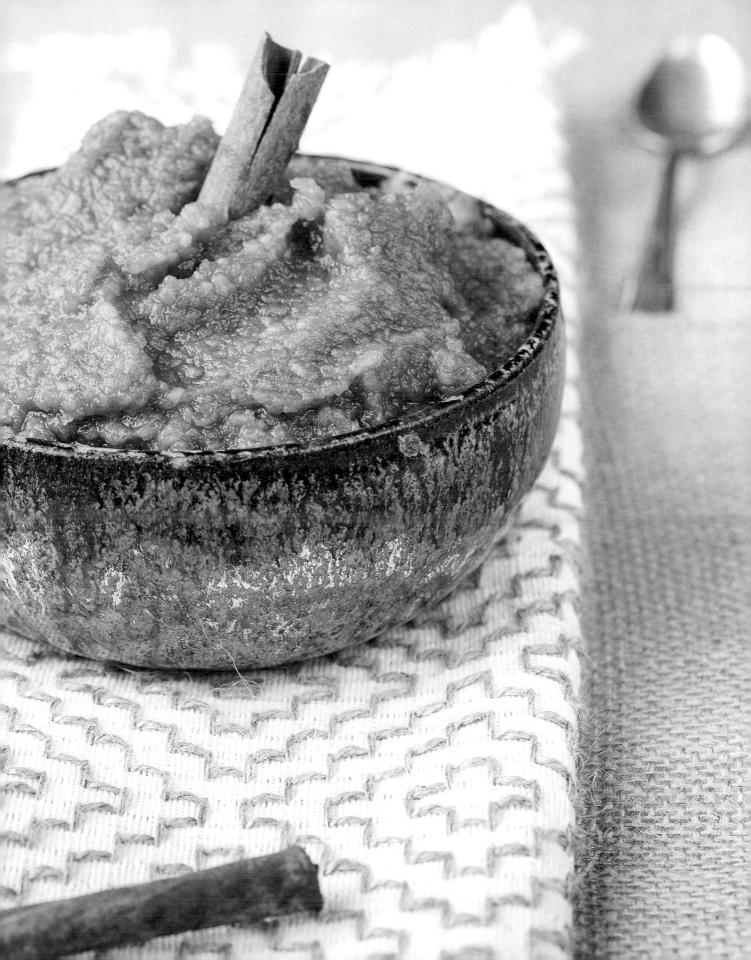

mini-meatloaf muffins

prep time: 20 minutes   cooking time: 30 minutes   yield: 6 servings

Classic American meatloaf becomes child-friendly when disguised as muffins that are perfect for little hands to hold. To appeal to extremely picky eaters, chop the vegetables really fine in a food processor and top the muffins with sweet homemade Tomato Ketchup and Mashed Cauliflower "frosting"!

ingredients

- 1 teaspoon coconut oil
- ½ cup minced yellow onion
- 2 medium carrots, finely chopped
- 1 clove garlic, minced
- 1 pound ground beef
- ½ pound lean ground pork
- ½ cup tomato puree
- ½ cup almond meal
- 1 egg, beaten
- 1 tablespoon fish sauce
- 1 tablespoon tomato paste
- 2 teaspoons Dijon mustard
- 1 teaspoon apple cider vinegar
- ¾ teaspoon sea salt
- ½ teaspoon oregano
- ¼ teaspoon cracked black pepper

TOPPINGS
- Tomato Ketchup (page 328)
- Mashed Cauliflower (page 122)

method

1. Preheat the oven to 350°F.

2. Place the oil in a saucepan over medium-high heat. Add the onions, carrots, and garlic and sauté for 5 to 7 minutes, until tender. Set aside to cool.

3. Place the remaining muffin ingredients in a bowl. Mix for 30 seconds to combine well, then incorporate the vegetable mixture.

4. Divide the meatloaf evenly among the cups of a 12-cup muffin pan, filling each to the top. Press gently to pack the meat down.

5. Bake for 30 minutes, rotating the tray midway through.

6. Remove muffins from the pan and gently shake off any fat and grease that has accumulated on the bottoms. Top artistically with Ketchup and Mashed Cauliflower.

tidbits:

This recipe can also be used to make a standard meatloaf. Press the meat into a 9-by-5-inch loaf pan and bake for 50 minutes.

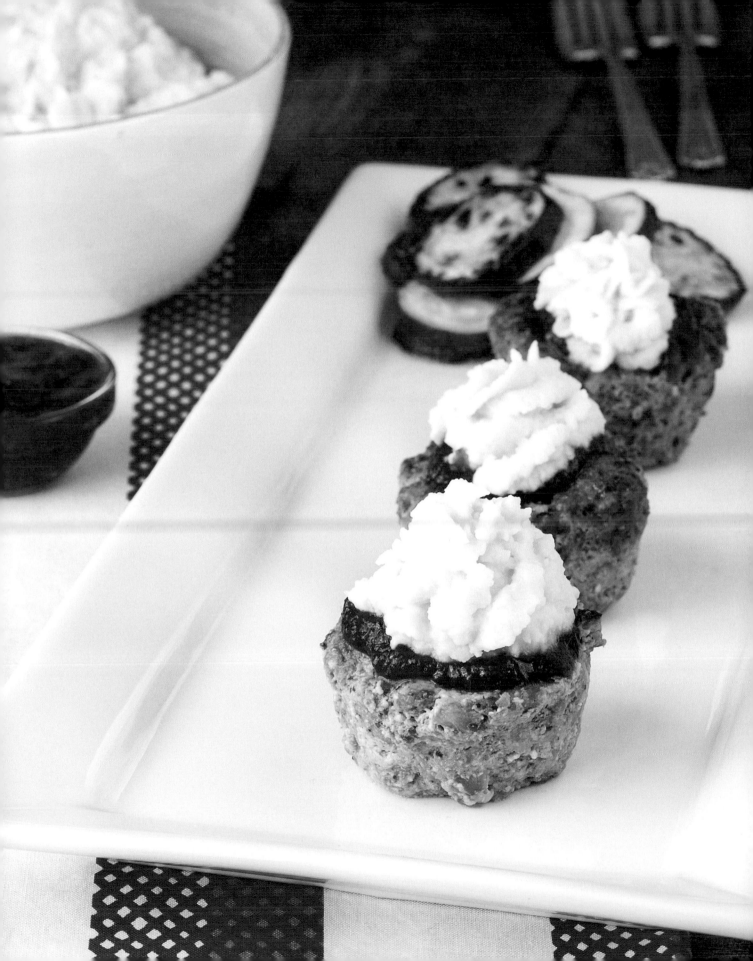

chewy honey graham crackers

prep time: 15 minutes   cooking time: 16 minutes   yield: 1 dozen crackers

*for the kid
in all of us*

These nut-free crackers are incredibly versatile. They make the perfect sandwich for ice cream or can be spread with sunflower seed butter and raisins for a satisfying snack. Follow the recipe and cut into rectangles or create fun shapes with your favorite cookie cutters.

ingredients

- ½ cup coconut flour, sifted
- ½ teaspoon cinnamon
- ¼ teaspoon salt
- ¼ teaspoon baking soda
- 2 egg whites
- ¼ cup coconut oil, softened
- ¼ cup honey
- 1 teaspoon pure vanilla extract

method

1. Preheat the oven to 350°F.

2. Place the dry ingredients in a small bowl and mix. Place the wet ingredients in the bowl of a stand mixer and mix, or use a hand mixer. Add the dry ingredients to the wet and mix until combined.

3. Form the dough into a ball and roll it out between 2 pieces of parchment paper to ¼-inch thickness.

4. Use a pizza cutter to cut the dough into rectangles, reserving dough scraps to reroll for more crackers.

5. Carefully slide the paper with the crackers onto a baking sheet. Place in the refrigerator for 20 minutes.

6. Gently separate the rectangles, spacing them evenly around the pan. Use a toothpick to prick holes all over the crackers.

7. Bake for 16 minutes, turning the crackers over halfway through. Cool on a wire rack.

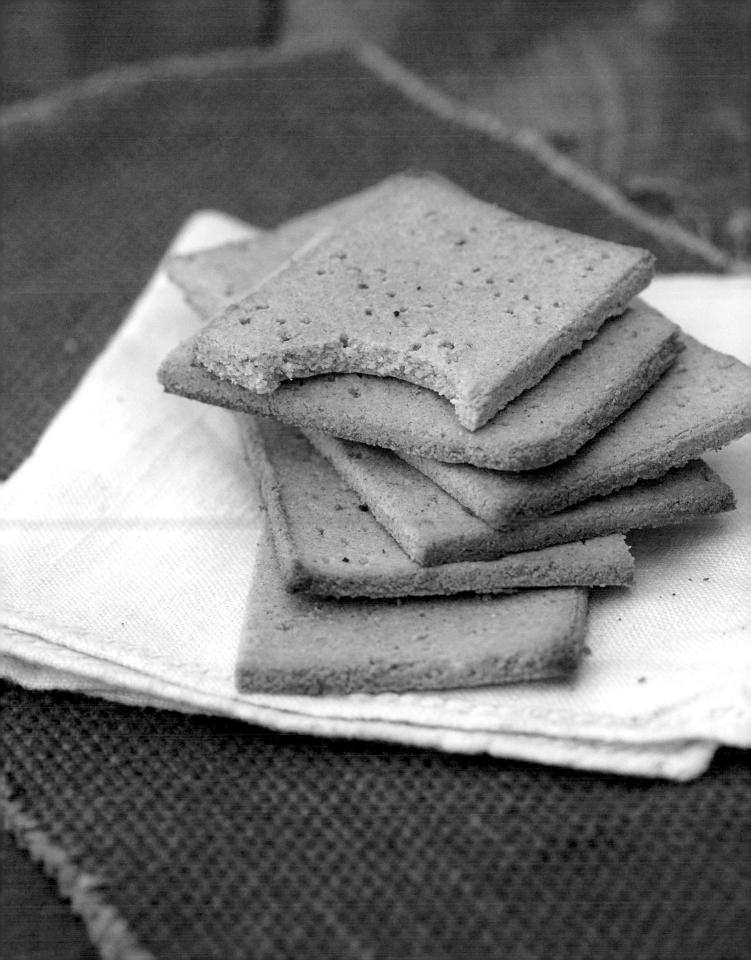

fruit juice gelatin shapes

prep time: 15 minutes + 8 hours chilling time

cooking time: 8 minutes   yield: 8 servings

Every time I was hospitalized for ulcerative colitis, an endless flow of unnaturally green Jell-O seemed to stream into my room, regardless of whether I ate it or not. But Jell-O doesn't have to be synonymous with the chemically-packed version we are all familiar with. Grass-fed, unflavored gelatin supports healthy skin, nails, and hair and also aids in joint recovery and pain. It's also beneficial for those with digestive diseases and to speed the recovery from colds or flus.

ingredients

- 4 cups unsweetened fruit juice
- 2 tablespoons + 2 teaspoons unflavored gelatin

method

1. Pour 1 cup of juice into a bowl. Sprinkle the gelatin over it and set aside.

2. Place the remaining juice in a saucepan over medium heat for 10 minutes. Do not boil.

3. Whisk hot juice into the gelatin until dissolved. Pour into a shallow baking dish or rimmed baking sheet. Place in the refrigerator overnight.

4. Briefly plunge the bottom of the dish or tray into hot water to make releasing the shapes easier. Use cookie cutters to create shapes or cut into cubes. Gently lift out shapes with a soft spatula. Keep refrigerated until ready to serve.

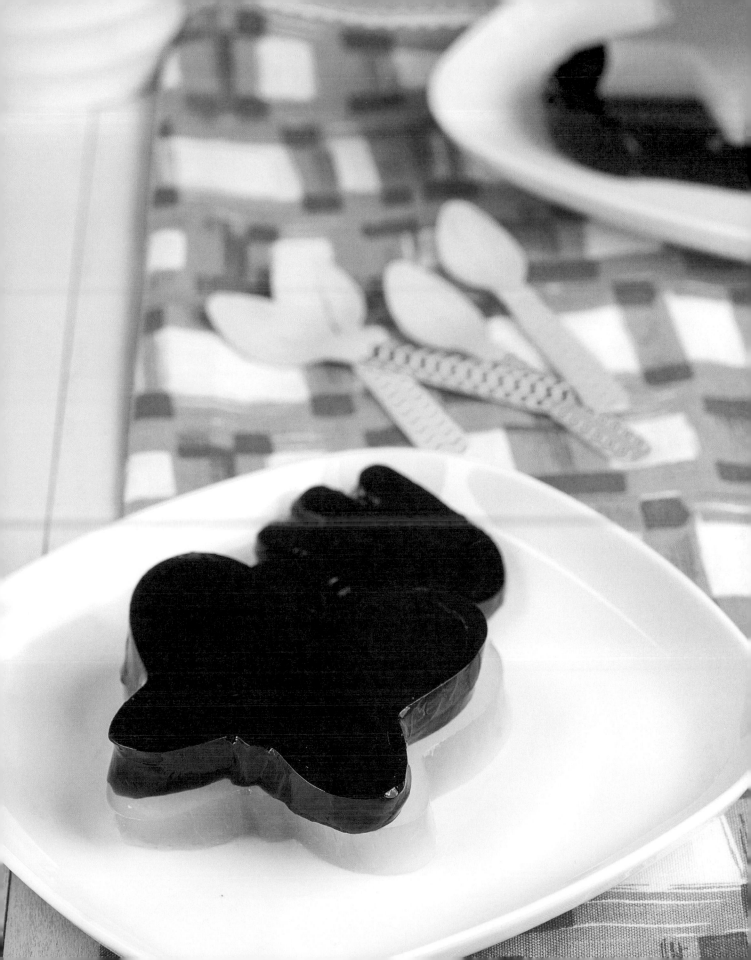

toddler-approved vegetable curry

prep time: 5 minutes   cooking time: 20 minutes   yield: 4 servings

*for the kid
in all of us*

What started as a quick and healthy lunch for me on days where I was too busy being a new mom to cook much for myself, this curry has now become one of Asher's favorite dishes! I always tended to give him food on the bland side, until one day he asked for a bite of my lunch and ended up finishing the entire thing. He even loves to help me measure out the different spices. Now I don't underestimate his palate and ask him to try everything at least once. You just never know until you try!

ingredients

- 2 teaspoons coconut oil
- 4 cups broccoli florets
- 1 cup shredded carrots
- 1 cup sliced zucchini
- 2 cups snow peas
- 2 cloves garlic, minced
- 1 teaspoon grated fresh ginger
- 2 tablespoons fish sauce
- 4 kaffir lime leaves, fresh or dried
- 1 tablespoon coconut aminos
- 1 teaspoon cumin
- 1 teaspoon turmeric
- ½ teaspoon coriander
- ¼ teaspoon nutmeg
- ¼ teaspoon cayenne
- 1 cup coconut milk

method

1. Place the oil in a skillet and heat over medium-high heat. Add the vegetables, garlic, and ginger and sauté for 5 minutes.

2. Add the fish sauce, kaffir leaves, coconut aminos, and spices and simmer for 10 minutes, until the vegetables are cooked but still firm.

3. Pour in the coconut milk, cover, and steam for 5 minutes. Remove the kaffir leaves before serving.

tidbits:

Reduce or omit the cayenne for young children sensitive to spice. Try substituting cubed butternut squash for the zucchini for a rich winter twist!

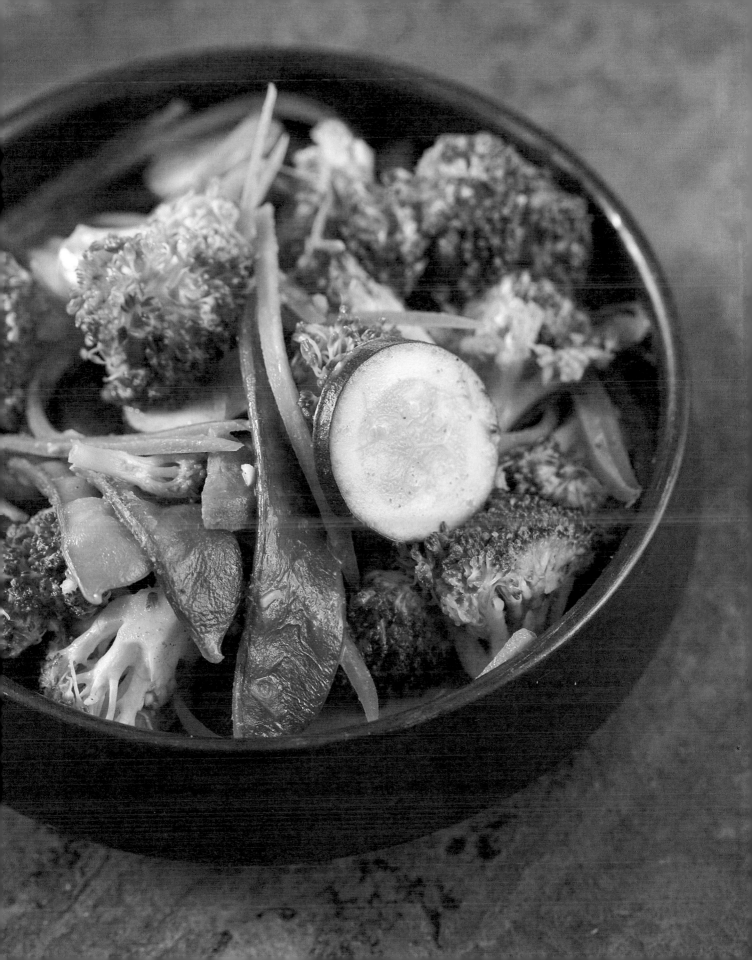

almond crisps

prep time: 15 minutes   cooking time: 10 minutes   yield: 3 dozen crackers

A remake of cheese crackers is one of the most frequent recipe requests on my blog, but it's been a challenge to come up with a dairy-free version. So I finally turned to a fairly untraditional ingredient in the Against All Grain kitchen: nutritional yeast. We love to eat them plain or dip them in guacamole. They also stay crunchy for days in a sealed container.

ingredients

- 2 cups blanched almond flour
- 2½ tablespoons nutritional yeast
- 4 teaspoons coconut oil, melted
- 4 teaspoons cold water
- 4 teaspoons egg whites
- ½ teaspoon baking soda
- ¼ teaspoon sea salt

method

1. Preheat the oven to 350°F.

2. Place all the ingredients in the bowl of a stand mixer. Mix until a loose dough forms, about 30 seconds.

3. Form the dough into a ball and roll it out between 2 sheets of parchment paper to about ¼-inch thickness.

4. Remove the top sheet of parchment paper. Use a pizza cutter or fluted pastry cutter to cut the dough into 1-inch squares. Save the scraps to reroll for more crackers.

5. Transfer the parchment paper to a baking sheet and carefully separate the crackers, spacing them evenly around the tray. Use a small round object, like the end of a skewer, to indent a circle in the centers.

6. Bake for 10 minutes, rotating the pan once, until golden around the edges. Let cool completely before serving.

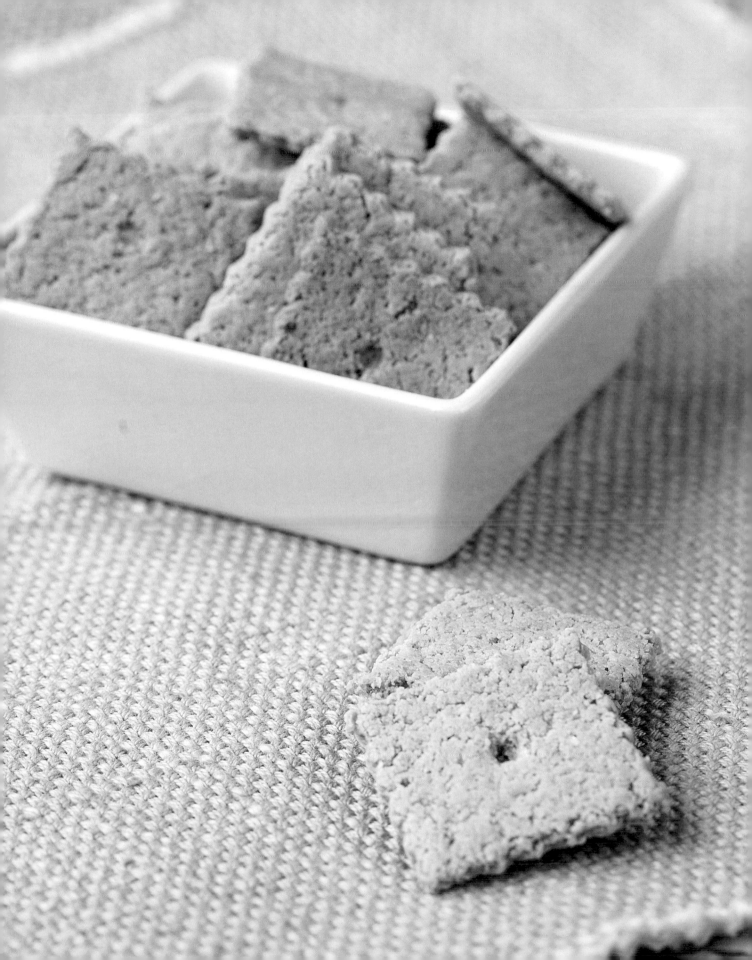

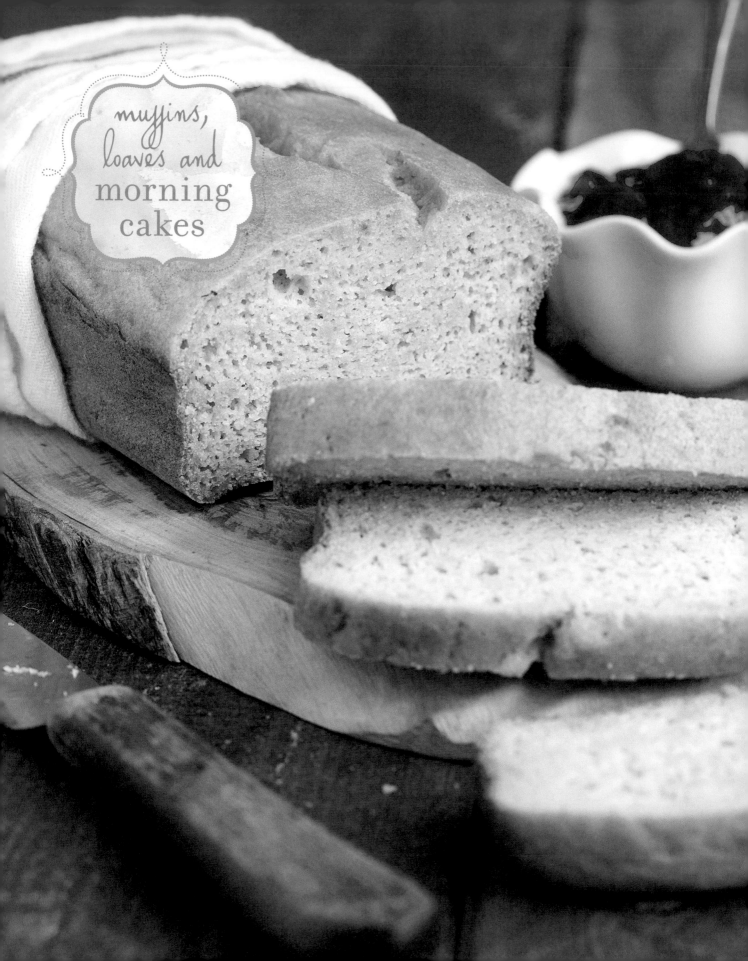

muffins,
loaves and
morning
cakes

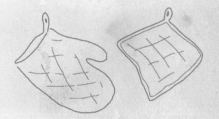

cinnamon-raisin coffee cake

prep time: 15 *minutes*   *cooking time:* 35 *minutes*   *yield:* 6 *servings*

Coffee cakes are a lovely and simple treat to bring to brunch gatherings, and those with tree–nut allergies should not have to miss out. This cinnamon and raisin swirled cake is made with coconut flour and is moist and delicious!

ingredients

BATTER

- 2 tablespoons coconut oil, melted plus ½ teaspoon for greasing pan
- 5 eggs at room temperature
- ½ cup honey
- 2 tablespoons coconut milk
- ¾ cup coconut flour, sifted
- ¾ teaspoon baking soda
- ½ teaspoon sea salt
- ¼ cup raisins

SWIRL

- 1 tablespoon coconut oil, melted
- 1 tablespoon honey
- 2 teaspoons cinnamon

method

1. Preheat the oven to 325°F.

2. Grease the sides of a 8-by-8-inch square baking dish with ½ teaspoon coconut oil.

3. Place the eggs, honey, 2 tablespoons coconut oil, and milk in a food processor and process for 30 seconds.

4. Add the coconut flour, baking soda, and salt. Process for 15 seconds to incorporate.

5. Stir in the raisins by hand.

6. Make the swirl. Place the coconut oil, honey, and cinnamon in a small bowl and stir to combine well. Mix into the batter by hand, stirring just a few times to create a ribbon through the batter.

7. Pour the batter into the prepared pan, spreading evenly. Bake for 25 minutes, until a toothpick inserted into the center comes out clean. Cool on a wire rack for 20 minutes.

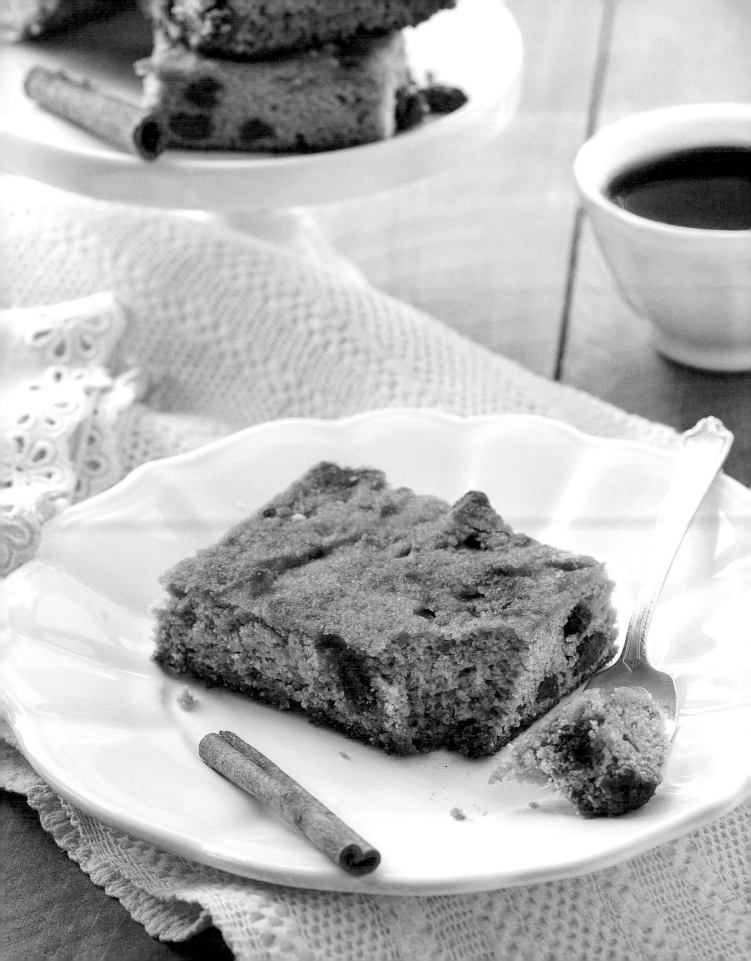

banana bread

prep time: 15 minutes   cooking time: 40-45 minutes   yield: 1 loaf

I can still recall the delicious aromas filling the house when my mom baked a loaf of banana bread. The same heavenly scents now waft out of my kitchen, but from grain-free ingredients. Be sure to use very ripe bananas with a lot of brown spots for the most sweetness, as the recipe calls for only a minimal amount of honey.

ingredients

- 2 tablespoons coconut oil, melted, plus more for greasing the pan
- 4 large eggs
- 3 tablespoons honey
- 1 teaspoon pure vanilla extract
- ½ teaspoon apple cider vinegar
- ½ cup coconut flour, sifted
- ¼ cup blanched almond flour, sifted
- 1 teaspoon baking soda
- ½ teaspoon sea salt
- ½ cup coconut milk
- 3 large ripe bananas
- Optional add-ins: ¼ cup dairy-free chocolate chips*, walnuts, dried cranberries, or raisins

method

1. Preheat the oven to 350°F.
2. Grease the sides and bottom of an 8½-by-4½-inch loaf pan, then place a piece of parchment paper on the bottom.
3. Place the 2 tablespoons coconut oil, eggs, honey, vanilla, and vinegar in the bowl of a stand mixer and beat on high for 30 seconds.
4. Combine the coconut flour, almond flour, baking soda, and sea salt in a bowl, then add them to the wet ingredients, beating on high until combined.
5. Place the coconut milk and bananas in a separate bowl and mash until the mixture resembles baby food.
6. Add the banana mixture to the batter and beat on medium until thoroughly combined.
7. Mix in the optional add-ins, if desired.
8. Pour the batter into the prepared loaf pan and bake for 40 to 45 minutes, until a toothpick inserted into the center comes out clean.
9. Remove from the oven and allow the loaf to cool in the pan for 15 minutes. Remove loaf and cool completely on a wire rack.

*For SCD, do not use.

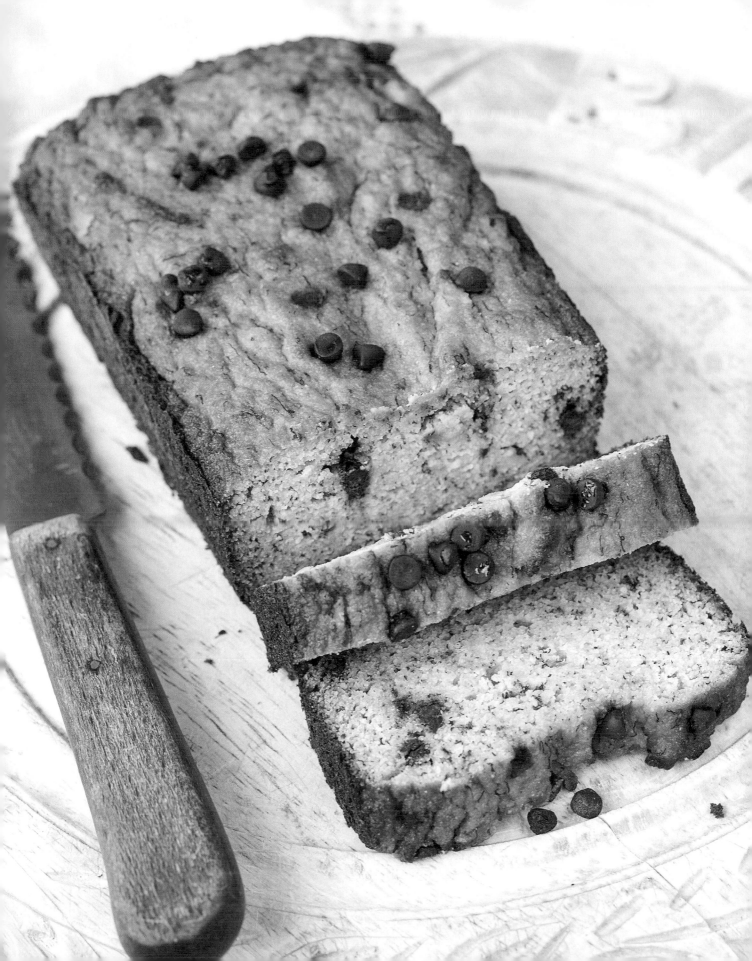

world-famous sandwich bread

prep time: 20 minutes   cooking time: 50 minutes   yield: 1 loaf

This is the bread that took my blog global. It is my most viewed and shared recipe of all time and has never received a negative comment, except about the cleanup! You can toast it to accompany eggs in the morning, send an almond butter and jam sandwich to school with your kids, or grill it Panini-style.

ingredients

- Coconut oil for greasing pan
- 4 large eggs, separated
- 1 cup smooth, raw, unsweetened cashew butter
- 1 tablespoon honey
- 2½ teaspoons apple cider vinegar
- ¼ cup almond milk
- ¼ cup coconut flour
- 1 teaspoon baking soda
- ½ teaspoon sea salt

method

1. Preheat the oven to 300°F. Place a small heatproof dish of water on the bottom rack while the oven heats.

2. Line the bottom of an 8½-by-4½-inch loaf pan with parchment paper, then grease the sides of the pan with a very thin coating of coconut oil.

3. Place the egg whites in the bowl of a stand mixer and beat until soft peaks form, or use a hand mixer.

4. Beat the egg yolks and cashew butter in a separate bowl until combined, then mix in the honey, vinegar, and milk.

5. Sift the coconut flour, baking soda, and salt into the cashew butter mixture. Beat until combined.

6. Add 2 tablespoons of the whipped egg whites to the cashew butter mixture and beat until smooth. Add the remaining egg whites and beat on low until just combined. Do not over mix.

7. Pour the batter into the prepared loaf pan, then immediately put it into the oven.

8. Bake for 45 to 50 minutes, until the top is golden brown and a toothpick inserted into the center comes out clean.

9. Remove from the oven, then let cool for 15 to 20 minutes. Use a knife to free the sides from the loaf pan, then flip the pan upside down to release the loaf onto a cooling rack. Cool right side up for an hour before serving.

tidbits:

- *The steam from the dish of water helps the loaf rise and keeps it a nice white color.*

- *While beating the egg whites separately is not required, it helps the loaf rise to almost twice the size as adding the eggs whole.*

- *Use homemade cashew butter made from unsalted raw cashews or purchase raw, unsweetened cashew butter in a jar.*

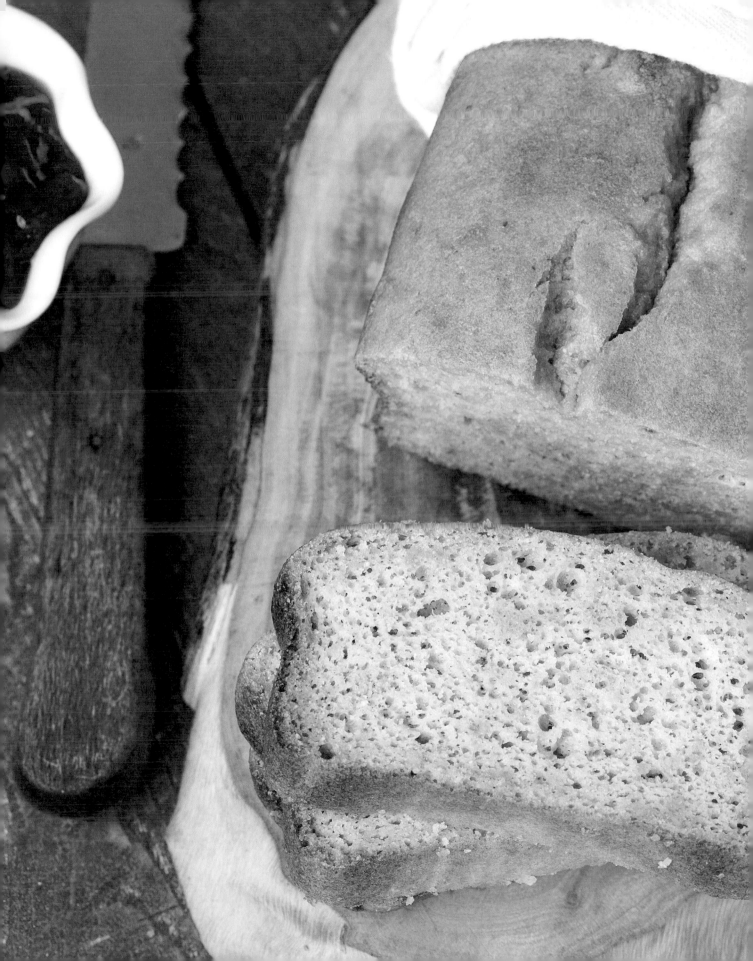

spiced pumpkin muffins

prep time: 15 minutes   *cooking time:* 25 minutes   *yield:* 12 muffins

Full of autumnal spices and ambrosial pumpkin puree, these muffins make for a quintessential autumn snack.

ingredients

- 2 cups blanched almond flour
- 3 tablespoons coconut flour
- 1 teaspoon baking soda
- 2 teaspoons cinnamon
- ¾ teaspoon nutmeg
- ¼ teaspoon ground ginger
- ¼ teaspoon cardamom
- ¼ teaspoon cloves
- ¼ teaspoon sea salt
- ¾ cup pumpkin puree, fresh or canned
- ⅓ cup pure maple syrup or honey
- 2 large eggs at room temperature
- 2 tablespoons coconut oil, melted
- 1 teaspoon pure vanilla extract
- Optional add-ins: ¼ cup dairy-free chocolate chips* or 2 tablespoons chopped pepitas

method

1. Preheat the oven to 350°F.
2. Line a muffin tin with baking cups.
3. Place the almond flour, coconut flour, baking soda, spices, and salt in a small bowl and mix to combine.
4. Place the remaining wet ingredients in the bowl of a stand mixer and beat on high until combined, or use a hand mixer.
5. Slowly incorporate the dry ingredients into the wet, mixing until smooth.
6. Gently mix in the chocolate chips or pepitas, if desired.
7. Pour the batter into the prepared muffin tin, filling each cup ⅔ of the way full.
8. Bake for 25 minutes, until a toothpick inserted into the center of a muffin comes out clean.

*For SCD, do not use.

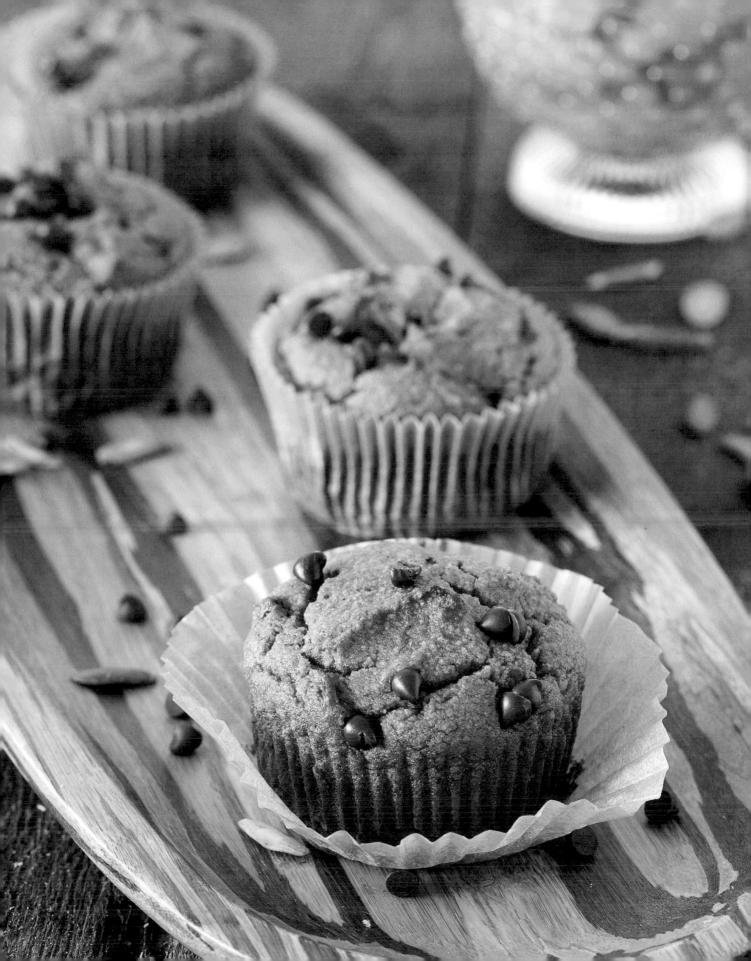

orange-cranberry muffins

prep time: 10 minutes   cooking time: 20-25 minutes   yield: 12 muffins

muffins, loaves, and morning cakes

These muffins are speckled with crimson cranberries and have a hit of orangey tanginess. They come together in a flash with only a blender or food processor—no mixing bowls!—which makes cleanup a snap as well. A steam bath increases the rise and keeps the almond flour from browning while baking, resulting in a moist and fluffy muffin.

ingredients

- 2 eggs at room temperature
- ¼ cup orange juice
- 2½ cups blanched almond flour
- ½ cup honey
- ½ cup palm shortening
- 1 tablespoon coconut flour
- 2 teaspoons pure vanilla extract
- 1 teaspoon orange zest
- ¾ teaspoon baking soda
- ½ teaspoon nutmeg
- ¼ teaspoon sea salt
- 1½ cups whole fresh cranberries

method

1. Preheat the oven to 350°F.

2. Place a heatproof dish filled with 2 cups of water on the very bottom rack and position another rack in the center of the oven.

3. Place all the ingredients, except the cranberries, in a high-speed blender or food processor in the order listed and blend for 30 seconds. Scrape down the sides, then blend again until very smooth.

4. Stir in the cranberries by hand.

5. Grease a 12-cup muffin tin or line with paper cups. Spoon the batter into the cups, filling each ⅔ of the way full.

6. Place the muffins in the oven on the center rack and bake for 20 to 25 minutes, or until a toothpick inserted into the center of a muffin comes out clean.

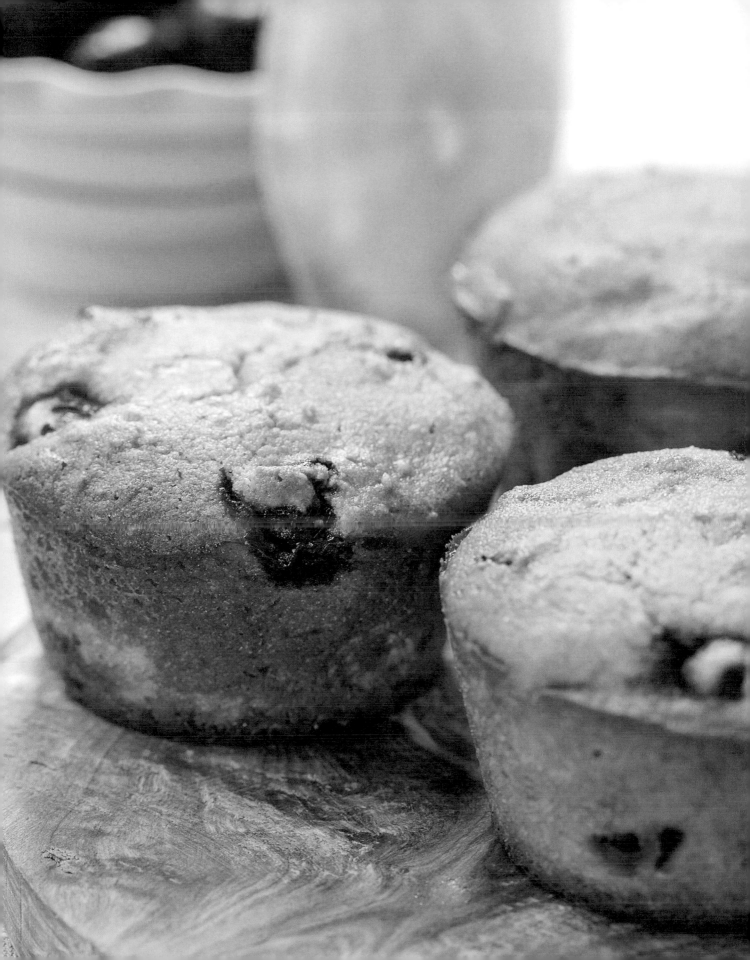

currant scones

prep time: 20 minutes   cooking time: 20 minutes   yield: 6 scones

I will never forget going to the UK with my parents and husband, Ryan, years ago. In southern England, my mom was relentless in seeking out the cutest tearooms and indulging in the scones, clotted cream, and lemon curd in every establishment. I must have eaten dozens of scones in just a few days! I'd be lying if I said I didn't utterly enjoy those dainty little biscuits, which is why I wanted to recreate a grain-free version we could savor together back home. These traditionally round pastries are mildly sweet and don't make you feel guilty the way the ginormous frosted ones that often beckon from coffee shop counters in the States do.

ingredients

- 1¾ cups blanched almond flour, sifted
- 3 tablespoons coconut flour, sifted, plus more for rolling out the dough
- ¼ cup honey
- 1 egg
- 2 tablespoons coconut milk
- 1 tablespoon fresh lemon juice
- ½ teaspoon baking soda
- ¼ teaspoon sea salt
- 3 tablespoons palm shortening
- ¼ cup dried currants
- Topping: 1 teaspoon coconut milk plus 1 teaspoon coconut crystals (omit for SCD)

method

1. Preheat the oven to 350°F.

2. Place the flours, honey, egg, coconut milk, lemon juice, baking soda, and salt in the bowl of a stand mixer and mix on medium until a loose dough forms.

3. Switch to a dough hook or use a pastry cutter to blend in the palm shortening, leaving pea-size bits of the shortening visible in the dough. Gently stir in the currants.

4. Lightly sprinkle coconut flour on a sheet of parchment paper. Gather the dough into a ball and form into a 1-inch-thick circle, using your hands to flatten it.

5. Use a round biscuit cutter to cut circular pieces of dough, gathering the remaining dough into a ball and repeating the process until it has all been used up.

6. Place the scones on a parchment-lined baking sheet. If desired, brush the tops with the coconut milk and sprinkle with coconut crystals.

7. Bake for 18 to 20 minutes, turning the tray once midway through. Cool on a wire rack before serving. These are best served immediately but may be stored in an airtight container and re-warmed later.

tidbits:
Serve with Lemon Curd (page 286) or Blueberry Preserves (page 330).

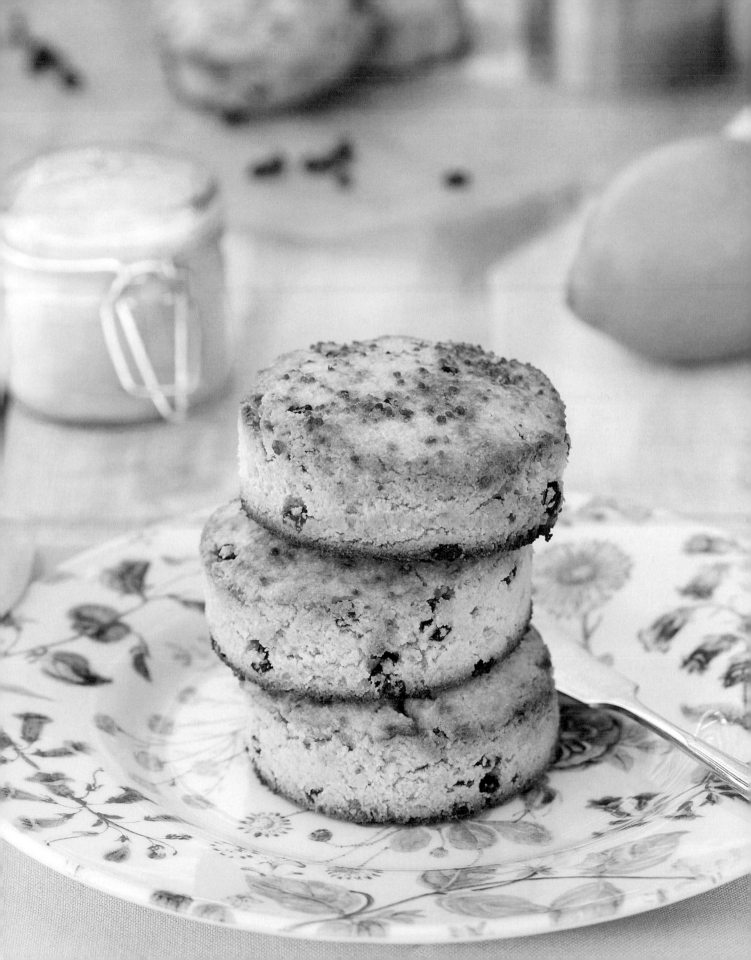

glazed lemon poppy seed pound cake

prep time: 20 minutes   *cooking time:* 40 minutes   *yield:* 8 servings

My husband's favorite treat with his coffee is a slice of glazed lemon pound cake. I've always enjoyed the pleasant flavor of lemon in cakes and the slight sweet crunch of poppy seeds, so I set out to recreate his favorite treat. The lemon glaze complements the rich, moist flavor of this delicate cake.

ingredients

CAKE

- ⅓ cup palm shortening, softened, plus more for greasing pan
- 3 tablespoons coconut flour, plus 1 teaspoon for dusting pan
- ¾ cup honey
- ⅔ cup unsweetened almond milk
- ¼ cup lemon juice
- 1 teaspoon pure vanilla extract
- 3 cups blanched almond flour
- 1 teaspoon baking soda
- ¼ teaspoon sea salt
- 5 large eggs at room temperature
- 2 tablespoons poppy seeds
- 1 tablespoon grated lemon zest

GLAZE

- 2 tablespoons plus 2 teaspoons finely ground cashews
- 2 teaspoons lemon juice
- 1 tablespoon coconut oil, melted
- 2 teaspoons honey, melted
- 1 tablespoon coconut milk

method

1. Preheat the oven to 325°F.
2. Make the cake. Grease a Bundt pan very well with palm shortening, then dust with 1 teaspoon coconut flour, carefully ensuring that every crack and surface is covered.
3. Place the first 9 ingredients in a food processor or high-speed blender and process for 15 seconds, until smooth.
4. Add 1 egg at a time, blending in-between, until all the eggs have been incorporated.
5. Gently stir the poppy seeds and lemon zest in by hand.
6. Pour the batter into the prepared pan, place in the oven, and bake for 40 minutes, until a toothpick inserted into the center comes out clean.
7. Let the cake cool for 15 minutes on a wire rack, then invert it onto the rack to cool completely. If necessary, use a rubber spatula to gently release the cake from the pan.
8. Whisk together the glaze ingredients in a bowl and drizzle over cooled cake before serving.

tidbits:
This batter also works well as a loaf. Bake for 90 minutes in a 8½ -by- 4½-inch loaf pan.

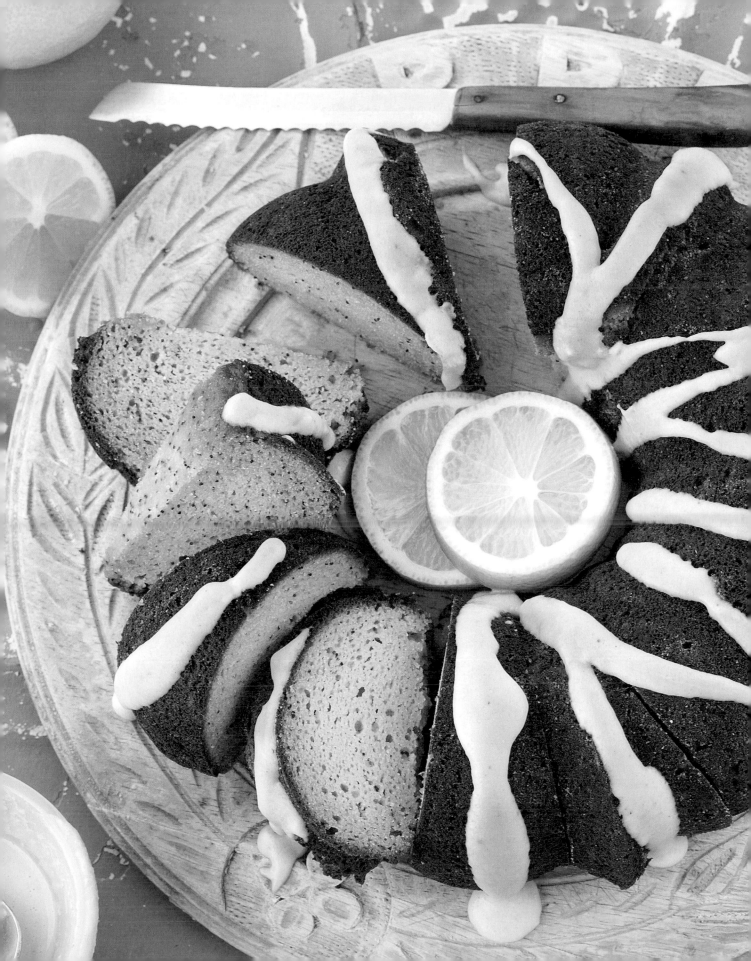

zucchini bread

prep time: 12 minutes   cooking time: 40 minutes   yield: 1 loaf or 12 muffins

Zucchini gives this quick bread incredible moistness. The sweet hints from the zucchini and banana plus the subtle spice from the cinnamon and nutmeg make this snacking bread utterly irresistible!

ingredients

- Coconut oil for greasing the pan
- 1 cup shredded zucchini
- 1½ cups blanched almond flour
- 2 teaspoons cinnamon
- ¾ teaspoon baking soda
- ½ teaspoon sea salt
- ½ teaspoon nutmeg
- 3 eggs, beaten
- ¼ cup honey
- 1 ripe banana

method

1. Preheat the oven to 350°F. Lightly grease an 8½ -by-4½-inch loaf pan and place a piece of parchment paper on the bottom.

2. Press the zucchini between 2 paper towels, squeezing lightly to release excess moisture.

3. Place the dry ingredients in a small bowl.

4. Place the eggs, honey, and banana in the bowl of a stand mixer and beat on medium for 1 minute, until frothy and fully combined. Add the zucchini and beat again to incorporate, about 15 seconds.

5. With the mixer running, slowly add the dry ingredients until they have all been incorporated.

6. Spoon the batter into the prepared pan or a 12-cup muffin pan lined with paper cups, filling each cup ⅔ full.

7. Bake the loaf for 40 minutes, until the middle is set and a toothpick inserted into the center comes out clean. Bake muffins for 30 to 35 minutes.

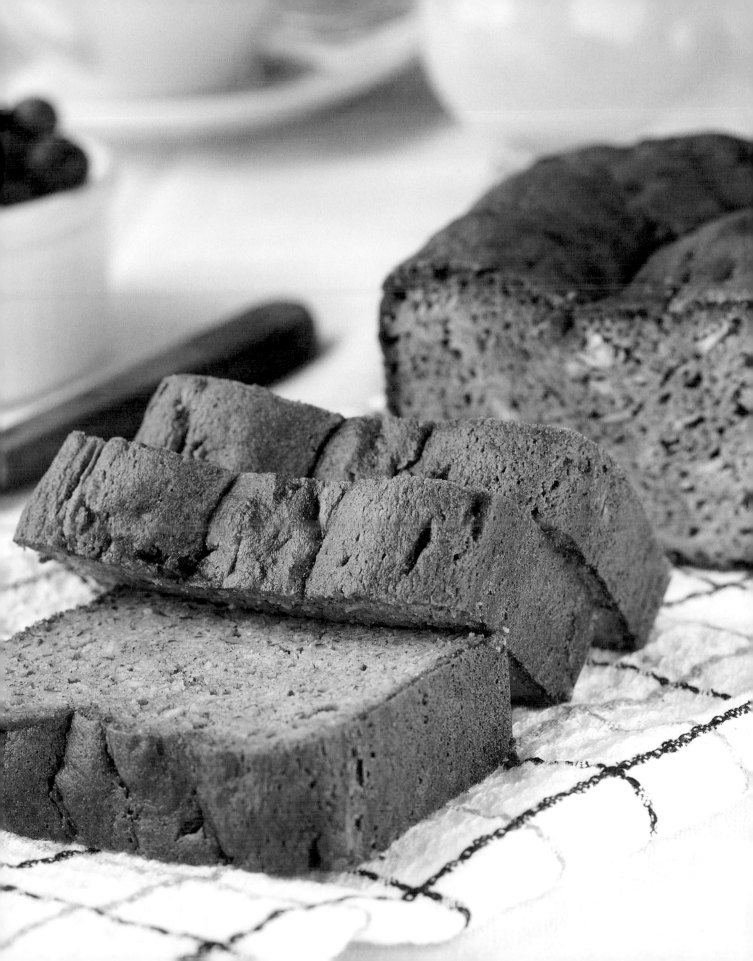

sun-dried tomato rosemary scones

prep time: 15 minutes   cooking time: 18 minutes   yield: 8 scones

muffins, loaves, and morning cakes

A savory bread to serve alongside salads or pasta, this scone can also double as sandwich bread or be crumbled into soups and stews.

ingredients

- 1¾ cups blanched almond flour
- 3 tablespoons coconut flour
- ½ teaspoon baking soda
- ½ teaspoon sea salt
- 2 tablespoons extra-virgin olive oil
- 1 teaspoon apple cider vinegar
- 2 tablespoons coconut milk
- 1 egg
- ¼ cup chopped sun-dried tomatoes
- 1 tablespoon chopped fresh rosemary

method

1. Preheat the oven to 350°F.

2. Place the flours, baking soda, salt, oil, vinegar, coconut milk, and egg in a food processor. Process until a ball of dough forms, about 30 seconds.

3. Add the sun-dried tomatoes and rosemary and pulse 3 or 4 times to incorporate.

4. Gather the dough into a ball and form into a circle on a piece of parchment paper. Use a sharp knife to cut 8 triangles. Separate the triangles and place on a parchment-lined baking sheet. Bake for 18 minutes, turning tray once midway through. Serve warm or store tightly wrapped for later use.

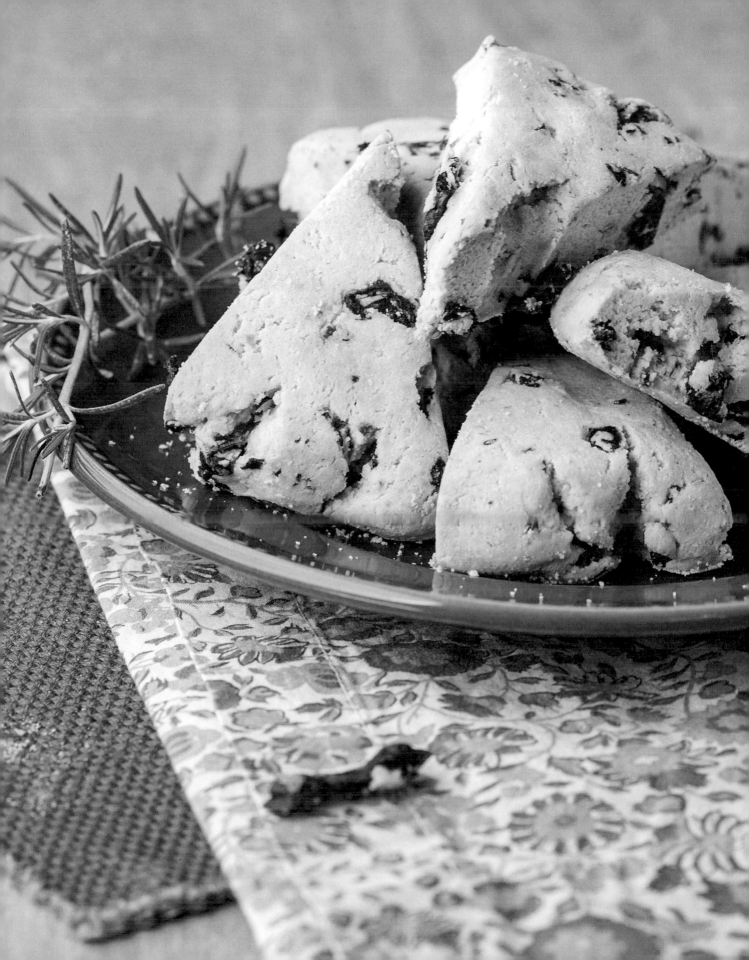

rosemary breadsticks

prep time: 15 minutes   cooking time: 12 minutes   yield: 10 breadsticks

Our family loves these breadsticks because they are soft and chewy with a hint of woody rosemary and garlic. Asher thinks they're fun because they are tall and skinny, and he especially loves to dip them in his leftover spaghetti sauce.

ingredients

- 1¼ cups blanched almond flour
- 1 egg
- 2 teaspoons extra-virgin olive oil
- 1 teaspoon honey
- 1 teaspoon chopped fresh rosemary
- ¼ teaspoon sea salt
- ¼ teaspoon garlic salt
- ¼ teaspoon baking soda

method

1. Preheat the oven to 350°F.

2. Place all the ingredients in the bowl of a stand mixer and mix on medium until a ball of dough forms. Divide the dough into 10 equal parts and roll them into golf-ball-sized pieces.

3. Roll each piece of dough out into a pencil shape with fingertips, about 12 inches long. If the dough begins to crack, wet fingertips slightly and continue rolling. Place the breadsticks on a baking sheet lined with parchment paper, spacing evenly.

4. Bake for 12 minutes, turning over halfway through.

tidbits:

For an even deeper flavored breadstick, brush with melted ghee and sprinkle with garlic salt before baking.

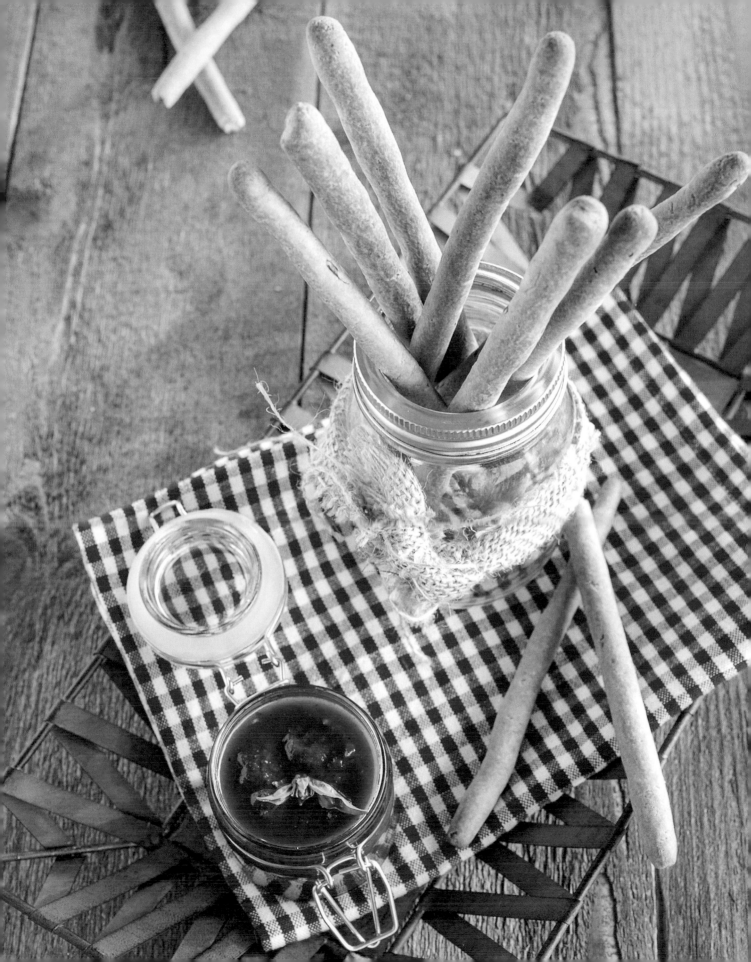

hamburger buns

prep time: 15 minutes   baking time: 25 minutes   yield: 4 buns

Lettuce-wrapped burgers and other sandwiches are wonderful when you want a lighter meal, but there are just certain times when you want to be able to pick up your sandwich and feel the heft of it.

ingredients

- 1½ cup raw cashews
- 3 eggs
- ¾ teaspoon apple cider vinegar
- ¼ cup unsweetened almond milk
- ¼ cup palm shortening or ghee, softened
- ⅓ cup coconut flour
- ⅓ cup blanched almond flour
- 1 teaspoon sea salt
- 1 teaspoon baking soda
- 1 egg yolk
- 2 teaspoons coconut milk
- 1 teaspoon sesame seeds

method

1. Preheat the oven to 325°F.

2. Place the cashews in a food processor and process for 10 seconds, until ground into coarse flour.

3. Add the eggs, vinegar, milk, and shortening. Process until very smooth, about 30 seconds.

4. Add the flours, salt, and baking soda. Process again until a smooth and sticky dough has formed.

5. Using wet hands, shape the dough into 4 buns. Rewet hands as needed to keep the dough from sticking and to achieve a smooth surface.

6. Place the egg yolk and coconut milk in a small bowl and whisk. Brush the dough tops with the egg wash and sprinkle with sesame seeds.

7. Place the buns on a baking sheet lined with parchment paper, place in the oven, and bake for 25 minutes.

tidbits:

As with all grain- and starch-free breads, these will crumble a bit more than their gluten counterparts but still do the trick! These are best eaten within a day, but can be frozen and toasted for later use.

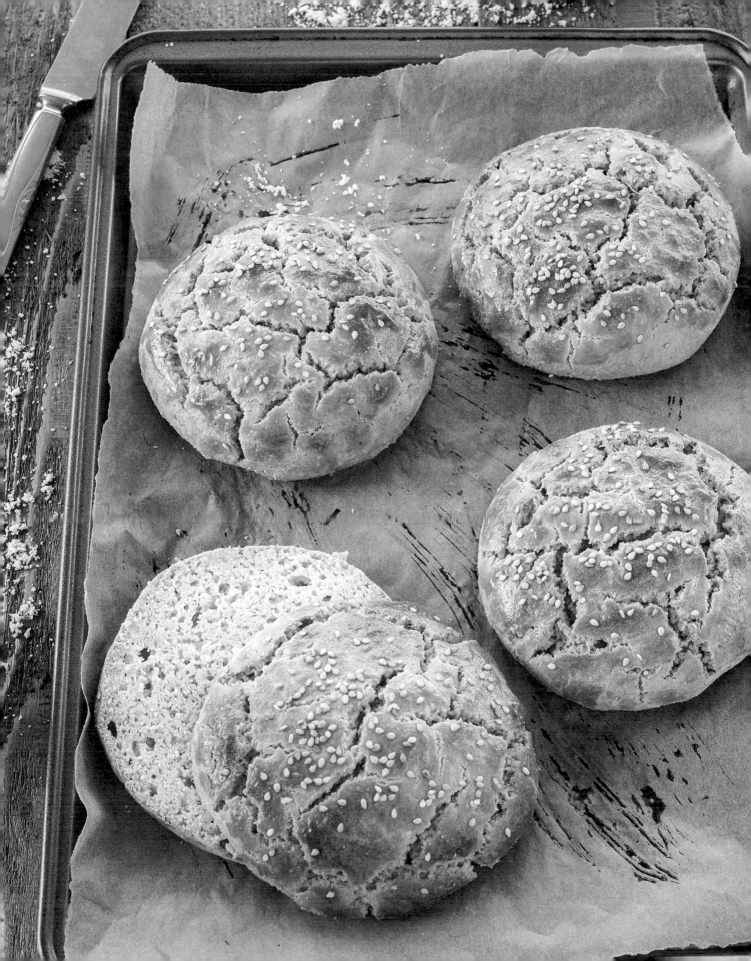

peach streusel coffee cake

prep time: 20 minutes   cooking time: 55 minutes   yield: 8 servings

Coffee cakes always remind me of my grandma. She would order one from the bakery and proudly bring it to every holiday gathering. I'm sure she would have loved my homemade rendition of the cakes she was so fond of. Infused with cinnamon, vanilla, cardamom, and ginger and topped with a coconut–pecan streusel, this coffee cake melts in your mouth.

ingredients

STREUSEL

- ⅓ cup raw pecan halves
- 1 tablespoon shredded, unsweetened coconut
- 1 tablespoon cold coconut oil
- 1 tablespoon blanched almond flour
- 1 tablespoon coconut crystals or honey
- ¾ teaspoon cinnamon
- 1 large date, pitted
- Pinch sea salt

CAKE

- ¼ cup coconut oil, melted, plus more for greasing the pan
- 3 large yellow peaches
- 4 large eggs at room temperature
- ½ cup honey
- 1 teaspoon pure vanilla extract
- 2¼ cups blanched almond flour
- 1 teaspoon baking soda
- ¾ teaspoon cardamom
- ½ teaspoon ground ginger
- ¼ teaspoon cinnamon
- Pinch sea salt

method

1. Make the streusel. Place all the streusel ingredients in a small food processor. Process until finely chopped and sticky, about 30 seconds. Set aside.

2. Make the cake. Preheat the oven to 325°F. Lightly grease a 9-inch-round springform pan or 9-inch cake pan with coconut oil.

3. Peel the peaches. Thinly slice 2 peaches and set on a paper towel to absorb excess moisture. Dice the third peach and set aside.

4. Place the eggs, honey, coconut oil, and vanilla in a high-speed blender and blend for 30 seconds, until frothy and smooth.

5. Add the almond flour, baking soda, cardamom, ginger, cinnamon, and salt. Blend on low for 30 seconds. Use a spatula to scrape the sides of the container. Blend again for 30 seconds on high.

6. Gently mix in the reserved diced peaches by hand. Spoon the batter into the prepared pan. Arrange the peach slices in a circular pattern on top, slightly overlapping each slice. Sprinkle the streusel over the entire top of the cake.

7. Bake for 55 minutes, until a toothpick inserted into the middle comes out clean.

8. Let cake cool for 10 minutes. Remove the sides of the springform pan and let cool completely on a wire rack.

tidbits:

If using a cake pan, reduce the oven temperature to 315° and serve directly from the pan.

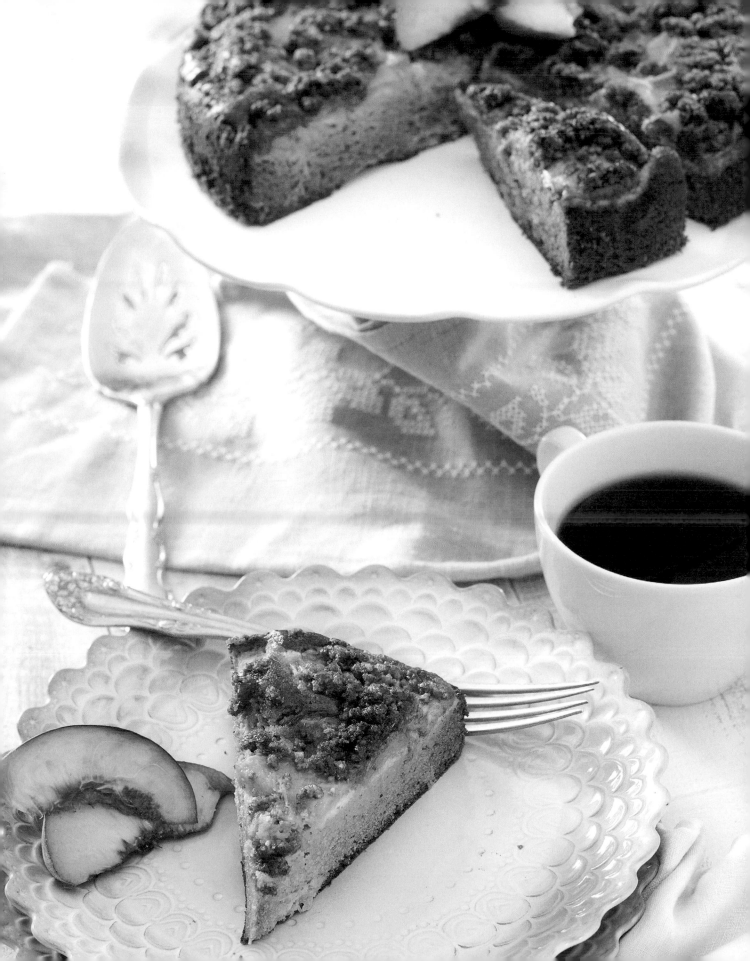

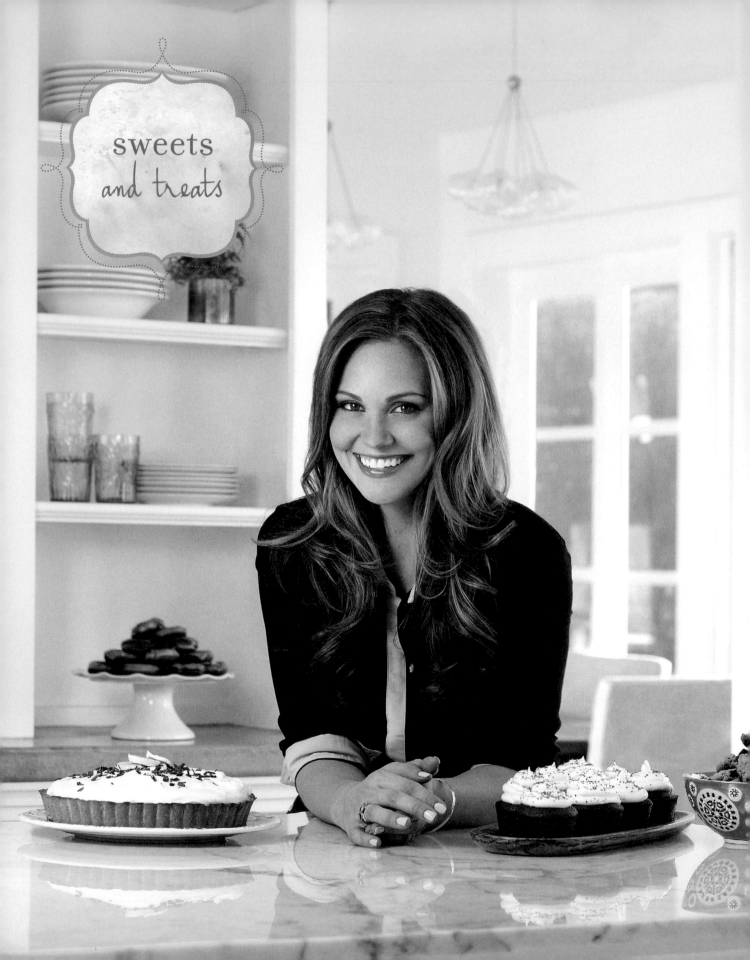

sweets
and treats

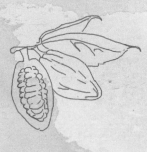

chocolate layer cake

prep time: 40 minutes   cooking time: 30 minutes   yield: 8 to 10 servings

A layer cake is a labor of love, but the end result is always worth the effort. A birthday comes only once a year, and everyone deserves a decadent delight on his or her special day. This four-tiered confection is layered with a vanilla frosting and encased in a dark chocolate buttercream frosting.

ingredients

- 6 eggs at room temperature
- ½ cup honey
- ¼ cup coconut oil, melted, plus more for greasing the pans
- ¼ cup coconut milk
- 1½ teaspoons pure vanilla extract
- ¾ cup blanched almond flour
- ⅓ cup coconut flour
- ⅓ cup cocoa powder
- 1 teaspoon baking soda
- ½ teaspoon sea salt
- ¼ cup dairy-free chocolate chips
- 1 recipe Vanilla Frosting (page 298)
- 1 recipe Chocolate Swiss Meringue Buttercream (page 296)

method

1. Preheat the oven to 325°F.

2. Place the eggs, honey, oil, coconut milk, and vanilla in a food processor and process until fully combined.

3. Sift the flours, cocoa powder, baking soda, and salt into a bowl, then add to the wet ingredients. Process again until smooth, about 30 seconds. Let the batter rest for 10 minutes. Stir in the chocolate chips.

4. Grease 2 6-inch cake pans. Cut 2 circles of parchment paper and fit them to the bottoms of the pans.

5. Evenly divide the batter between the two pans, lightly smoothing the tops with a spatula. Bake, rotating the pans halfway through, until a cake tester inserted in the centers comes out clean, 28 to 30 minutes. Transfer the pans to a wire rack for 20 minutes to cool. Invert the cakes onto the rack, releasing them from the pans; peel off the parchment. Cool the cakes right-side-up until room temperature.

6. Assemble the cake. Slice each cake in half horizontally. Set aside the best-looking dome for the top of the cake. Use the other dome for the bottom layer of the cake and place it dome side down on a cake stand or plate. Top with ¼ cup of Vanilla Frosting, spreading evenly. Place the second cake layer on top and spread with another ¼ cup of frosting. Repeat with the third layer; top with the final dome.

7. Spread the Chocolate Swiss Meringue over the entire cake, swirling with a knife to create a decorative finish or piping with a pastry bag. Serve immediately, or cover and refrigerate. If chilled, let sit at room temperature for about 20 minutes before serving.

tidbits:

- *The cakes can be baked up to 3 days in advance. Store tightly wrapped in the refrigerator. Frost up to 1 day in advance for the best quality and to prevent the cake from getting too moist.*

- *Bake as cupcakes for 20 minutes.*

- *Use 1 8-inch cake pan and bake for 35 to 40 minutes.*

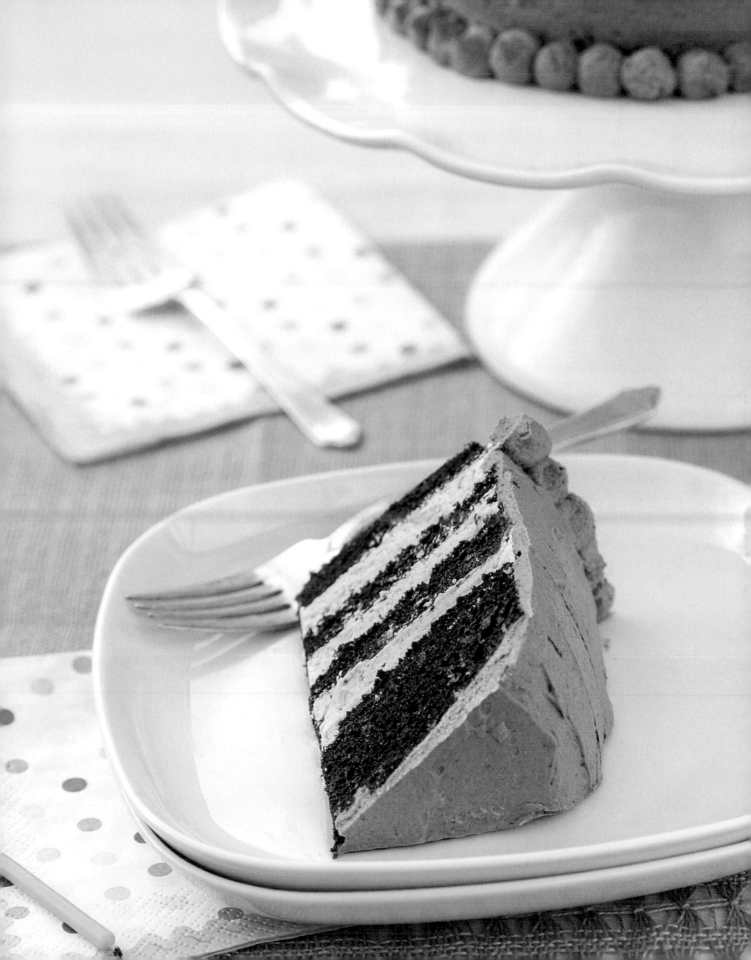

snickerdoodle cupcakes

prep time: 15 minutes   cooking time: 18 minutes   yield: 8 cupcakes

Every body is unique, but it is thankfully fairly uncommon for people with nut allergies to experience symptoms from consuming coconut products. Playing off the intense cinnamon flavor of snickerdoodles, these tree nut–free cupcakes are made with coconut flour, speckled with cinnamon, and topped with a marshmallow–like frosting.

ingredients

- 4 eggs at room temperature
- ½ cup honey
- 1 tablespoon coconut milk at room temperature
- 3 tablespoons melted raw cacao butter
- 2 teaspoons pure vanilla extract
- ½ cup coconut flour, sifted
- 1½ teaspoons cinnamon, plus more for dusting
- ½ teaspoon baking soda
- ¼ teaspoon sea salt
- 1 recipe Italian Meringue Frosting (page 294)

method

1. Preheat the oven to 350°F. Line a 12-cup muffin pan with baking cups.

2. Place the wet ingredients in the bowl of a stand mixer and beat on medium until frothy and fully incorporated.

3. Add the dry ingredients, beating until combined.

4. Spoon the batter into the prepared muffin pan, filling each cup ⅔ full.

5. Bake for 18 minutes. Cool completely on a wire rack before frosting.

6. Pipe or spread frosting on cupcakes, then dust with cinnamon.

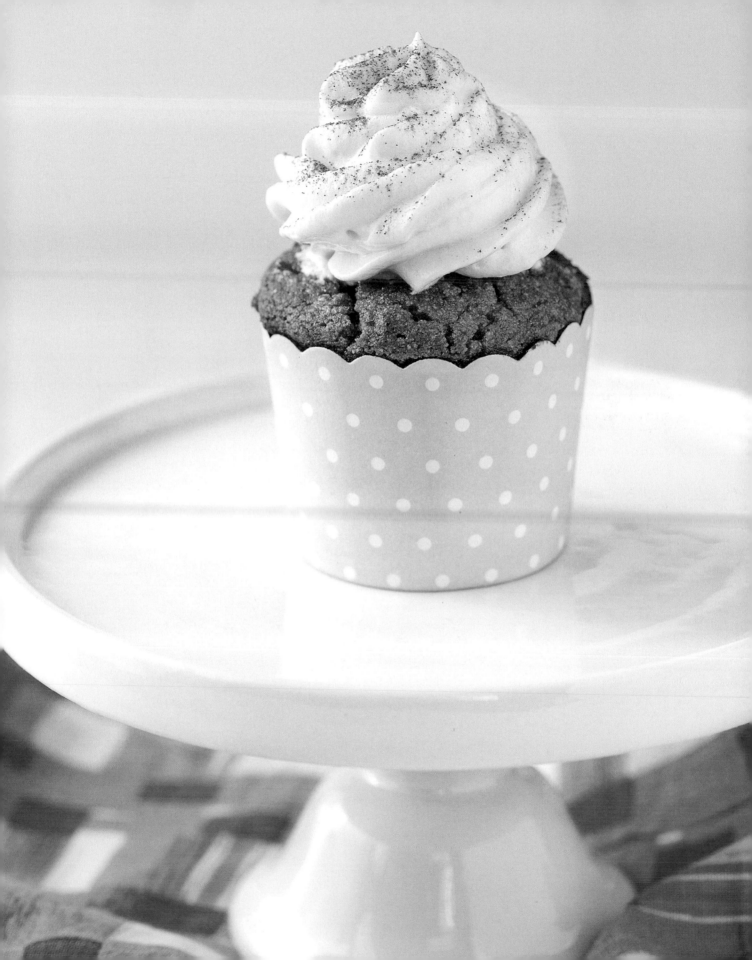

strawberry cake
with lemon cream filling

prep time: 30 minutes   cooking time: 30 minutes   yield: 8 servings

A little taste of spring, this cake is filled with lemon creaminess and gets a dose of fresh strawberries both inside and out. Make sure to chill a can of coconut milk and make the lemon curd 24 hours before making the cake!

ingredients

CAKE

- ⅔ cup melted coconut oil, plus more for greasing the pans
- 5 cups blanched almond flour
- 8 eggs at room temperature
- 1⅓ cups honey
- 1 tablespoon lemon juice
- 1 tablespoon pure vanilla extract
- 1½ teaspoons baking soda
- ½ teaspoon sea salt
- 1 cup chopped strawberries

FROSTING

- 2 13.5-ounce cans full-fat coconut milk, refrigerated for 24 hours
- ¾ cup Lemon Curd (page 286)
- 10-12 strawberries, hulled and halved

method

1. Make the cake. Preheat the oven to 325°F. Lightly grease 2 9-inch cake pans. Cut 2 circles of parchment paper and fit them to the bottoms of the pans.

2. Place the oil, flour, eggs, honey, lemon juice, and vanilla in a food processor. Process for 45 seconds, until smooth. If necessary, scrape down the sides and process again.

3. Add the baking soda, salt, and strawberries. Process for 15 seconds, to create a smooth batter.

4. Divide the batter evenly between the prepared pans, place in the oven on the center rack, and bake for 28 to 30 minutes, until a toothpick inserted into the center comes out clean.

5. Let cool on a wire rack for 20 minutes, then loosen the sides and invert onto the rack. Remove parchment paper. Cool completely right side up before frosting.

6. Meanwhile, make the frosting. Scoop off the cream from the top of each can of coconut milk. Place in a chilled bowl and beat on high with chilled beaters for 10 minutes, until thick and soft peaks form. Gently fold in the Lemon Curd. Place the frosting in the refrigerator while the cakes cool.

7. If both cakes have a domed top, use a sharp knife to slice off the dome of one of the cakes to create a flat surface for layering.

8. Spread half of the lemon cream on top, then place the other cake on top, dome side up.

9. Spread the remaining lemon cream on top of the cake. Surround the cake with sliced strawberries. Serve immediately or refrigerate.

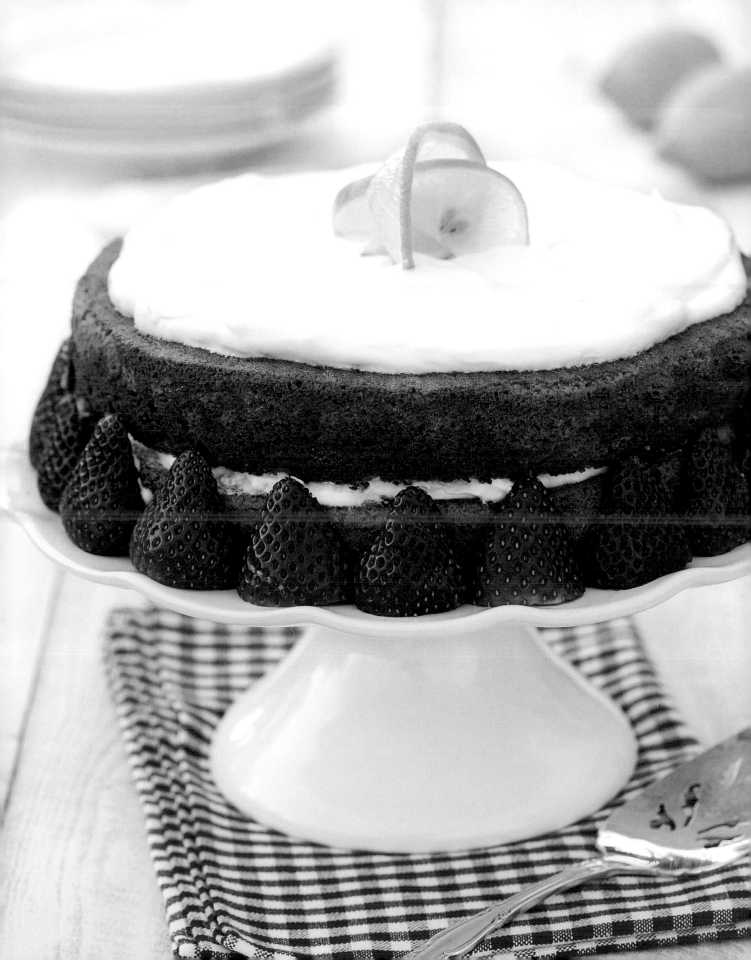

dark chocolate cake brownies

prep time: 15 minutes   cooking time: 35-40 minutes   yield: 10 to 12 servings

I frequently receive requests for a brownie recipe, and while brownies are one of my favorite desserts (especially hot with vanilla coconut milk ice cream!), I was never able to create one that rivaled the wheat-flour version. But I knew I had to master a brownie recipe for this book, and to satisfy all those requests, so here it is, roughly 20 tries later. These deep-chocolaty squares are perfect as solo indulgences, but feel free to turn them into the base of an ice cream sundae!

ingredients

- ½ cup palm shortening plus more for greasing the pan
- 3 ounces unsweetened chocolate
- 5 large eggs
- ¾ cup honey
- ⅓ cup coconut flour, sifted
- ¼ cup cocoa powder
- 1 teaspoon pure vanilla extract
- ¾ teaspoon baking soda
- Pinch of sea salt
- ¼ cup dairy-free chocolate chips

method

1. Preheat the oven to 325°F.

2. Lightly grease a 9-by-13-inch baking pan with palm shortening.

3. Place the shortening and chocolate in a small bowl over a pot of simmering water and whisk until melted and smooth. Be careful not to boil. Set aside.

4. Place the eggs and honey in the bowl of a stand mixer and beat on medium. Add the coconut flour, cocoa powder, vanilla, baking soda, and salt. Beat on low until incorporated, then on high until smooth.

5. Add the melted chocolate mixture and beat on medium until batter thickens, about 15 seconds. Stir in the chocolate chips by hand.

6. Pour the batter evenly into the prepared pan, smoothing the top with the back of a spoon.

7. Bake for 30 to 35 minutes, until a toothpick inserted into the center comes out clean. Cool in pan for 10 minutes.

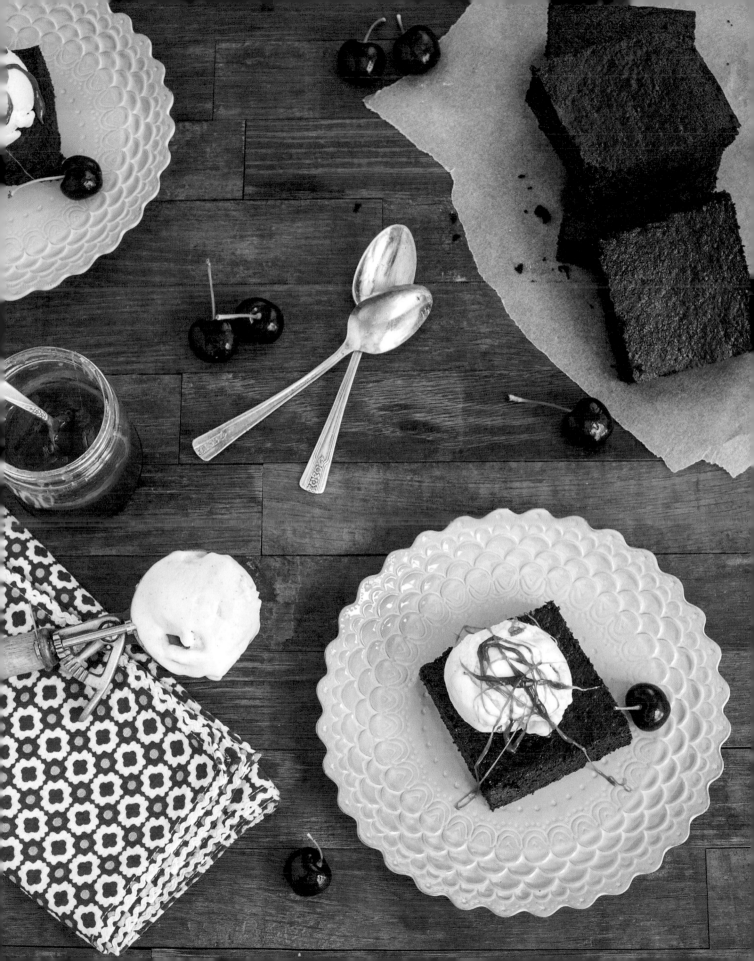

pumpkin donuts
(with maple-bacon glaze or chocolate frosting)

prep time: 25 minutes   *cooking time:* 20 minutes   *yield:* 1 dozen doughnuts

These cake doughnuts are reminiscent of the old-fashioned variety I used to love. Dense, satisfying, and rich; they also have two crunchy and sweet topping options—maple-bacon or dark chocolate. With each bite, you'll taste all the flavors of fall: pumpkin, cinnamon, nutmeg, ginger, cardamom, and clove.

ingredients

DOUGHNUTS

- Palm shortening for greasing the pan
- 5 large eggs
- ½ cup coconut milk
- ½ cup pumpkin puree (canned or fresh)
- ½ cup maple syrup*
- ¼ cup coconut oil, melted
- 1 teaspoon pure vanilla extract
- ¾ cup blanched almond flour
- ½ cup coconut flour
- 1 teaspoon baking soda
- 2 teaspoons pumpkin pie spice
- ¼ teaspoon sea salt

DARK CHOCOLATE FROSTING

- ¼ cup dark chocolate, chopped and melted
- 1½ teaspoons coconut oil, melted
- 1 teaspoon honey

MAPLE-BACON GLAZE (SCD)

- 1 tablespoon raw cacao butter, chopped
- 2 teaspoons palm shortening
- 2½ teaspoons cold maple syrup
- ½ teaspoon pure vanilla extract
- ¼ teaspoon cinnamon
- 1 strip bacon, fried crisp and finely chopped

method

1. Make the doughnuts. Preheat the oven to 350°F and grease 1 12-cavity doughnut pan or 2 6-cavity pans really well.

2. Place the eggs, coconut milk, pumpkin, maple syrup, oil, and vanilla in a blender or food processor and blend until frothy, about 15 seconds.

3. Add the dry ingredients and blend on low for 10 seconds, then on high for about 20 seconds.

4. Pour the batter into the pan, filling each cavity ⅔ full.

5. Bake for 20 minutes. Let cool for 10 minutes before gently removing the doughnuts from the pan. Cool completely on a cooling rack.

6. **To frost with chocolate frosting:** Place all the ingredients in a shallow bowl and whisk until smooth. Dip the top of each doughnut in the frosting, then gently rotate to let the excess drip off. Return to the cooling rack. Let set for 5 minutes, then refrigerate for 15 minutes, or until the glaze has hardened.

7. **To frost with maple-bacon glaze:** Place the cacao butter in the top of a double boiler over 1-inch of boiling water. Once it has completely melted, remove it from the heat and whisk in the palm shortening. Add the cold maple syrup, vanilla, and cinnamon and whisk until smooth. Dip each doughnut into the glaze, then gently rotate to allow the excess to drip off. Return to the cooling rack and sprinkle with bacon bits. Allow to sit at room temperature for 5 minutes, then place in the refrigerator for 15 to 20 minutes, or until the glaze has hardened.

*For SCD, use honey in place of the maple syrup.

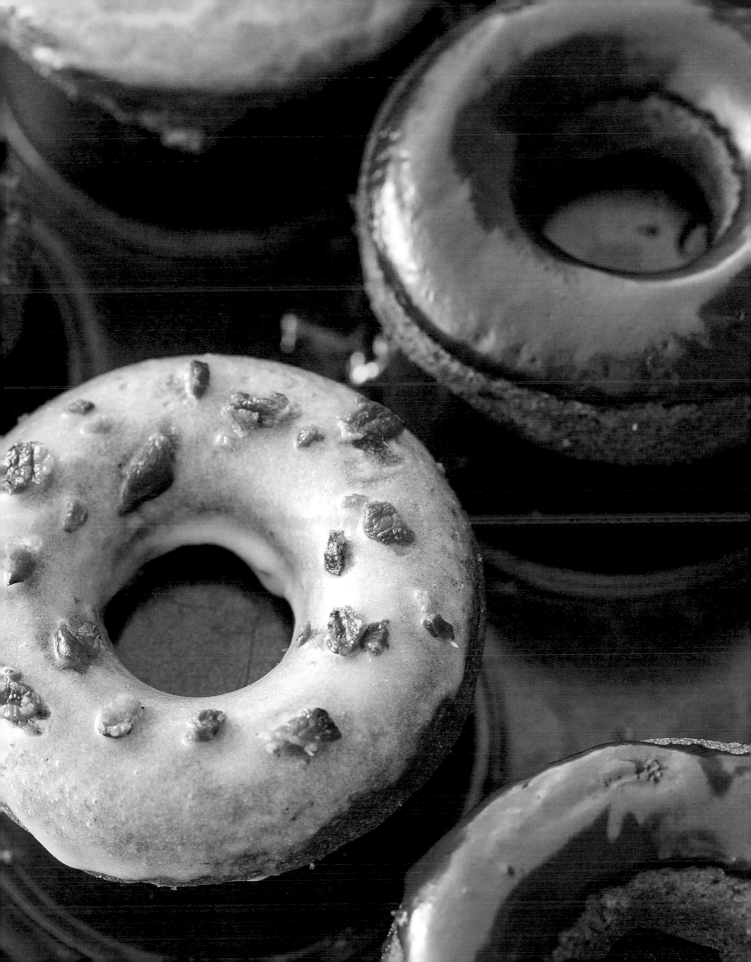

real-deal chocolate-chip cookies

prep time: 12 minutes   cooking time: 10 minutes   yield: 1 dozen

sweets and treats

An all-time favorite with my blog fans, these cookies have earned the reputation as the mother of all Paleo chocolate chip cookies and the closest you can get to the ones you grew up on. In fact, the reviews continue to insist that they far surpass those old cookies. Try them at your own risk: you will probably become addicted after the first bite and have to ban them from your kitchen as I have!

ingredients

- ¼ cup palm shortening
- 1 egg at room temperature
- ¼ cup coconut crystals
- 2 tablespoons honey
- 2 teaspoons pure vanilla extract
- 1½ cups blanched almond flour
- 2 tablespoons coconut flour
- ½ teaspoon baking soda
- ½ teaspoon sea salt
- ¼ cup dark-chocolate pieces
- ¼ cup dairy-free chocolate chips

method

1. Preheat the oven to 350°F.

2. Place the shortening and egg in a food processor and process for 15 seconds.

3. Add the coconut crystals, honey, and vanilla extract. Process again until combined.

4. Add the flours, baking soda, and salt and process for 30 seconds.

5. Scrape down the sides and pulse again if necessary to fully incorporate the dry ingredients.

6. Stir the chocolate in by hand.

7. Use a large tablespoon to scoop balls of the dough, placing them on a baking sheet lined with parchment paper. Lightly press them down to flatten, making disks about ½-inch thick.

8. Bake for 10 minutes, until the cookies are browned around the edges. Cool on a wire rack.

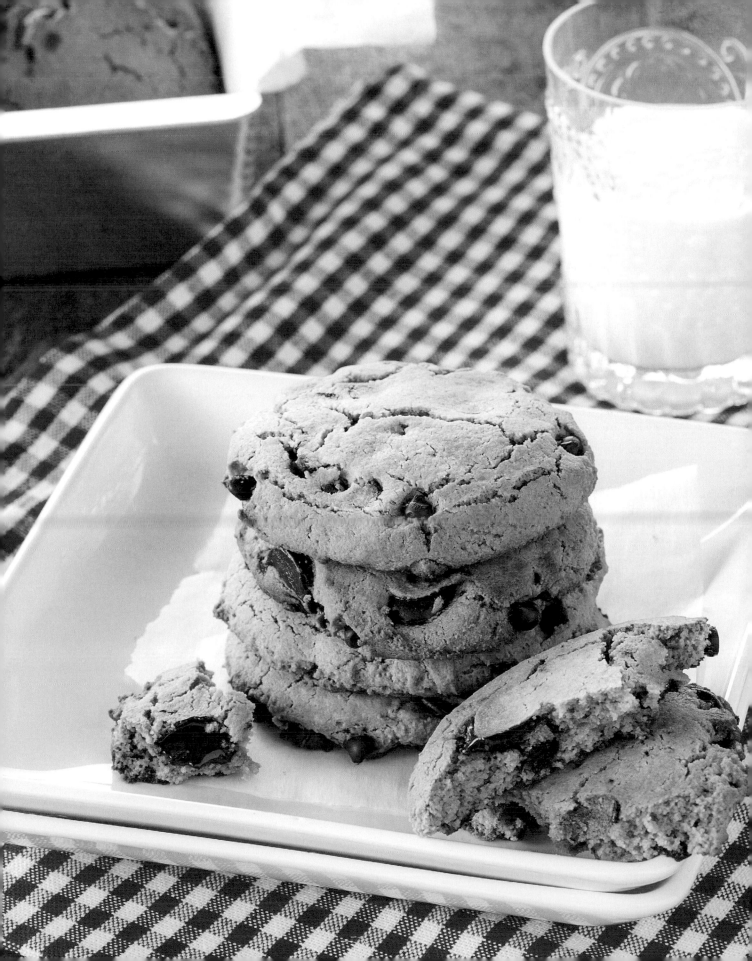

n'oatmeal raisin cookies

prep time: 15 minutes   cooking time: 12 minutes   yield: 1 dozen cookies

Chewy and moist, and with the texture of the oatmeal cookies you remember, but without the grain! You can dress these up by adding other dried fruits, chopped nuts, or chocolate chips.

ingredients

- ¼ cup palm shortening
- 1 large egg at room temperature
- ⅓ cup honey
- 1 teaspoon pure vanilla extract
- 4 teaspoons cinnamon
- ¾ teaspoons nutmeg
- 1 cup blanched almond flour
- 2 tablespoons coconut flour
- ½ teaspoon baking soda
- ½ teaspoon sea salt
- 2 teaspoons finely ground flaxseeds*
- ¾ cup finely shredded, unsweetened coconut
- ½ cup raisins

method

1. Preheat the oven to 350°F.

2. Place the shortening and egg in the bowl of a stand mixer and cream for 1 minute on high. Alternatively, use an electric hand mixer.

3. Add the honey and vanilla and mix for another minute, until creamy.

4. Place the cinnamon, nutmeg, flours, baking soda, salt, and flaxseeds in a small bowl and stir to combine.

5. Slowly add the dry ingredients to the wet and mix for another minute, until combined. Scrape down the sides of the bowl, then mix again for 30 seconds.

6. Add the coconut and raisins, then mix again for a minute.

7. Using an ice cream scoop or a large spoon, drop balls of dough the size of a golf ball onto a baking sheet lined with parchment paper.

8. Place another piece of parchment paper over the cookies, then use a spatula to gently press them down into circles about ¼-inch thick.

9. Bake for 12 minutes, until the edges are lightly browned.

*Omit for SCD.

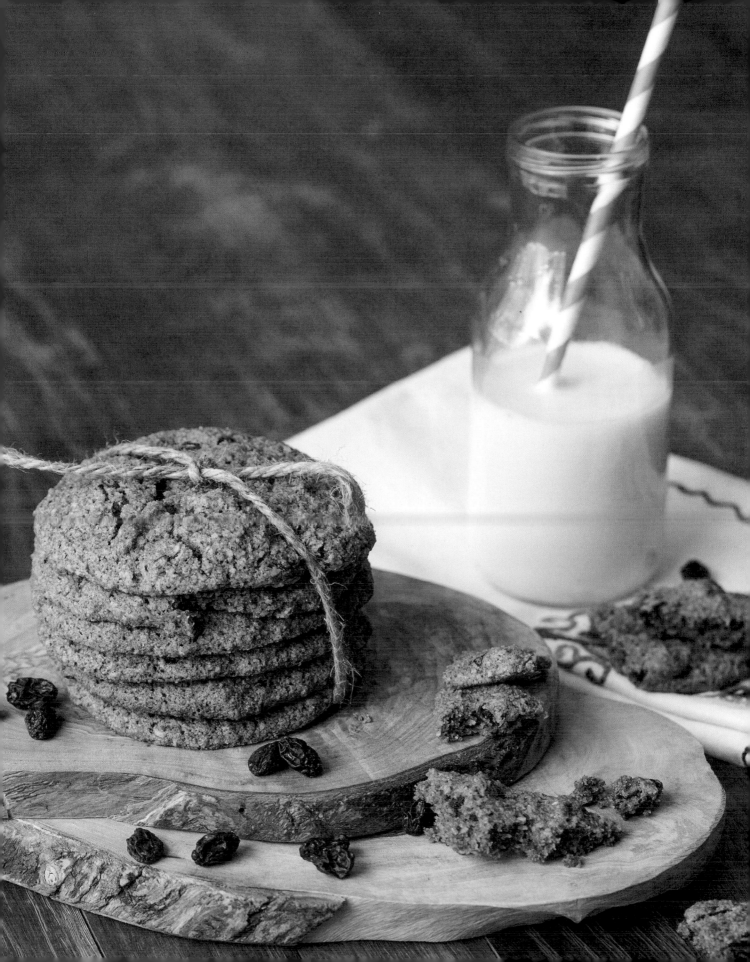

"peanut butter" cookies

prep time: 12 minutes   cooking time: 10 minutes   yield: 1 dozen

In this nut-free alternative to the classic peanut butter cookies, sunflower seed butter replaces the peanut butter, but I guarantee that you won't notice. Crisp on the outside and delightfully chewy on the inside, these cookies won't last long in allergy-free households!

ingredients

- ¼ cup palm shortening
- ¼ cup unsweetened sunflower seed butter
- 1 egg at room temperature
- ¼ cup honey
- 2 teaspoons pure vanilla extract
- ¾ teaspoon lemon juice
- ¼ cup coconut flour, sifted, plus more for flouring fork
- ¼ teaspoon baking soda

method

1. Preheat the oven to 350°F.

2. Place the shortening, sunflower seed butter, and egg in the bowl of a stand mixer fitted with the paddle attachment and cream for 1 minute on medium-high.

3. Add the honey, vanilla, and lemon juice. Mix on medium until combined.

4. Add the coconut flour and baking soda. Mix on medium for 30 seconds.

5. Scrape down the sides of the bowl and mix again for 30 seconds, until the dough has thickened.

6. Use a large spoon to drop balls of dough on a baking sheet lined with parchment paper. Dip a fork in coconut flour and lightly press the tines into the dough to flatten and make a grid pattern.

7. Place the cookies in the oven and bake for 10 minutes, until browned around the edges. Cool on a wire rack.

tidbits:

Be warned that certain brands of sunflower seed butter can turn baked goods a very bright shamrock green because of a harmless chemical reaction between small amounts of the chlorophyll in the seeds and the baking soda. The lemon juice is meant to neutralize the reaction, but do not be alarmed if you do end up with green cookies—they will still be delicious!

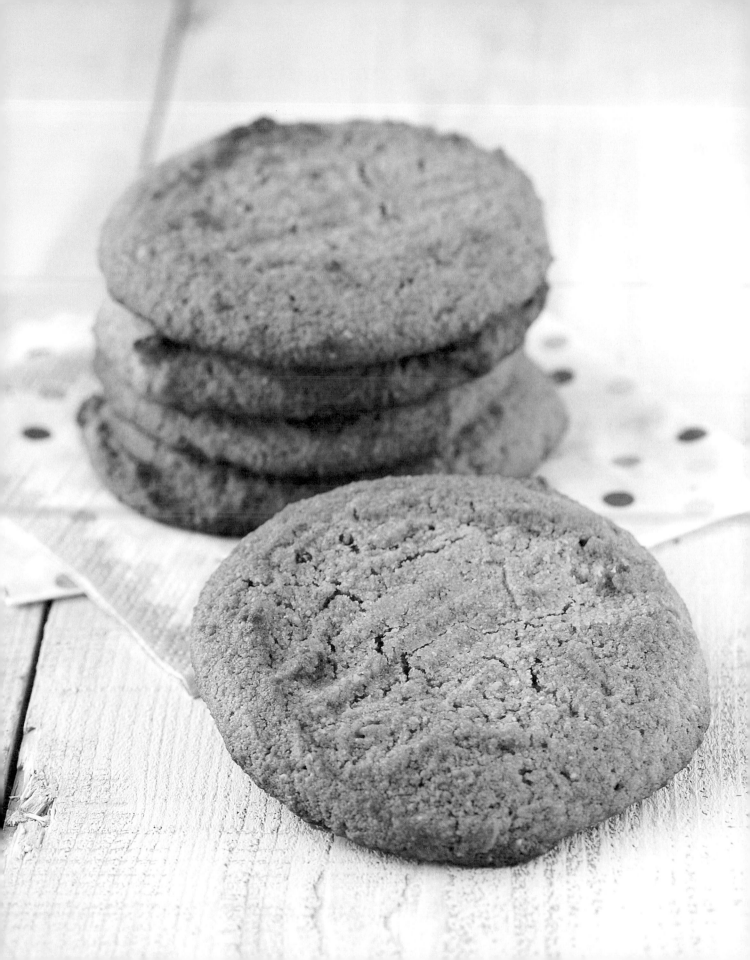

double-chocolate macaroons

prep time: 10 minutes   cooking time: 30 minutes   yield: 1 dozen

These rich, chocolat-y macaroons have a crisp outside and a chewy inside. They come together easily, and you probably already have the majority of the ingredients in your pantry.

ingredients

- 3 cups shredded, unsweetened coconut
- ½ cup unsweetened cocoa powder
- ½ cup honey
- ½ cup coconut milk
- ½ teaspoon cinnamon
- ¼ teaspoon pure vanilla extract
- 1 egg white
- Pinch sea salt
- ½ cup dark-chocolate chips, melted

method

1. Preheat the oven to 325°F.

2. Place the first 6 ingredients in a bowl and stir to combine.

3. Place the egg white in the bowl of a stand mixer, or use a hand mixer, and beat with a small pinch of salt for 1 to 2 minutes, until soft peaks form.

4. Fold the egg white into the coconut mixture by hand and mix gently until fully combined.

5. Using an ice cream scoop or tablespoon, scoop out balls of dough, packing them down tightly with your fingers.

6. Place the dough on a parchment-lined baking sheet, place in the oven, and bake for 30 minutes, rotating the tray halfway through. Cool on a wire cooling rack for 1 hour.

7. Dip the bottoms of the macaroons in the melted chocolate and set them on a rack lined with parchment paper. Allow cookies to set at room temperature for 1 hour or place in the refrigerator for 30 minutes.

tidbits:
I prefer Let's Do Organic brand shredded coconut for these cookies.

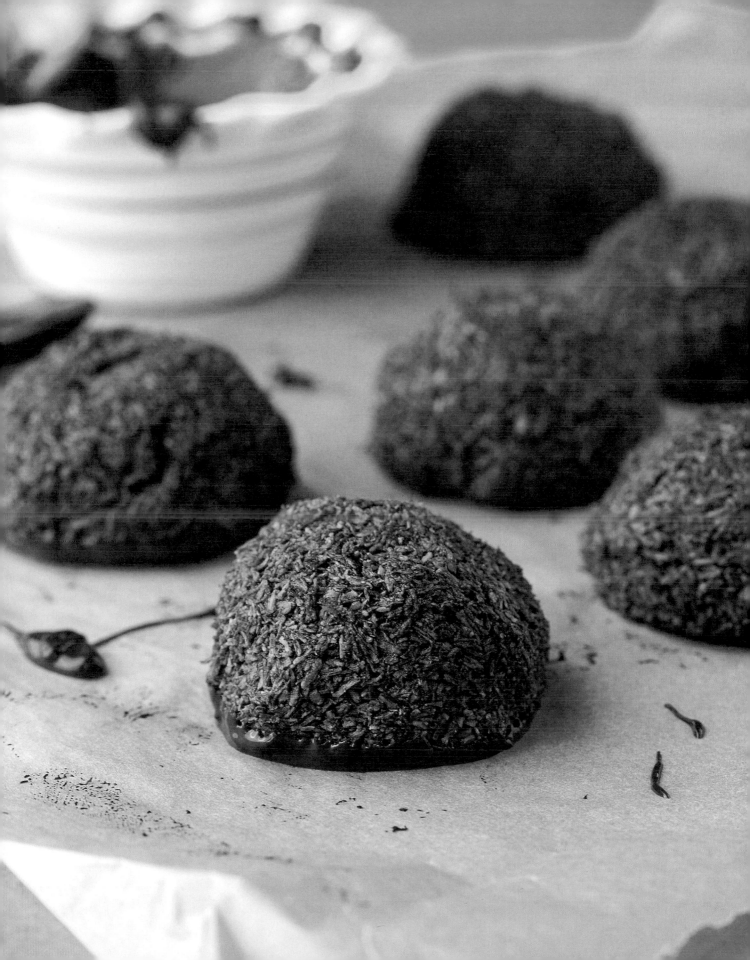

seven-layer bars

prep time: 1 hour   cooking time: 45 minutes

chilling time: 1 hour   yield: 1 dozen bars

These bars take a little work as every layer has to be prepared separately, but they are so worth the time and effort. An egg-free graham cookie crust is the base for a layer of rich chocolate ganache, followed by caramel sauce, then chopped walnuts, coconut cream, shredded coconut, and finally more chocolate.

ingredients

- 1 recipe for Caramel Sauce (page 290)

CRUST

- ⅓ cup plus 1 tablespoon coconut flour
- ¼ cup almond flour
- ¼ cup unsweetened applesauce
- 2 tablespoons coconut oil, softened
- 1 tablespoon honey
- ½ teaspoon pure vanilla extract
- ½ teaspoon apple cider vinegar
- ¼ teaspoon baking soda
- ¼ teaspoon cinnamon
- Pinch sea salt

GANACHE

- 3 ounces unsweetened chocolate
- 1 tablespoon coconut milk
- 3 tablespoons honey

COCONUT CREAM

- 3 tablespoons coconut butter
- 6 tablespoons coconut milk
- 2 tablespoons honey

TOPPINGS

- ½ cup chopped walnuts
- ¼ cup shredded, unsweetened coconut
- ¼ cup dairy-free chocolate chips

method

1. Make the caramel according to the instructions on page 290. Cool to room temperature.

2. Make the crust. Preheat the oven to 350°F. Place the crust ingredients in a bowl and mix until a dough forms. Press the dough into an 8-by-8-inch ovenproof dish. Bake for 10 minutes. Remove and cool on a wire rack for 15 minutes.

3. Make the ganache. Melt the chocolate slowly over a double broiler or in a bowl set over a pot of simmering water. Stir in the milk and honey. Spread the chocolate mixture over the crust.

4. Drizzle cooled caramel sauce over the chocolate layer.

5. Sprinkle chopped walnuts over the chocolate layer.

6. Make the coconut cream. Place the coconut cream ingredients in a small bowl, whisk, and then drizzle over the walnuts.

7. Sprinkle shredded coconut over the cream layer.

8. Finish with a layer of chocolate chips.

9. Place the bars in the oven and bake for 20 minutes. Cool on a wire rack for 15 minutes, then refrigerate for 1 hour to set. Cut into 12 even bars.

> tidbits:
> *Make the crust and caramel sauce the day before to save time. To make this confection nut-free, use the nut-free version of the Honey Graham Piecrust from page 270 as the base and omit the walnuts.*

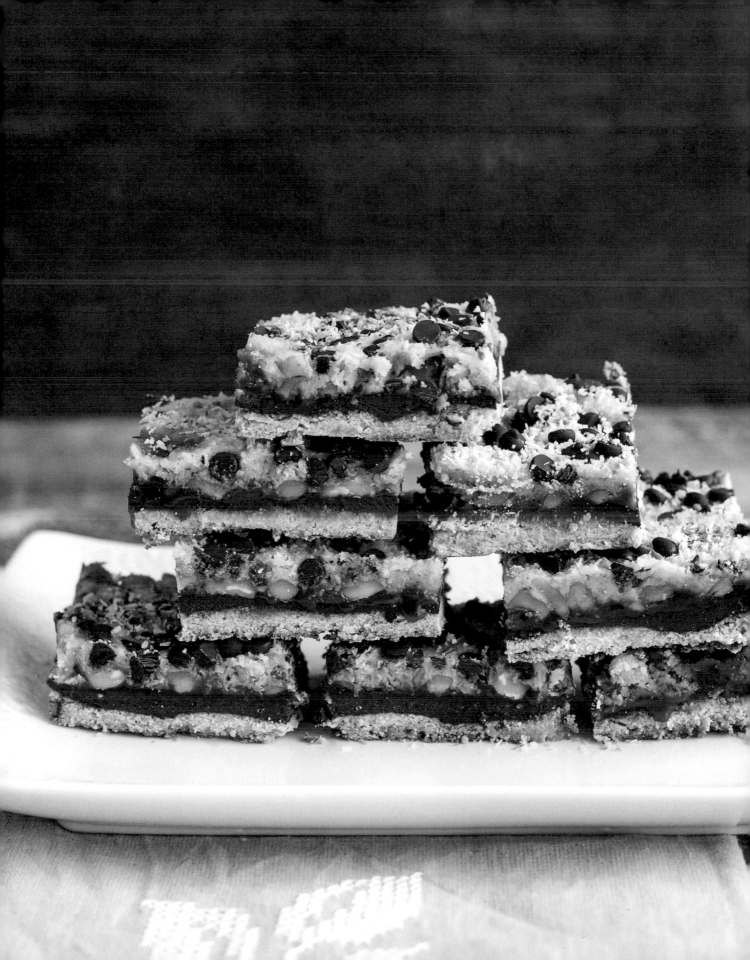

lemon vanilla bean macaroons

prep time: 20 minutes   cooking time: 20 to 25 minutes   yield: 1 dozen

Tangy lemon and fresh vanilla bean brighten up this version of a classic confection. Made with shredded coconut and coconut flour, these morsels are nut-free and a cinch to whip up. To make them sweeter, juice fresh Meyer lemons instead of conventional lemons.

ingredients

- ½ cup honey
- 3 cups shredded, unsweetened coconut
- ½ cup coconut milk
- ¼ cup fresh lemon juice
- 1 vanilla bean
- 1 egg white
- Pinch salt
- 3½ tablespoons coconut flour

method

1. Preheat the oven to 325°F.

2. Place the honey, coconut, coconut milk, and lemon juice in a bowl and mix. Slice the vanilla bean lengthwise and scrape out the seeds. Add them to the bowl and discard the pod or save for another use.

3. Place the egg white in the bowl of a stand mixer, or use a hand mixer, and beat with a small pinch of salt. Beat for 1 to 2 minutes, until soft peaks form.

4. Fold the beaten egg whites and coconut flour into the coconut mixture and mix gently until fully combined.

5. Using an ice cream scoop or tablespoon, scoop out balls of dough and pack them down by lightly knocking the scoop against the side of the bowl or using your fingers.

6. Place the cookies on a parchment-lined baking sheet, place in the oven, and bake for 20 to 25 minutes, until golden, rotating the tray halfway through.

7. Cool on a wire cooling rack for 1 hour before serving.

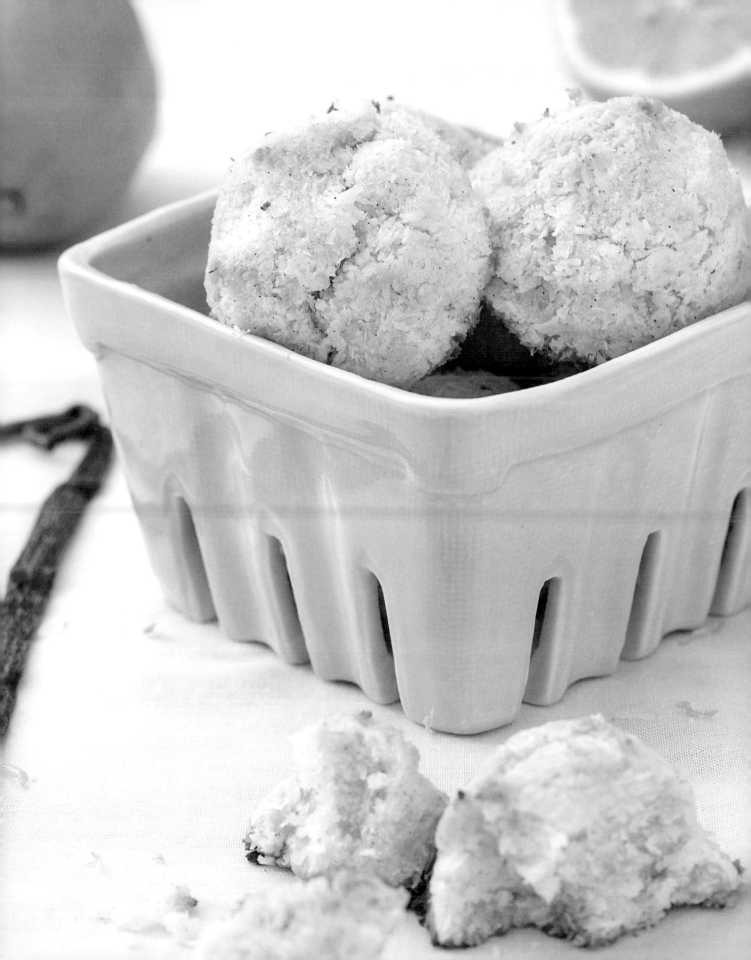

honey graham piecrust

prep time: 10 minutes   cooking time: 5-15 minutes   yield: 1 9-inch piecrust

This classic cookie crust is soft and chewy and will pair well with various sweet pie varieties.

ingredients

- ¼ cup blanched almond flour
- ½ cup plus 2 tablespoons coconut flour
- ¼ teaspoon sea salt
- ¼ teaspoon baking soda
- 1 teaspoon cinnamon
- ¼ cup coconut oil, softened
- ¼ cup honey
- 1 egg
- 1 teaspoon pure vanilla extract

NUT-FREE VERSION

- ½ cup coconut flour, sifted
- ¼ teaspoon sea salt
- ¼ teaspoon baking soda
- ½ teaspoon cinnamon
- ¼ cup coconut oil, softened
- ¼ cup honey
- 2 egg whites
- 1 teaspoon pure vanilla extract

method

1. Preheat the oven to 350°F.
2. Place the dry ingredients in a small bowl and mix.
3. Place the wet ingredients in the bowl of a stand mixer, or use a hand mixer, and beat to combine.
4. Add the dry ingredients to the wet and mix until combined.
5. Press the dough evenly into the bottom and up the sides of a 9-inch pie pan.
6. Cut a circle of parchment paper to fit over the bottom of the crust and fill with pie weights or dried beans.
7. Bake the crust for 15 minutes for pies that do not require additional baking. Cool completely, then add filling.
8. For pies that require a par-baked crust, bake the crust for 5 to 7 minutes, until it's a very light golden color. Place the crust in the freezer for 30 minutes, then add the filling and cover with a crust shield or foil to prevent the edges from burning. Return to the oven and bake according to the pie recipe instructions.

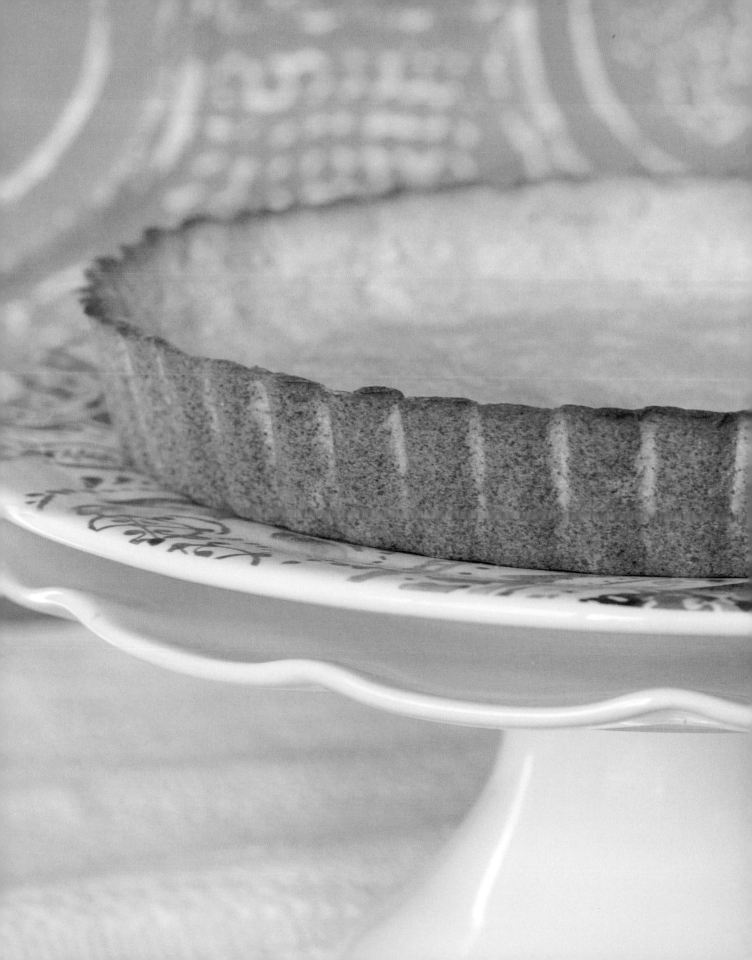

black-bottom banana cream pie

prep time: 30 minutes   cooking time: 8-15 minutes

chilling time: 6 hours   yield: 1 9-inch pie or tart

There are five layers to this scrumptious confection. Dairy-free fudge ganache smothers a graham cracker crust, followed by a layer of sliced bananas, then a velvety vanilla custard, which is topped with coconut whipped cream. There's no better combination than bananas and chocolate as far as I'm concerned. Except for maybe peanut butter and chocolate, but since legumes have been nixed from my diet, chocolate and bananas take the cake. Or the pie!

ingredients

- 1 recipe Honey Graham Piecrust (page 270), unbaked
- 2 large ripe bananas, sliced
- 1 cup Coconut Milk Whipped Cream (page 292)
- Dark chocolate shavings, optional

CUSTARD

- 4 teaspoons warm water
- 2½ teaspoons unflavored gelatin
- 2 cups coconut milk
- 5 large egg yolks
- ½ cup honey
- 1½ teaspoons pure vanilla extract

GANACHE

- 2 ounces unsweetened chocolate
- 2 tablespoons coconut milk
- 1 tablespoon coconut oil
- 3 tablespoons honey

tidbits:

To make this SCD-friendly, omit the ganache layer.

method

1. Preheat the oven to 350°F.

2. Bake the crust as directed on page 270, then cool on a wire rack before filling.

3. Meanwhile, make the custard. Pour the water into a small bowl and sprinkle the gelatin over it. Let it sit for 10 minutes to soften.

4. Place the coconut milk in a saucepan and bring to a simmer over medium-high heat.

5. Place the egg yolks and honey in a bowl, whisk to combine, then quickly add half of the hot coconut milk, whisking constantly to temper the eggs.

6. Pour the mixture into the saucepan. Stir over medium-high heat for 4 minutes, or until the mixture thickens enough to lightly coat the back of a spoon. Make sure it doesn't boil.

7. Add the gelatin mixture and whisk until fully dissolved, about 2 minutes.

8. Pour the custard into a glass bowl, then stir in the vanilla extract. Place in the refrigerator to chill.

9. Make the ganache. Gently melt all of the ingredients in a double boiler or a bowl set over a pot of simmering water. Spread on the bottom of the cooled piecrust. Let cool for 10 minutes.

10. Place a layer of sliced bananas over the chocolate in a circular pattern. Press the slices gently down into the ganache.

11. Pour the cooled custard over the bananas, spreading it evenly. Place the pie in the refrigerator to chill until set, about 6 hours.

12. Spread the whipped cream over the top and garnish with chocolate shavings if desired. Let sit at room temperature 15 minutes before serving.

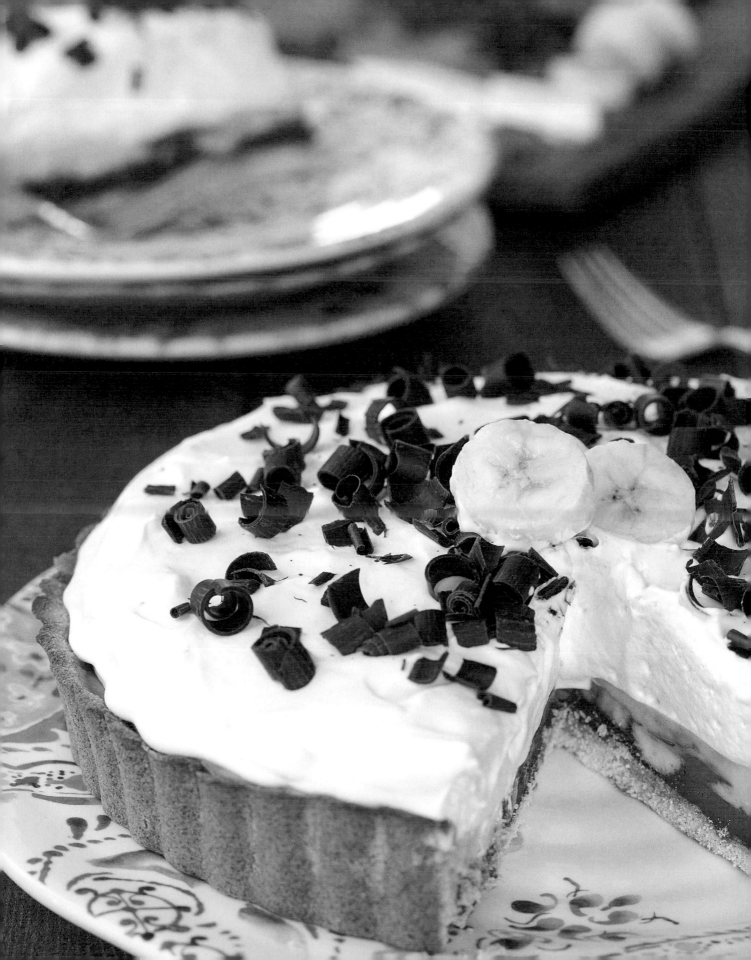

chocolate cream pie with chocolate-cookie crust

prep time: 30 minutes   *cooking time: 20 minutes*   *chilling time: 6 hours*   *yield: 1 9-inch pie*

This pie was one of the first desserts I created after going grain-free, but has been given a chocolate-cookie-crust upgrade for this book. I make this every year for the holidays, sometimes multiple times — it's my signature dessert offering for gatherings. I have never met anyone who didn't love it, so I know you will too. While a traditional cream or pudding pie uses cornstarch for thickening, this pie uses nutrient-rich gelatin.

ingredients

CRUST

- 2 cups blanched almond flour
- 2 tablespoons coconut flour
- ½ cup cocoa powder
- ½ teaspoon baking soda
- ¼ teaspoons sea salt
- ½ cup honey
- ¼ cup coconut oil
- 2 ounces unsweetened chocolate
- 2 teaspoons pure vanilla extract

FILLING

- 2 tablespoons water
- 2¾ teaspoons unflavored gelatin
- 2½ cups coconut milk
- 4 egg yolks
- ¾ cup grade B maple syrup
- ¼ teaspoon sea salt
- 4 ounces unsweetened chocolate, roughly chopped
- 1½ teaspoons pure vanilla extract
- 1 cup Coconut Milk Whipped Cream (page 292)
- Dark chocolate shavings, optional

tidbits:

This pie can be nut-free! Just use the nut-free Honey Graham Piecrust recipe on page 270.

method

1. Preheat the oven to 350°F.
2. Make the crust. Sift the dry ingredients into the bowl of a stand mixer or food processor.
3. Place the remaining ingredients in a saucepan set over low heat until melted.
4. Add the melted chocolate mixture to the dry ingredients. Beat in a stand mixer or food processor until fully combined.
5. Press the dough into a 9-inch pie pan, being sure to spread it evenly along the bottom and up the sides.
6. Bake for 12 minutes, then let cool.
7. Meanwhile, make the filling. Place the water in a small bowl and sprinkle the gelatin over it.
8. Place the coconut milk in a saucepan set over medium-high heat to warm.
9. Place the egg yolks, maple syrup, and salt in a mixing bowl and whisk to combine.
10. Temper the eggs by adding half of the heated milk into the bowl, whisking continuously.
11. Pour the mixture back into the saucepan and cook over medium heat for 6 minutes, stirring frequently. Do not let it boil or the yolks will curdle.
12. Whisk in the gelatin, then continue to cook for 2 minutes, whisking vigorously until the gelatin has dissolved entirely. The mixture should be thick enough to coat the back of a spoon.
13. Pour the custard through a mesh sieve into a bowl.
14. Add the chocolate pieces and vanilla, whisking until smooth.
15. Pour the custard into the cooled piecrust and cover with plastic wrap. Place in the refrigerator for 6 hours, until firm.
16. Let sit at room temperature for 20 minutes before serving. Top with whipped cream and sprinkle with chocolate shavings, if desired.

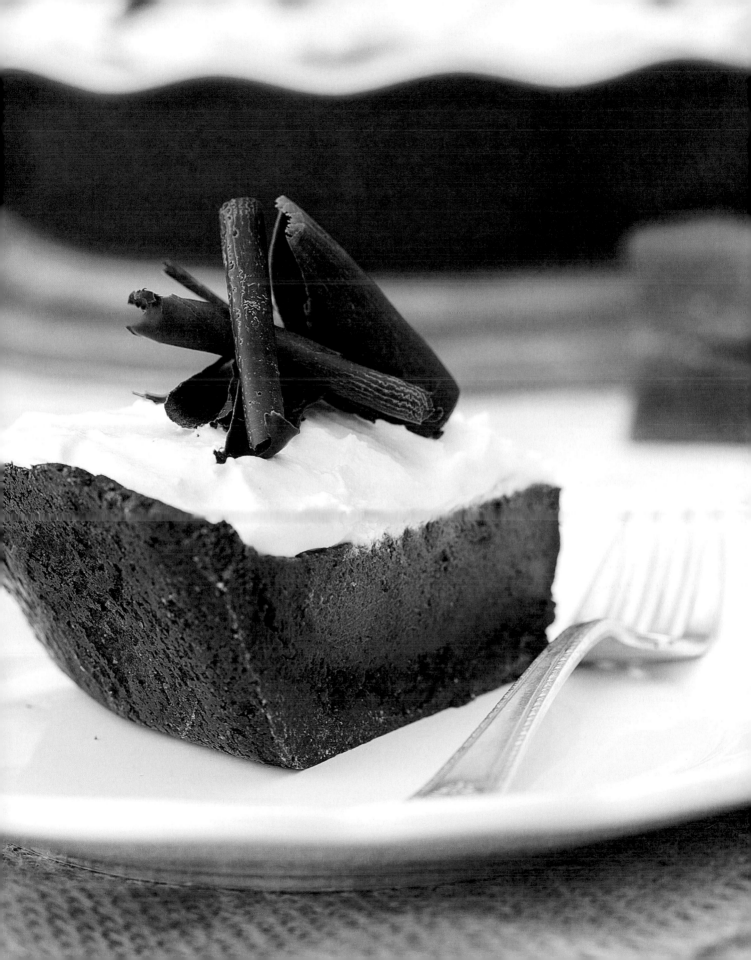

meyer lemon meringue pie

prep time: 45 minutes   cooking time: 20 minutes

chilling time: 6 hours   yield: 8 to 10 servings

I was never fond of lemon meringue pie growing up, but as it is a quintessential American dessert, I knew I had to include it in my first cookbook. I made sure to test it on all of my lemon-loving family and friends and even ordered a slice of conventional lemon meringue pie at a restaurant for the sake of research—oh, what I won't do for my readers! The survey results: This recipe is as good as, if not better than, the original and even I devoured it! Enjoy!

ingredients

FILING

- 1 Pastry Crust (page 310), baked and cooled
- ½ cup water plus 3 tablespoons at room temperature
- 2¾ teaspoons unflavored gelatin
- 1 cup fresh Meyer lemon juice
- ¾ cup honey
- Zest of 1 lemon, finely grated
- 6 large egg yolks
- 4 tablespoons palm shortening or ghee
- ¼ cup coconut milk
- Pinch sea salt

MERINGUE

- ⅓ cup honey
- 3 egg whites
- ¼ teaspoon fresh lemon juice
- Pinch sea salt

tidbits:

- *Regular lemon juice may be substituted.*
- *For a nut-free pie, use the nut-free Honey Graham Piecrust recipe on page 270.*
- *The crust and filling can be prepared up to 2 days ahead and refrigerated. Prepare the meringue right before serving.*

method

1. Place 3 tablespoons of the water in a bowl and sprinkle gelatin over it to soften.

2. Place the ½ cup water, lemon juice, honey, and lemon zest in a saucepan over medium heat for 5 minutes.

3. Place the egg yolks in a bowl and whisk. Temper the eggs by adding half of the heated mixture to the egg yolks, whisking continuously.

4. Pour the tempered egg yolks into the saucepan and cook while whisking frequently until the mixture has thickened, about 5 to 7 minutes. Remove from the heat and add the gelatin, whisking until dissolved. Add the shortening, coconut milk, and salt, whisking until fully combined.

5. Pour the lemon curd through a fine mesh sieve into a bowl and place in the refrigerator for 20 minutes to cool. Pour the cooled lemon curd into the piecrust and press a piece of plastic wrap directly onto the surface to prevent a skin from forming. Place the pie in the fridge to set for 6 hours.

6. Prepare the meringue. Place the honey in a small saucepan and bring to a boil. Place the egg whites in the bowl of a stand mixer and beat on medium until soft peaks form, about 3 to 4 minutes. With the mixer running, pour the boiling honey down the side of the bowl in a slow, steady stream. Add the lemon juice and salt and continue beating for 8 to 10 minutes, until the meringue has cooled and doubled in volume.

7. Spread the meringue over the chilled pie, ensuring that it touches the crust all the way around. Place the pie under the broiler for 30 seconds to toast the top of the meringue, watching closely to prevent burning. Serve at room temperature.

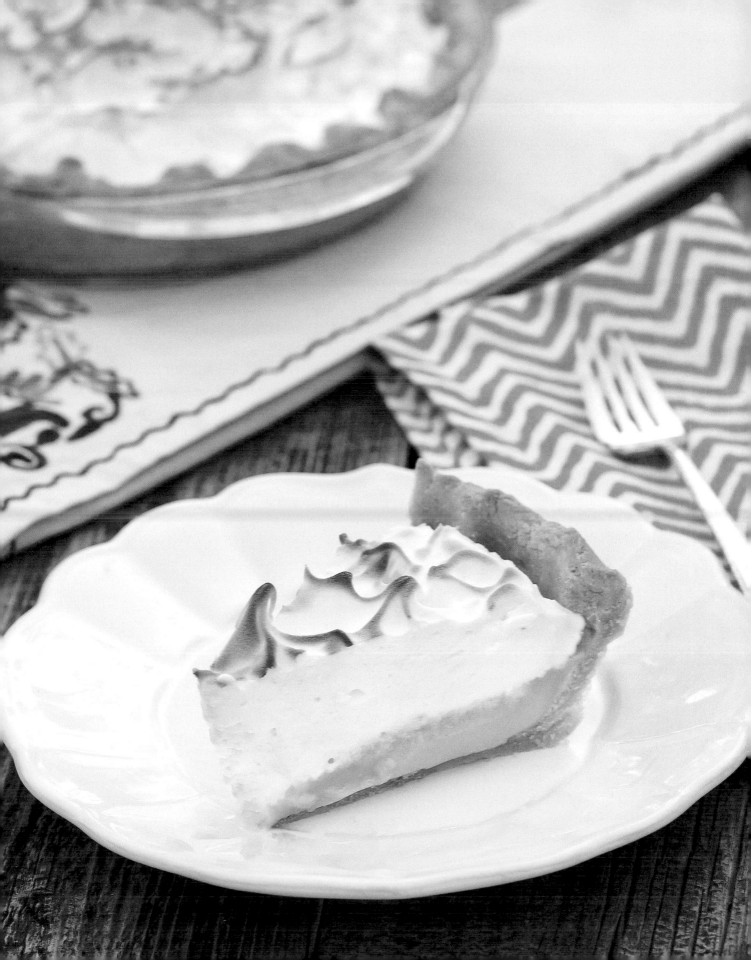

double-chocolate frozen yogurt with "peanut" butter fudge swirl

prep time: 20 minutes
cooking time: 12 minutes chilling time: 4 hours yield: 4 to 6 servings

Oh, ice cream. I love it and loathe it. Ice cream is where my self-control goes totally off-track, especially when it comes to this flavor combination. My trick is to make only half the recipe, so it's not hanging out in the freezer, sending me wicked vibes to eat just one more spoonful. The good news is that it's made with cultured yogurt, so at least you get your daily dose of gut-nourishing probiotics with each bite!

ingredients

FROZEN YOGURT

- 3 cups Coconut Milk Yogurt, divided (page 46)
- 1 cup coconut milk
- ¼ cup unsweetened cocoa powder
- ½ cup maple syrup
- ½ pound unsweetened chocolate, chopped
- 2 teaspoons coconut oil
- Pinch sea salt
- ½ teaspoon pure vanilla extract or bourbon

SWIRL

- 3 tablespoons sunflower seed butter, unsweetened
- 1 tablespoon coconut oil, melted
- 2 teaspoons maple syrup
- ¼ cup melted dark chocolate

method

1. Make the frozen yogurt. Place 2 cups of the yogurt and the coconut milk in a saucepan over medium-low heat for 5 to 7 minutes, whisking occasionally. Whisk in the cocoa powder, maple syrup, chocolate, salt, and oil. Continue heating for 5 more minutes, until the chocolate is melted and all the ingredients are incorporated. Do not allow the mixture to boil.

2. Remove from the heat and transfer to a glass bowl. Add the remaining yogurt and the vanilla and stir to combine. Press a piece of plastic wrap directly onto the mixture and place in the refrigerator for 2 hours, or until the mixture has cooled completely.

3. Meanwhile, prepare the swirl. Place the sunflower seed butter, oil, and maple syrup in a bowl and stir to combine.

4. Place the chilled yogurt mixture in an ice cream maker and process according to the manufacturer's instructions, until it reaches a soft-serve consistency.

5. Spoon ⅓ of the frozen yogurt into a container. Drizzle ½ of the sunflower seed butter over it, then drizzle ½ of the melted chocolate on top of the sunflower seed butter. Spread another ⅓ of the frozen yogurt on top of the chocolate and repeat with the remaining swirl ingredients. Top with the remaining frozen yogurt.

6. Place a sheet of plastic wrap directly on the surface of the frozen yogurt to prevent freezer burn. Cover and freeze until firm, at least 2 hours.

7. Allow the frozen yogurt to thaw at room temperature for 20 minutes before serving.

tidbits:

The gelatin in the homemade yogurt is what keeps this treat smooth and creamy after freezing.

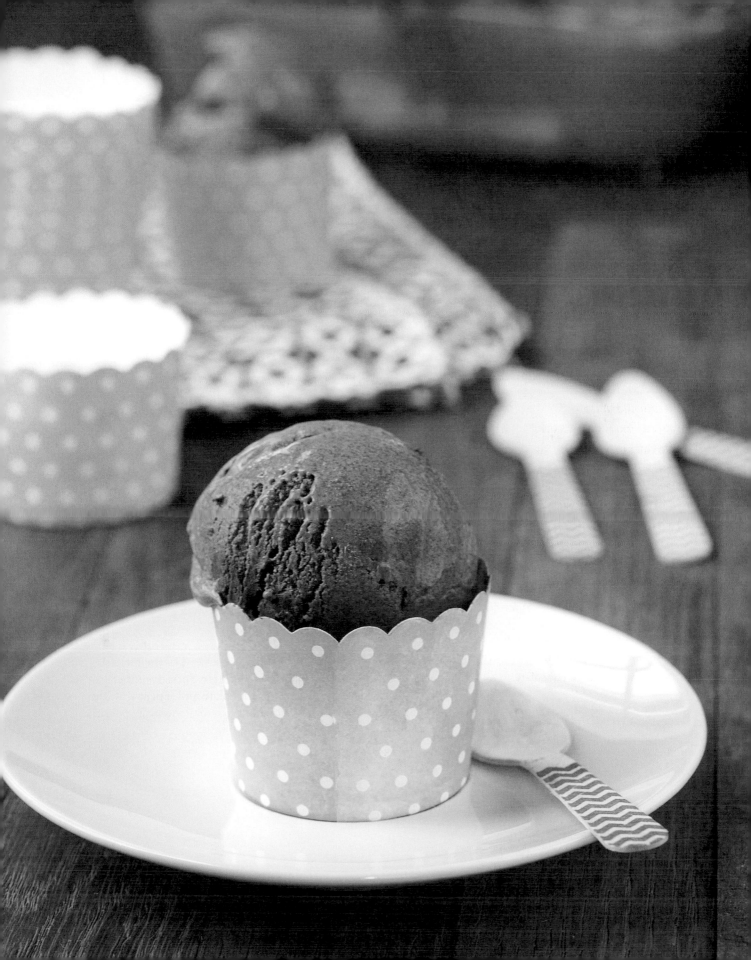

french vanilla ice cream

prep time: 15 minutes   cooking time: 15 minutes

chilling time: 6 hours   yield: 6 servings

This dairy-free rendition of a French vanilla ice cream, made with an egg-yolk custard and fresh vanilla beans, has an unbeatable sumptuous flavor and velvety consistency.

ingredients

- 2 13.5-ounce cans coconut milk
- ½ vanilla bean, split and seeds scraped from it
- ½ cup maple syrup or honey
- 4 egg yolks
- 1 teaspoon pure vanilla extract

method

1. Place the coconut milk, vanilla bean and its seeds, maple syrup, and egg yolks in a cold saucepan and whisk to combine the ingredients. Heat the mixture over medium-low heat, stirring constantly, until the mixture coats the back of a spoon, about 15 minutes. Be sure not to let it boil.

2. Transfer the mixture to a bowl and place in the refrigerator and chill for 30 minutes. Press a piece of plastic wrap directly on the liquid to prevent condensation. Continue chilling for 4 hours, until cold.

3. Remove the vanilla pod and mix in the vanilla extract. Pour the custard into an ice cream maker and process according to the manufacturer's instructions until the mixture has reached a soft-serve consistency.

4. Spoon the ice cream into an airtight container and press a piece of plastic wrap directly on top of the ice cream to prevent freezer burn. Place the lid to the container on top and freeze until firm, about 2 hours.

5. To serve, let sit at room temperature for 20 minutes until it is soft enough to scoop.

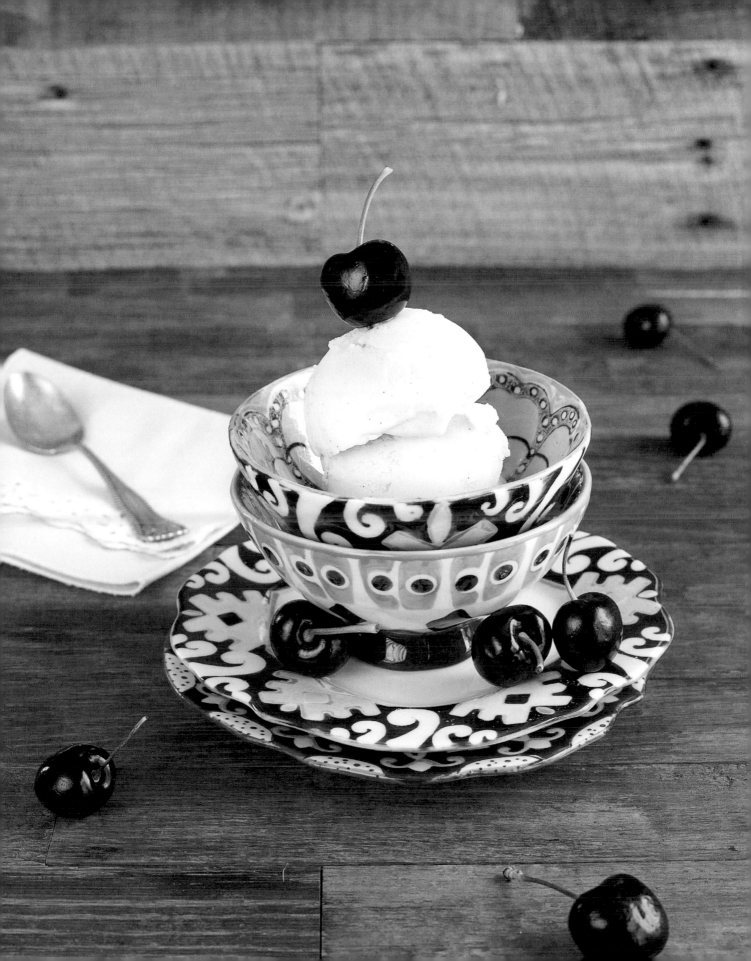

mint-chip ice cream

prep time: 15 minutes   cooking time: 5 minutes
chilling time: 6 hours   yield: 6 servings

My dad and I could easily polish off an entire container of mint-chip ice cream when I was growing up. It's still our favorite flavor so I created this dairy-free version so he and I could still enjoy a bowl together. Because this version has no eggs, it's suitable for those with egg allergies and also eliminates the extra step of making the custard that most ice cream recipes call for. Yet it's every bit as creamy and boasts a bold fresh mint flavor.

ingredients

- 1 13.5-ounce can coconut milk
- ½ cup fresh mint leaves, roughly chopped
- ½ cup honey
- 2 cups cold almond milk
- ¾ teaspoon peppermint extract
- ⅓ cup diced avocado
- 1 tablespoon melted coconut oil
- 10 drops liquid chlorophyll for coloring, optional
- ½ cup dark chocolate*, chopped

method

1. Place the coconut milk and mint leaves in a saucepan over medium-high heat for 10 minutes.

2. Place the warm coconut milk, mint, and honey in a bowl and mix until the honey has dissolved. Stir in the almond milk and peppermint extract. Cover and place in the refrigerator for 4 hours.

3. Pour the mixture into a blender and add the avocado, coconut oil, and coloring if desired. Blend until smooth.

4. Place in an ice cream maker and process according to the manufacturer's instructions until the mixture has reached a soft-serve consistency.

5. Stir the chocolate in by hand. Spoon the ice cream into an airtight container and press a piece of plastic wrap directly on top of the ice cream to prevent freezer burn. Place the lid to the container on top and freeze until firm, about 2 hours.

6. Serve immediately, or slightly defrost the ice cream in the refrigerator for 1 hour for later serving.

*For SCD, omit or substitute with chopped pistachios.

tidbits:
Don't skip the avocado! It's what makes this ice cream extremely creamy and rich.

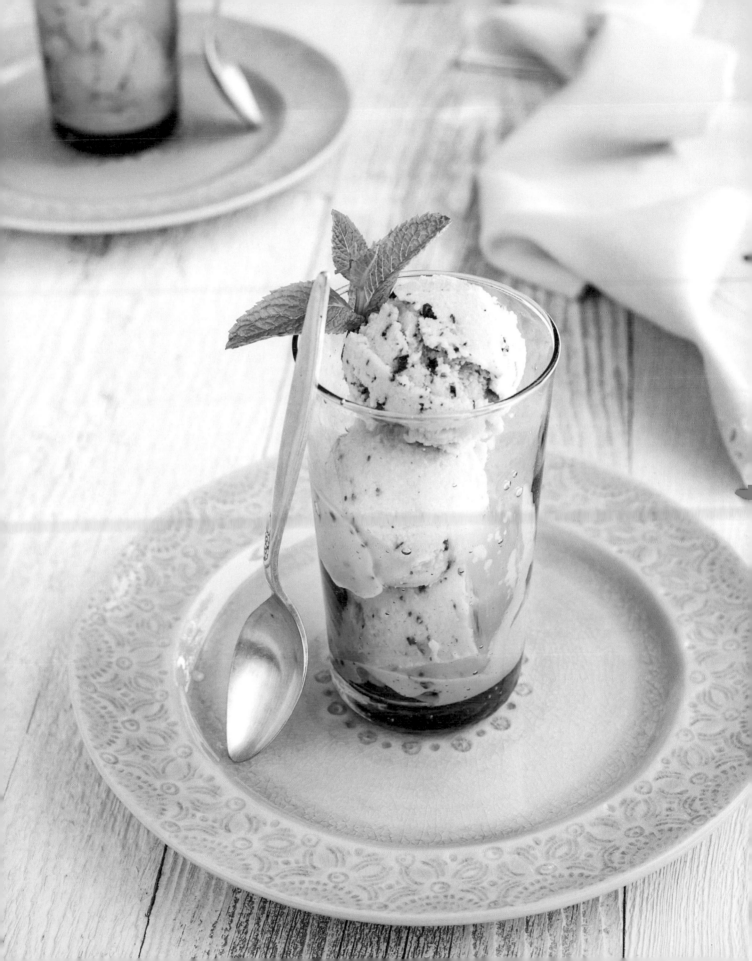

ganache tart with toasted hazelnuts

prep time: 15 minutes   cooking time: 20 minutes

chilling time: 3 hours   yield: 12 servings

This tart is so rich and creamy you'll be able to eat only a small sliver, but that just means you can continue to enjoy alluring slices for days after your guests have departed.

ingredients

- 1 cup coconut milk
- 1½ tablespoons cacao butter, chopped
- ½ cup honey or maple syrup
- 2 teaspoons brewed coffee
- 1 vanilla bean, split, seeds scraped
- ½ teaspoon sea salt
- 12 ounces unsweetened chocolate, chopped
- 2 tablespoons raw hazelnuts

method

1. Place the coconut milk in a saucepan over medium heat for 5 minutes. Stir in the cacao butter, honey, coffee, and vanilla bean pod and seeds. Cook for 20 more minutes. Remove the vanilla pod and stir in the salt.

2. Place the chocolate in a large bowl. Pour the coconut milk mixture over it, whisking the ganache until smooth. Let sit at room temperature for 40 minutes.

3. Meanwhile, preheat the oven to 350°F.

4. Place the hazelnuts in the oven on a cookie sheet for 15 minutes to toast. Wrap the hot nuts in a towel and steam for 1 minute to loosen the skins. Vigorously rub the towel between your hands to remove the skins. Coarsely chop the skinned nuts.

5. Pour the ganache into a 14-by-4.5-inch rectangular (or 9-inch round) tart mold with a removable bottom. Sprinkle with the chopped hazelnuts. Place in the refrigerator to chill for 2 hours, or until set.

6. Let the tart sit at room temperature for 15 minutes then gently slide a knife around the edges to release before serving.

tidbits:

You can reserve 2 tablespoons of the ganache at room temperature for drizzling on top of the tart decoratively after it has set, right before serving.

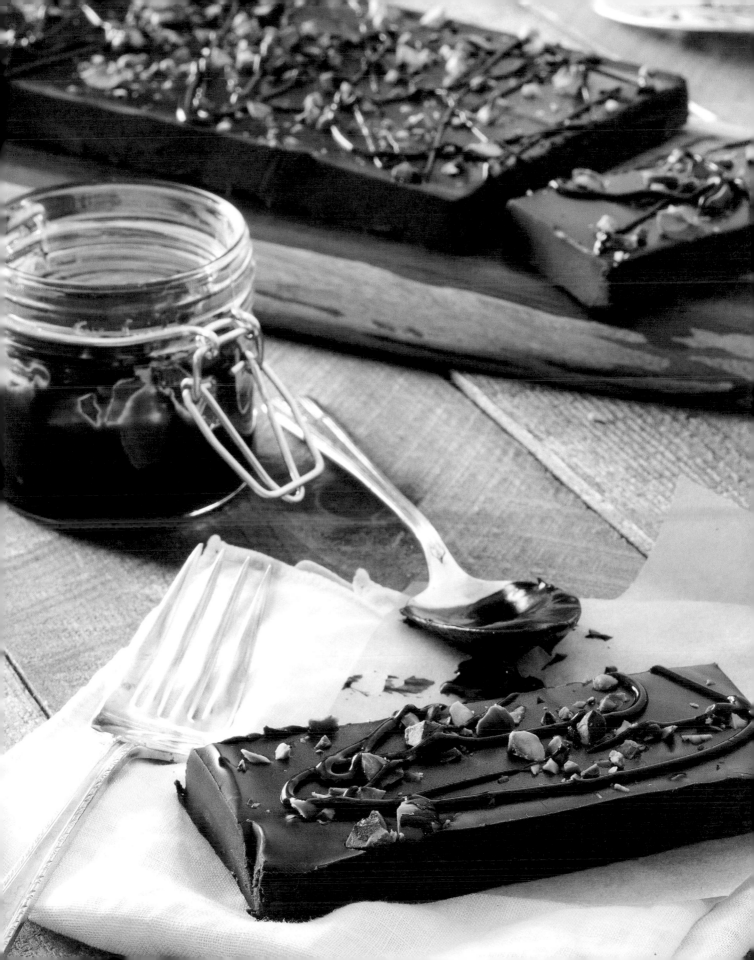

lemon curd

prep time: 5 minutes   cooking time: 5 minutes
chilling time: 1 hour   yield: 3/4 cup

This lemon curd is rich and velvety and can be stored in the refrigerator for several days. Spread on a scone or fill a pastry shell with a dollop and top with fresh berries.

ingredients

- ½ cup honey
- 2 teaspoons grated lemon zest
- ½ cup fresh lemon juice
- 6 egg yolks
- Pinch sea salt
- 4 tablespoons palm shortening

method

1. Place the honey, lemon zest, lemon juice, egg yolks, and salt in a medium saucepan and whisk to combine. Place the saucepan over medium heat and bring to a simmer, whisking constantly, until the mixture has thickened, 4 to 5 minutes.

2. Strain through a fine sieve into a bowl. Whisk in the shortening and place in the refrigerator to chill for 15 minutes. Press a piece of plastic wrap directly onto the surface to prevent a skin from forming, and continue chilling until cold, at least 1 hour or up to overnight.

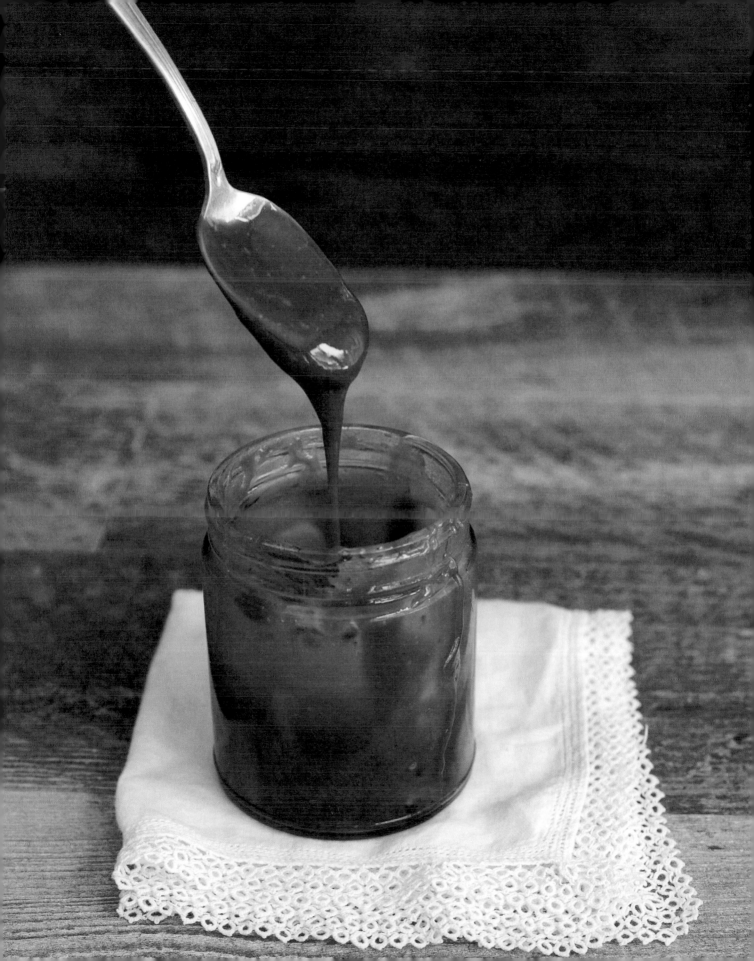

coconut milk whipped cream

prep time: 15 minutes   yield: 2 cups

I use this dairy-free topping on more cakes than I can count or to dollop on a grain-free fruit crisp.

ingredients

- 2 13.5-ounce cans coconut milk, refrigerated at least 24 hours
- 2 teaspoons honey, optional

method

1. Place a glass or metal bowl and beaters in the freezer to chill for at least 30 minutes.

2. Carefully remove the coconut milk from the fridge so as not to disturb the separation of cream from the water that has taken place. Scoop off the cream that has risen to the top and place in the chilled bowl. Save the thinner coconut water for shakes or other uses.

3. Beat the cream on high until peaks form. If desired, drizzle in honey with the beaters running and mix until incorporated.

tidbits:

Every so often, you will open a can that has chilled the appropriate amount of time but will not have separated. To avoid being caught with this dilemma, I often place an extra can or 2 in the refrigerator as a precaution.

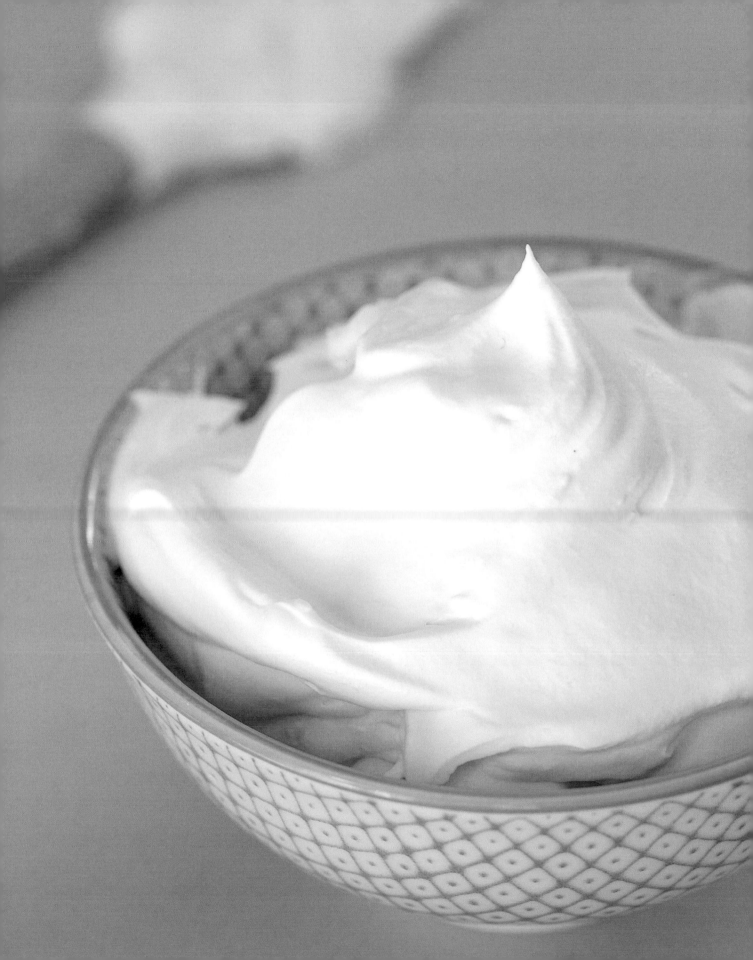

italian meringue frosting

prep time: 15 minutes   cooking time: 5 minutes

yield: 3 cups, enough to frost 2 9-inch cakes or 1 dozen cupcakes

A cross between marshmallow and whipped cream, this fluffy frosting can be used on top of any cake or cupcake, or even dolloped into a mug of Vanilla Bean Hot Cocoa (page 340). Meringue is typically an intimidating recipe for new cooks, but it doesn't have to be. It is quick to prepare, and if you follow my foolproof instructions, you won't fail!

ingredients

- 2 egg whites
- ⅓ cup honey
- ¼ teaspoon lemon juice
- Small pinch sea salt

method

1. Place the honey in a saucepan over medium-high heat and bring to a boil.

2. Meanwhile, place the egg whites in the bowl of a stand mixer, or use a hand mixer, and beat on high until soft peaks form. Add the lemon juice and salt and beat to combine.

3. With the beaters or mixer on medium, pour the boiling honey into the bowl in a slow, steady stream. Continue beating for 6 to 8 minutes, until stiff peaks form and meringue is cool to the touch and has doubled in volume.

meringue making tips:

- *Eggs will separate easier when cold, but let them sit at room temperature for at least 30 minutes before whipping. Make sure no trace of egg yolk gets into the whites: this will prevent them from whipping.*

- *Use a clean bowl and whisk.*

- *Use or toast meringue immediately after preparing it.*

- *Make meringue on a dry day if possible. The humidity from rainy days causes weepy meringue.*

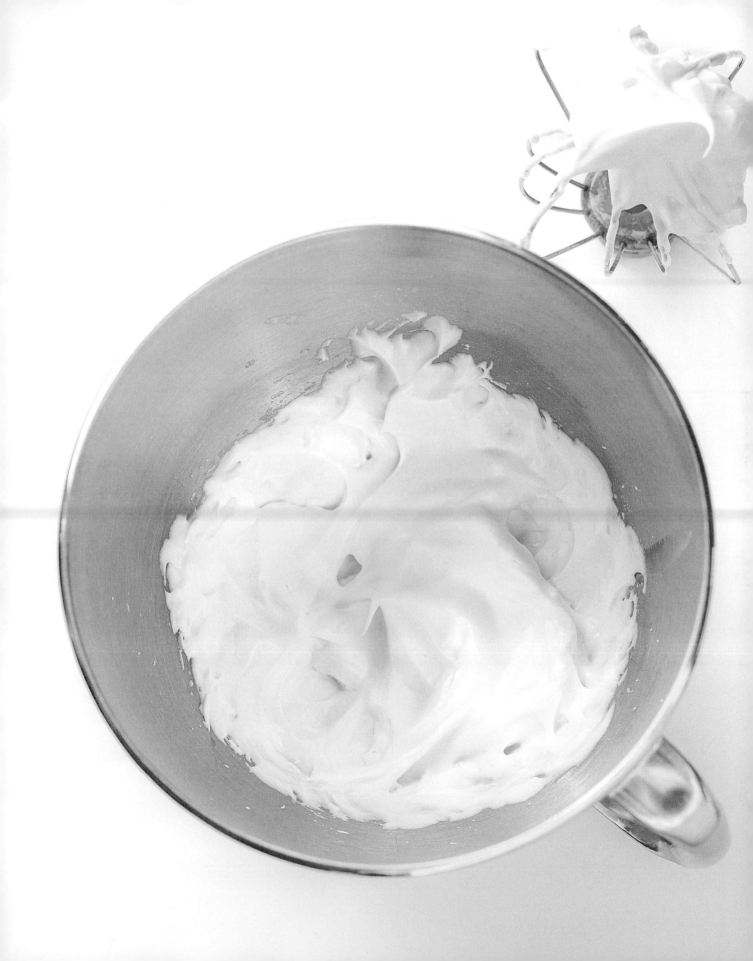

chocolate swiss meringue buttercream

prep time: *15 minutes*   cooking time: *5 minutes*

yield: *3 cups*

*A light and fluffy chocolate frosting that you can use on all types of cakes
and cupcakes.*

ingredients

- ¾ cup honey
- 4 large egg whites, about ½ cup
- ¼ teaspoon sea salt
- ¼ teaspoon lemon juice
- 2 tablespoons unsweetened cocoa powder, sifted
- ¾ cup palm shortening, softened
- ¾ teaspoon pure vanilla extract
- 3½ ounces dark chocolate, melted and cooled to room temperature

method

1. Place 2 inches of water in a saucepan and bring to a simmer. Place the honey, egg whites, and salt in a large heatproof mixing bowl and stir to combine. Set the bowl over (not in) the simmering water, and whisk until whites are warm to the touch and honey is incorporated, 4 to 6 minutes, or until a candy thermometer reads 150°F.

2. Transfer to a stand mixer, or use a hand mixer, and beat on low until foamy. Add the lemon juice, and beat on medium-high until stiff, glossy peaks form and the mixture has cooled completely, about 12 minutes.

3. Mix in the sifted cocoa powder.

4. Reduce the speed to medium-low and add the shortening a spoonful at a time, beating to incorporate fully after each addition. The buttercream will appear curdled at this point but will become smooth again with continued beating. After all the shortening has been incorporated, add the vanilla and continue beating for 10 to 15 minutes. Place the frosting in the refrigerator for 20 minutes.

5. Remove from the refrigerator and return the bowl to the mixer. With the machine still running, slowly drizzle in the chocolate. Beat until smooth and the frosting has thickened.

tidbits:

If the frosting is still too thin, it is likely because the meringue or chocolate were still warm and melted the shortening. Place the mixing bowl back in the refrigerator for 30 minutes, then beat again until smooth.

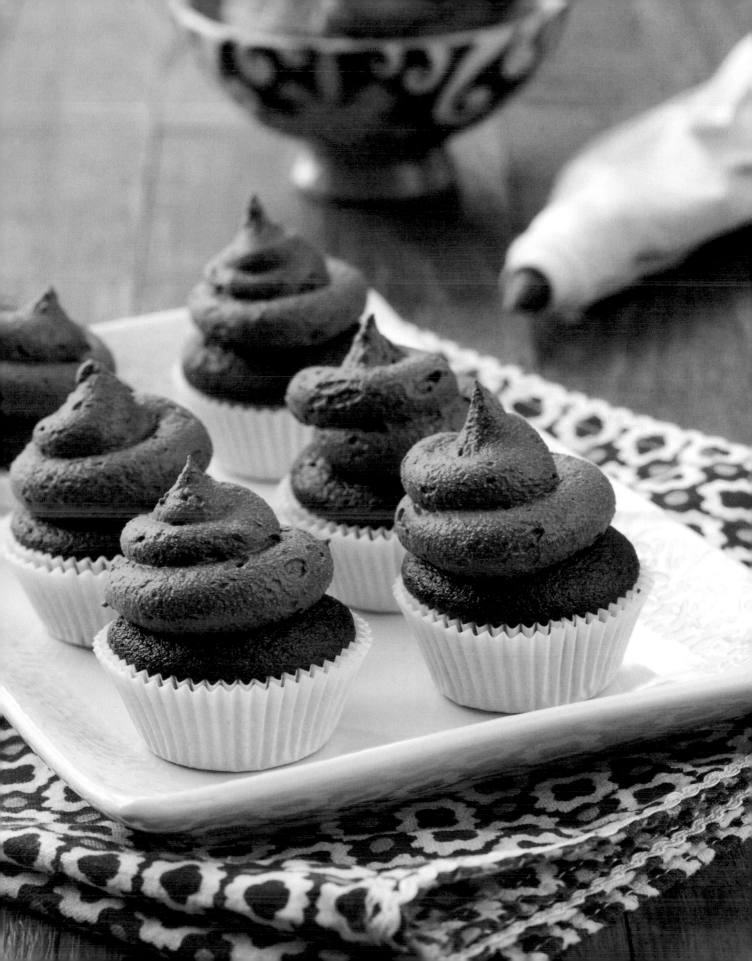

vanilla frosting

prep time: 15 minutes   yield: 2 cups

This dairy free vanilla frosting sets up nicely and even holds up in warmer weather!

ingredients

- ¾ cup palm shortening
- 1 13.5-ounce can coconut milk, refrigerated overnight
- ½ cup honey
- 3 teaspoons coconut flour, sifted
- 1 teaspoon vanilla extract

method

1. Gently open the can of coconut milk and scoop off ½ cup of the cold cream that has risen and solidified at the top of the can. In a stand mixer or using electric hand beaters, beat the shortening and cream on medium high until thick, about 5 minutes.

2. Add the honey, coconut flour, and vanilla, and beat again until incorporated. Refrigerate for 20 minutes before spreading or piping onto cooled cakes, cookies, or cupcakes.

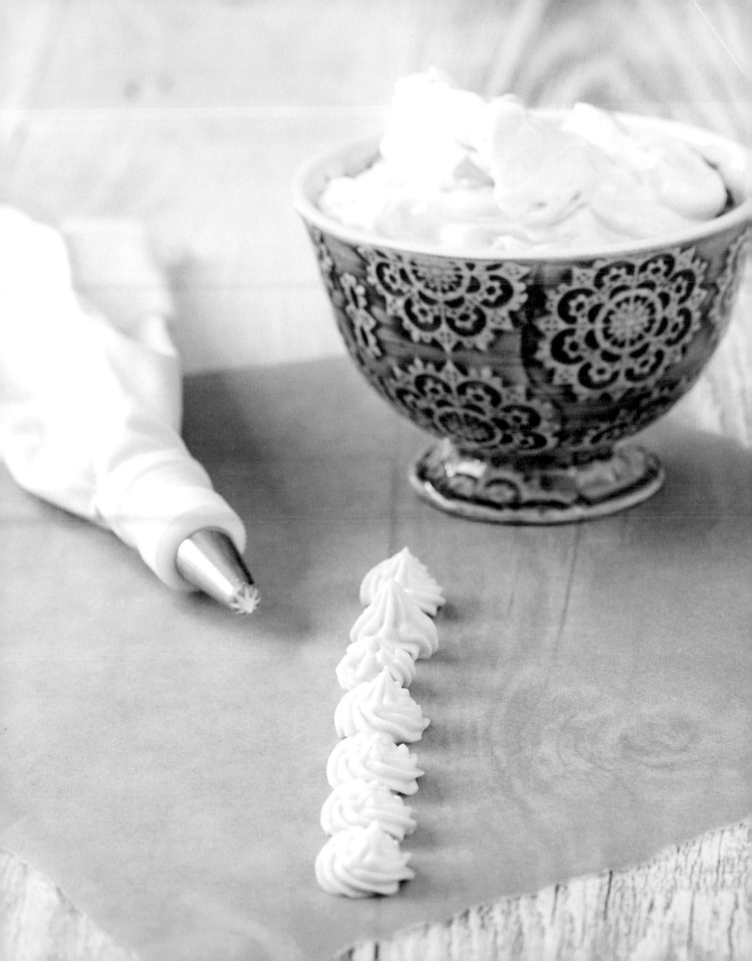

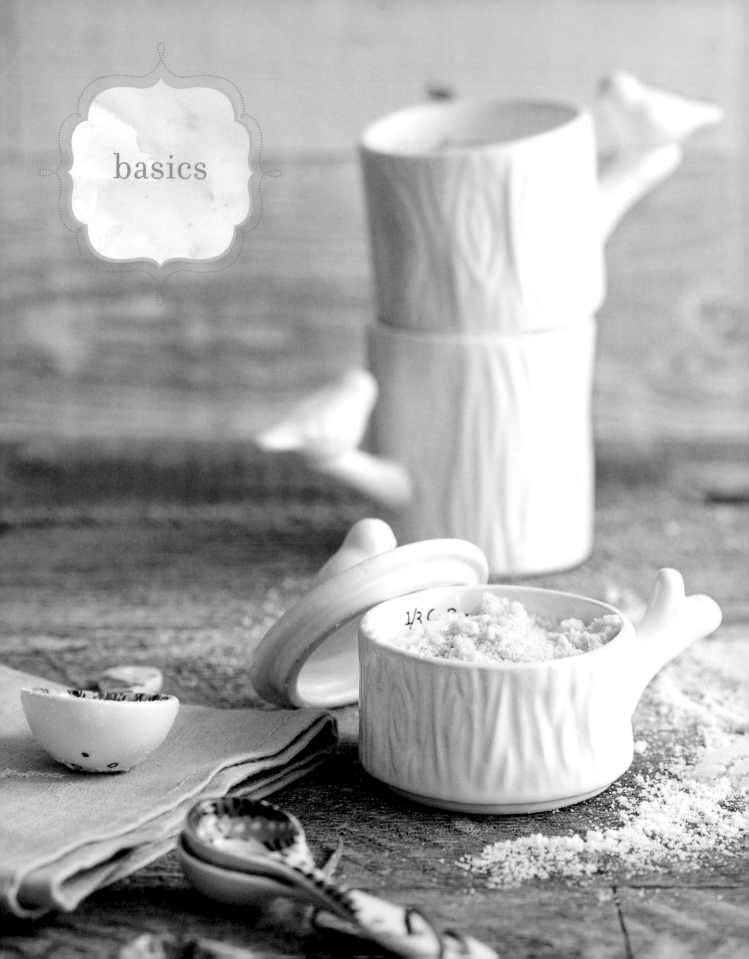

basics

crepes

prep time: 5 minutes cooking time: 15 minutes yield: 10 crepes

These crepes are incredibly versatile and easy to make. Stuff them with sweet fillings like berries and coconut whipped cream, or use them as tortillas for enchiladas or quesadillas, even as lasagna noodles.

ingredients

- 6 large eggs
- 1 cup unsweetened almond milk or other nondairy milk
- 3 tablespoons coconut flour, sifted
- 2 teaspoons coconut oil, melted plus 2 tablespoons for the pan
- ¼ teaspoon sea salt

method

1. Whisk together the crepe ingredients in a bowl. Let sit for 10 minutes while the pan heats so the coconut flour can absorb the liquid, then whisk again.

2. Heat a crepe pan or enameled skillet over medium-high heat.

3. Place 1 tablespoon of the coconut oil in the pan, swirling to coat the bottom and sides.

4. Pour ¼ cup of the batter into the hot pan, turning the pan in a circular motion with one hand so the batter spreads thinly around the pan. Alternatively, very quickly use a spatula to spread the batter. Fill any holes with a drop of batter, making sure the pan is fully covered.

5. Cook for 1 minute, until the edges start to lift. Gently work a spatula under the crepe and flip it over. Cook on the second side for 15 seconds and turn out onto a plate.

6. Continue with the remaining batter, stacking the crepes on the plate as you work. Add a little more oil to the pan after about every 3 or 4 crepes or if they begin to stick.

crepe fillings:

- *Almond butter and banana slices*
- *Smoked salmon, arugula, capers, and Hollandaise Sauce (page 30)*
- *Berries, Coconut Milk Whipped Cream (page 292), lemon juice, and honey*
- *Ham, scrambled eggs, and sautéed vegetables*
- *Melted ghee, cinnamon, and coconut crystals*

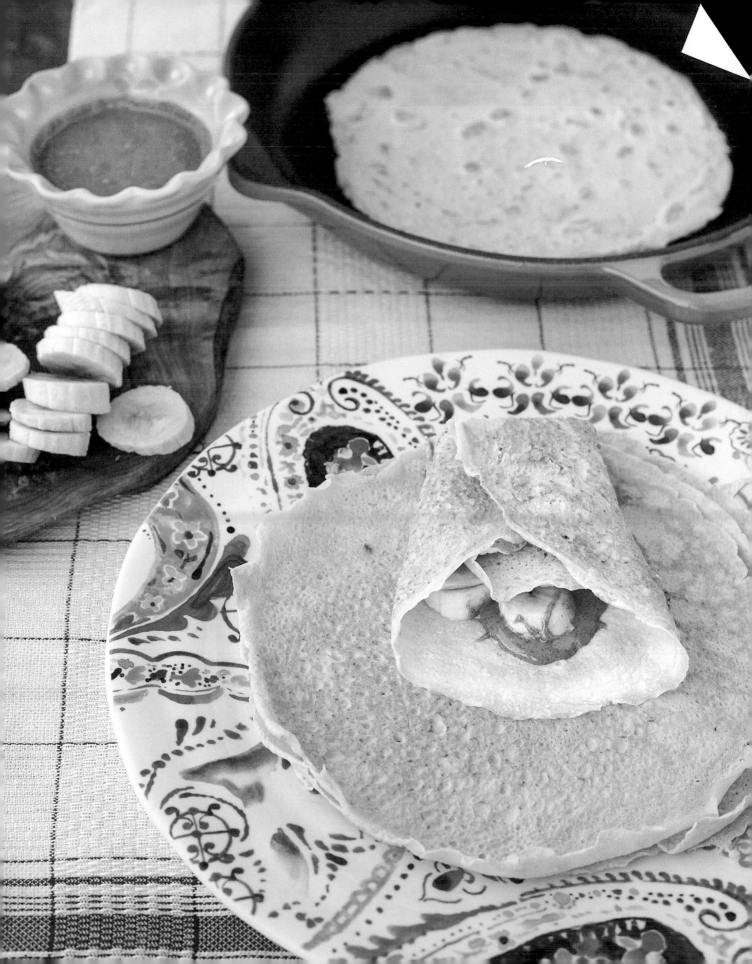

basic nut cheese

soak time: 24 hours   prep time: 15 minutes   yield: 2 cups

I still occasionally cook with grass-fed, raw dairy, but I really wanted the recipes in this book to appeal to people who are both grain- and dairy-free. That meant modifying some of our family favorites like lasagna and enchiladas—Nut Cheese to the rescue! This is an impressive ricotta substitute and also lends itself well to other uses.

ingredients

- 1 cup blanched skinless almonds, raw cashews, or raw macadamia nuts
- ½ teaspoon sea salt, plus a pinch for soaking
- 3 tablespoons water
- 2 tablespoons extra-virgin olive oil
- 4 teaspoons lemon juice

method

1. Place the nuts in a large bowl and fill with filtered water and a pinch of salt. Cover and soak the almonds for 24 hours, cashews or macadamia nuts for 6.

2. Drain the nuts and rinse thoroughly, until the water runs clear.

3. Place the nuts in a food processor or high-speed blender with the remaining ingredients.

4. Process until smooth and the mixture resembles ricotta cheese. Store in the refrigerator up to 5 days.

tidbits:

You can use almonds with skins, but they will have to be removed after soaking.

variations:

- *Add 1 teaspoon chopped rosemary, 1 teaspoon chopped parsley, and 1 teaspoon minced garlic to the mixture. Form into a ball and refrigerate until firm. Serve with crackers or crudité.*

- *Spread the cheese in a very thin layer on a baking sheet lined with parchment paper. Bake at 200°F for 30 minutes, until dry and crunchy. Break off pieces and sprinkle on salads or on top of pasta.*

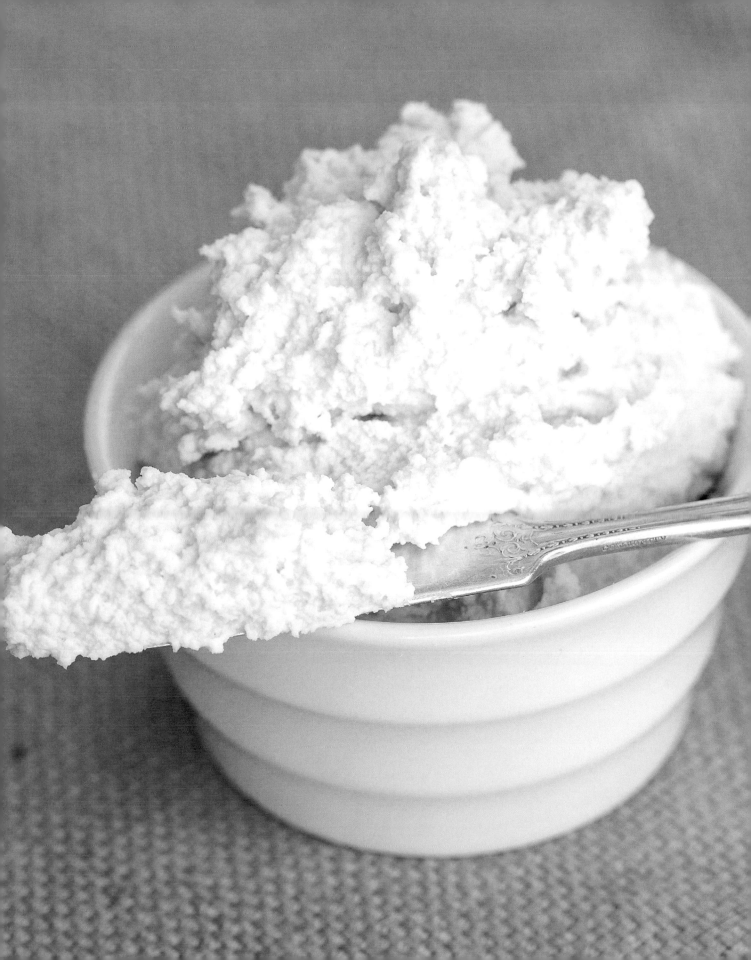

marinara sauce

prep time: 15 minutes   *cooking time:* 50 minutes   *yield:* 1 quart

Easy to prepare and incredibly versatile, this sauce can be used in lasagna, as a dip for breadsticks, or ladled over a simple bowl of zucchini noodles. Add ground beef for a hearty Bolognese sauce or chopped vegetables for a vegetarian version.

ingredients

- ¼ cup extra-virgin olive oil
- ½ small onion, sliced into thick chunks
- 1 26-ounce box or jar tomato puree
- 1 26-ounce box or jar chopped tomatoes
- 2 cloves garlic, crushed
- 1 tablespoon sea salt
- ½ tablespoon black pepper
- 6 fresh basil leaves

method

1. Place the oil in a medium saucepan over medium-high heat. Add the onion and sauté until translucent. Remove the onion using a slotted spoon, keeping as much of the fragrant oil in the pan as possible.

2. Add the remaining ingredients and bring to a boil. Reduce the heat to low and simmer the sauce for 40 minutes. Adjust the seasoning to taste. If tomato pieces are prominent, put the sauce through a strainer to remove large chunks or purée in a blender.

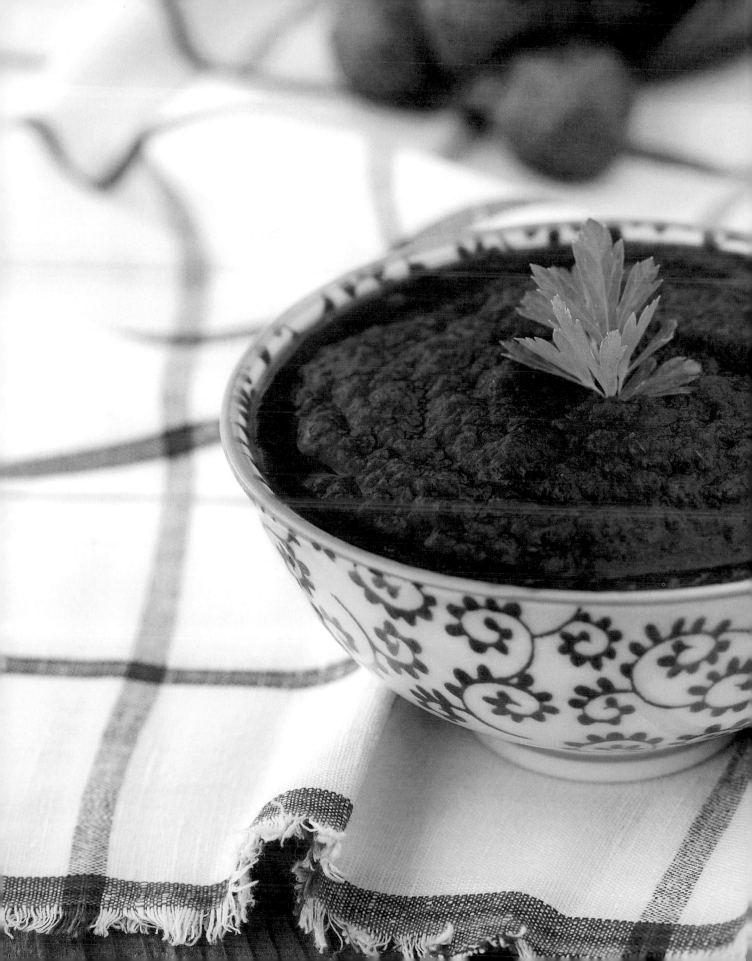

mayonnaise

prep time: 12 minutes   yield: ¾ cup

Homemade mayonnaise takes virtually no time to make and ensures that you are not ingesting canola oil or white sugar. You'll never want to go back to store-bought once you taste this delicious version using healthy macadamia oil.

ingredients

- 1 large egg yolk
- 1 teaspoon lemon juice
- 1 teaspoon white vinegar
- ½ teaspoon honey
- ½ teaspoon sea salt
- ¼ teaspoon Dijon mustard
- ¾ cup macadamia nut oil

Add some flare to your mayonnaise by puréeing the ingredients for these combinations:

- CHIPOTLE MAYO:
  ½ cup Mayo plus 2 chipotle chilies in adobo sauce plus 1 teaspoon adobo sauce

- ROASTED RED PEPPER MAYO:
  ½ cup Mayo plus 1 roasted red pepper

- ROASTED-GARLIC MAYO:
  ½ cup Mayo plus 4 cloves roasted garlic

- WASABI MAYO:
  ½ cup Mayo plus 1 teaspoon wasabi powder plus ¼ teaspoon lime juice plus ⅛ teaspoon salt

- PESTO MAYO:
  ½ cup Mayo plus 3 basil leaves plus 1 garlic clove plus 1 teaspoon extra-virgin olive oil

method

1. Place the first 6 ingredients in a small blender or mini food processor and blend on low until combined.

2. With the blender on medium-low, add the oil 1 drop at a time until the mixture resembles mayonnaise. Begin adding the oil in a slow steady stream with the blender still running, until all the oil has been incorporated.

3. Cover and chill. Can be stored in the refrigerator for 5 days.

tidbits:

- *Macadamia nut oil is used for its mild flavor, but other oils, such as olive, avocado, or almond, may also be used.*

- *A small blender or mini food processor is essential for the method above, however, mayonnaise can also be made by hand. Place the first 6 ingredients in a medium bowl and whisk to combine. Add ¼ cup of the oil in increments of ½ teaspoon of oil at a time, whisking vigorously. Gradually add the remaining ½ cup oil in a slow, steady stream, whisking constantly, until thick, about 5 to 7 minutes.*

* Take caution in consuming raw eggs because of the slight risk of salmonella or other food-borne bacteria. To reduce this risk, use only fresh, properly refrigerated, clean grade A or AA eggs with intact shells and avoid contact between the yolks or whites and the outer shell.

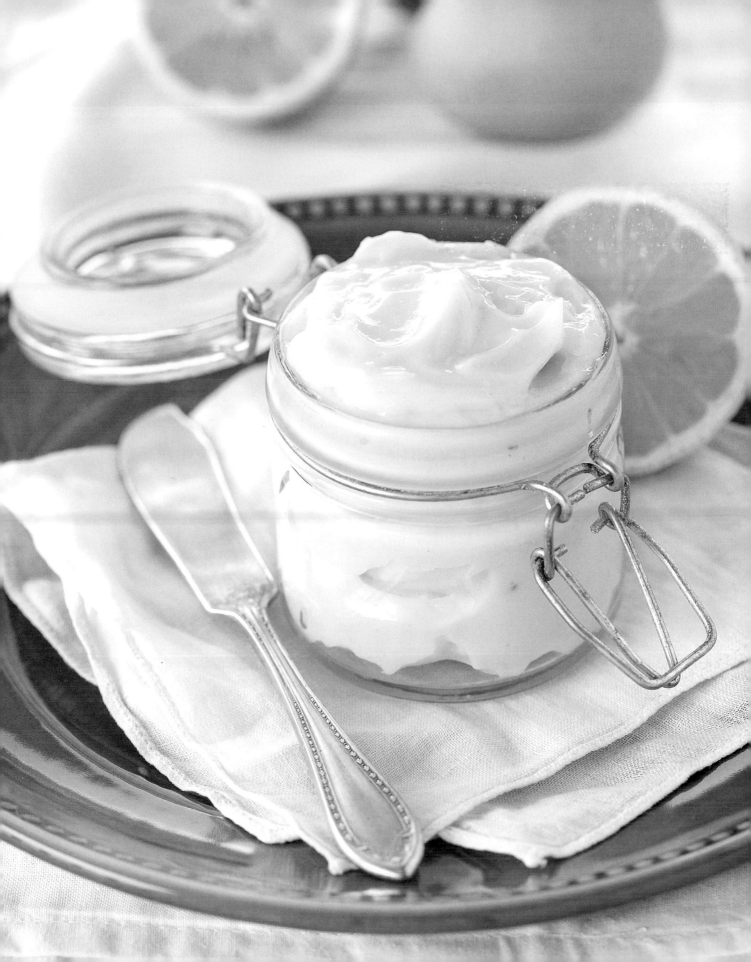

pastry crust

prep time: 10 minutes   cooking time: 15 minutes   yield: 1 9-inch piecrust

This satisfyingly buttery piecrust will serve as a sturdy foundation for whatever your imagination wants to fill it with, whether a savory quiche or sweet lemon meringue pie.

ingredients

- 2½ cups blanched almond flour
- 1 tablespoon coconut flour
- 1 large cold egg
- 5 teaspoons ice water
- ¾ teaspoon sea salt
- 3½ tablespoons palm shortening

method

1. Preheat the oven to 325°F.

2. Place the first 5 ingredients in a food processor and process for 30 seconds. Add the shortening in small spoonfuls, spacing them out around the bowl. Pulse 4 or 5 times, just enough for the shortening to be mixed in and the dough to come together.

3. Press the dough into the bottom and up the sides of a 9-inch pie plate. Create fluted edges with fingers if desired.

4. Cut a circle of parchment and fit into the bottom of the pie shell. Fill with pie weights or dried beans. Bake until the edges begin to turn gold, about 10 minutes. Remove the pie weights and parchment paper and bake for 5 minutes more. Transfer to a wire rack and let cool.

tidbits:

Double this recipe for pies such as apple or potpies that require a top crust layer.

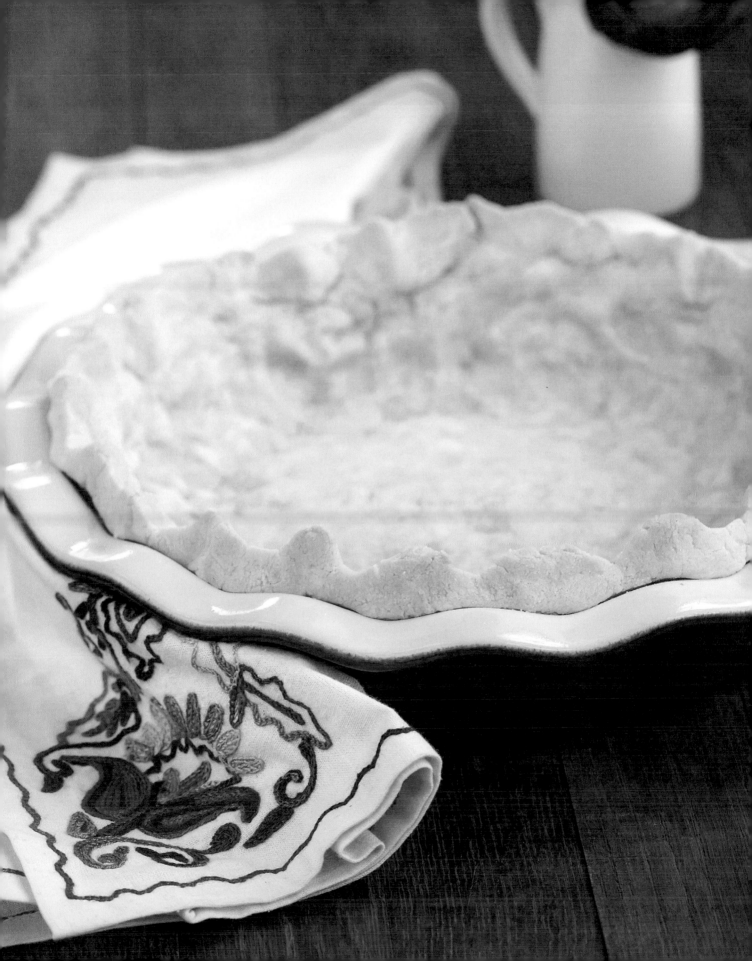

pizza crust

prep time: 10 minutes   cooking time: 12 minutes   yield: 1 9-inch crust

My family loves to pile this crust high with fresh toppings on Friday nights. I often make individual-size crusts so we can each personalize our own!

ingredients

- ¾ cup whole raw cashews, about 4 ounces
- 3 tablespoons blanched almond flour, plus more for rolling out the dough
- ¼ cup coconut flour
- ½ teaspoon baking soda
- ½ teaspoon sea salt
- 2 eggs
- 2 tablespoons almond milk
- ½ teaspoon apple cider vinegar
- 2 tablespoons palm shortening
- 1 tablespoon cold water
- ½ teaspoon chopped fresh parsley
- 1 fresh basil leaf

method

1. Preheat the oven to 350°.

2. Place the cashews, almond flour, and coconut flour in a food processor and pulse until a fine flour has formed, about 15 seconds.

3. Add the baking soda, salt, eggs, almond milk, vinegar, shortening, and water and process for 1 minute. Scrape down the sides of the bowl and pulse a few more times, until a very smooth but wet dough has formed.

4. Add the parsley and basil, and pulse 2 more times to incorporate the herbs.

5. Allow the dough to rest for 2 minutes to let the coconut flour absorb some of the liquid.

6. Sprinkle a piece of parchment paper with a little almond flour. Place the dough on top of it, then place another sheet of parchment paper over the dough. Roll the dough out between the 2 sheets of parchment paper into a circle about ¼-inch thick.

7. Remove the top piece of parchment and carefully slide the other piece with the crust onto a pizza pan.

8. Place the crust in the oven and bake for 12 minutes, or until it has puffed up and is golden brown around the edges. Top with desired toppings and bake for an additional 10 to 15 minutes, or until toppings are cooked through.

tidbits:

This crust works best with precooked toppings. Sauté vegetables or meat before adding them to the baked crust, then bake until just hot so as not to burn the crust.

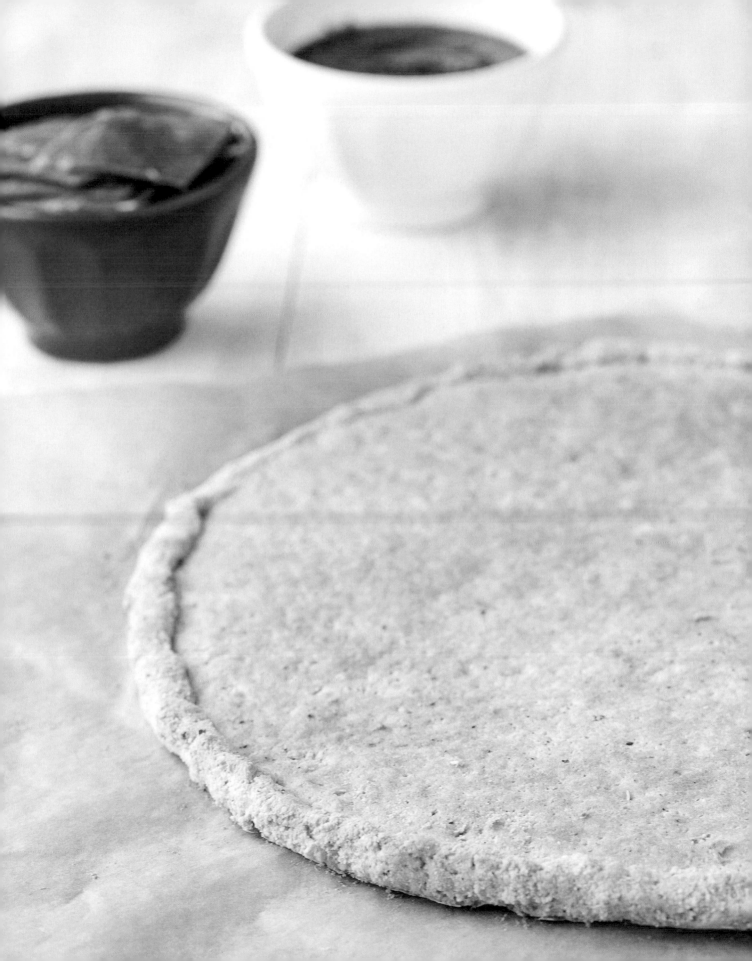

almond milk

prep time: 5 minutes   yield: 1 quart

Commercial almond milks are not only overpriced, but they are also full of additives. All you need is a blender and some cheesecloth to create healthy dairy-free milk alternatives.

ingredients

- 1 cup raw almonds
- 8 cups filtered water, divided
- ¼ teaspoon sea salt, divided
- 1 small date, pitted

method

1. Place almonds in a bowl with 4 cups of filtered water and ⅛ teaspoon of the salt and soak for 10 hours or overnight.

2. Drain the nuts and rinse well. Transfer them to a blender and fill with 4 cups filtered water. Add the date and the remaining ⅛ teaspoon salt and purée until smooth.

3. Strain the milk through a fine-mesh sieve, a nut milk bag, or doubled cheesecloth. Squeeze to remove all of the liquid. Store in the refrigerator for 5 days.

tidbits:

- *You can also make cashew, hazelnut, or brazil nut milk. Soak cashews for 4 hours. Hazelnuts and brazil nuts don't need to be soaked because they don't contain the enzyme inhibitors that prevent nuts from being digested properly—so you can make milk from those nuts at the drop of a hat.*

- *There are many uses for the leftover almond pulp, so be sure to save it and look online for ways to utilize it!*

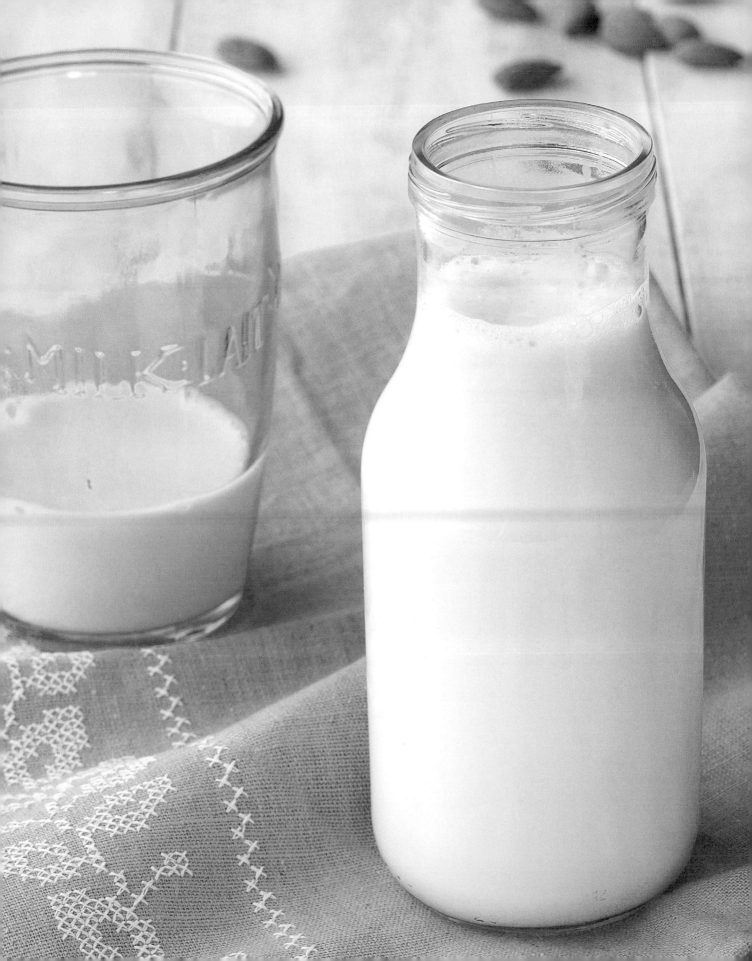

chicken broth

prep time: 20 minutes   cooking time: 14 hours 30 minutes

yield: 3 quarts

While commercial chicken broths and stocks are convenient, some of their ingredients aren't necessarily convenient to your health. Homemade stocks incorporate healing elements like gelatin, which are generally lost when food is processed. I make my broth with a whole chicken so that the flavor from both the bones and the meat seeps into the broth. Make a large batch and freeze it in pints or quarts so you have some on hand whenever you need it.

ingredients

- 12 cups filtered water
- 3 pounds bone-in chicken parts, and gizzards
- 1 tablespoon apple cider vinegar
- 1 yellow onion, peeled and quartered
- 3 large carrots, cut into large dice
- 4 cloves garlic, smashed
- 2 stalks celery with leaves
- 2 bay leaves
- 1 teaspoon sea salt
- ½ teaspoon cracked black pepper
- 1 bunch fresh parsley

method

1. Place the water and chicken parts in a slow cooker and cook on high for 2 hours. Skim off any foam from the surface and remove the chicken. Shred the meat off the bones, and set the meat aside. Return the bones to the pot.

2. Reduce slow cooker to low. Add all the remaining ingredients, except the parsley, to the pot and cook on low for 12 hours or on high for 6 hours. Turn off the pot, skim the fat off the top, stir in the parsley, and cover for 30 minutes.

3. Strain the broth through a fine-mesh sieve or cheesecloth. Store in the refrigerator or freezer for later use. Scoop off any solidified fat before using.

tidbits:

Broth and stock are often used interchangeably, but stock is typically made with more bones than meat and is left unseasoned so it is a blank canvas for soups or other uses. If purchasing store-bought broth or stock in place of homemade, opt for a low sodium variety to ensure a proper outcome in the recipes.

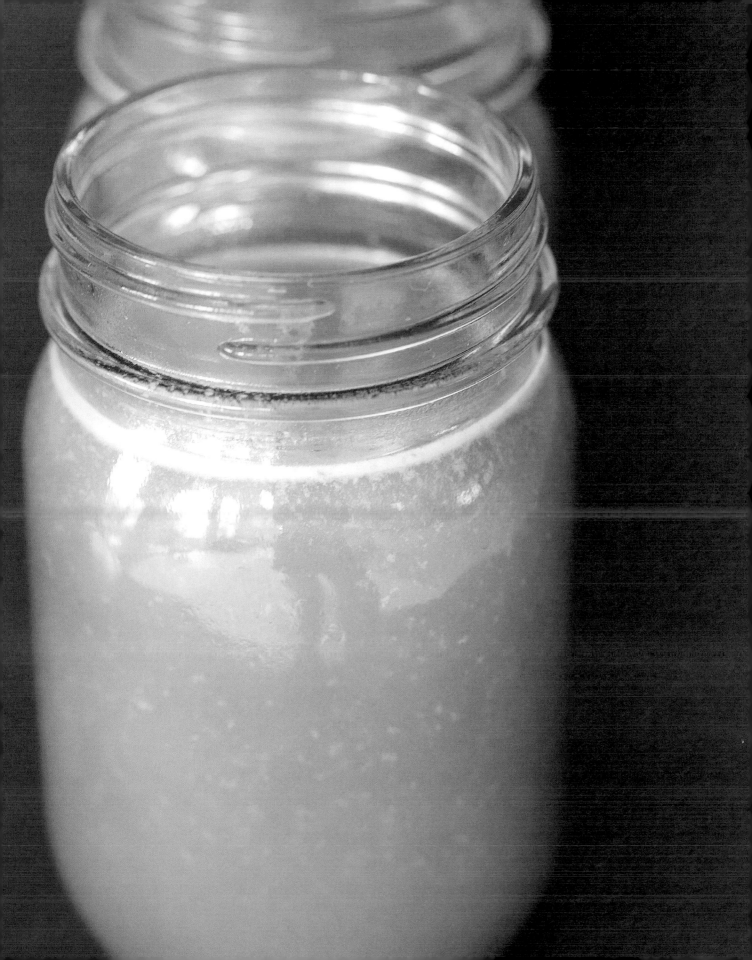

thai 'peanut' vinaigrette

prep time: 15 minutes   yield: 1 cup

The peanut sauces that often accompany Thai dishes inspired this dressing—a spunky vinaigrette to drizzle on salads or serve as a dipping sauce.

ingredients

- 1½ tablespoons almond butter or sunflower seed butter, unsweetened
- 1½ tablespoons cilantro
- 1 tablespoon coconut aminos
- 1 tablespoon apple cider vinegar
- 1 tablespoon fresh lime juice
- 2 teaspoons honey
- 1 teaspoon minced garlic
- 1-inch piece ginger, peeled
- ¼ teaspoon sea salt
- ¾ cup melted coconut oil

method

1. Place all the ingredients, except the oil, in a blender or small food processor and blend until smooth.
2. With the blender on low, slowly drizzle in the oil in a steady stream. Continue blending until emulsified.

tidbits:

The vessel of the blender or food processor needs to be small for the dressing to emulsify and not spread up the walls of the jar. If making by hand, mince the cilantro, garlic, and ginger ahead of time. Whisk together all of the ingredients except the oil, then whisk vigorously as you slowly drizzle in the oil. This dressing will harden when refrigerated, so gently warm over very low heat until it is pourable again.

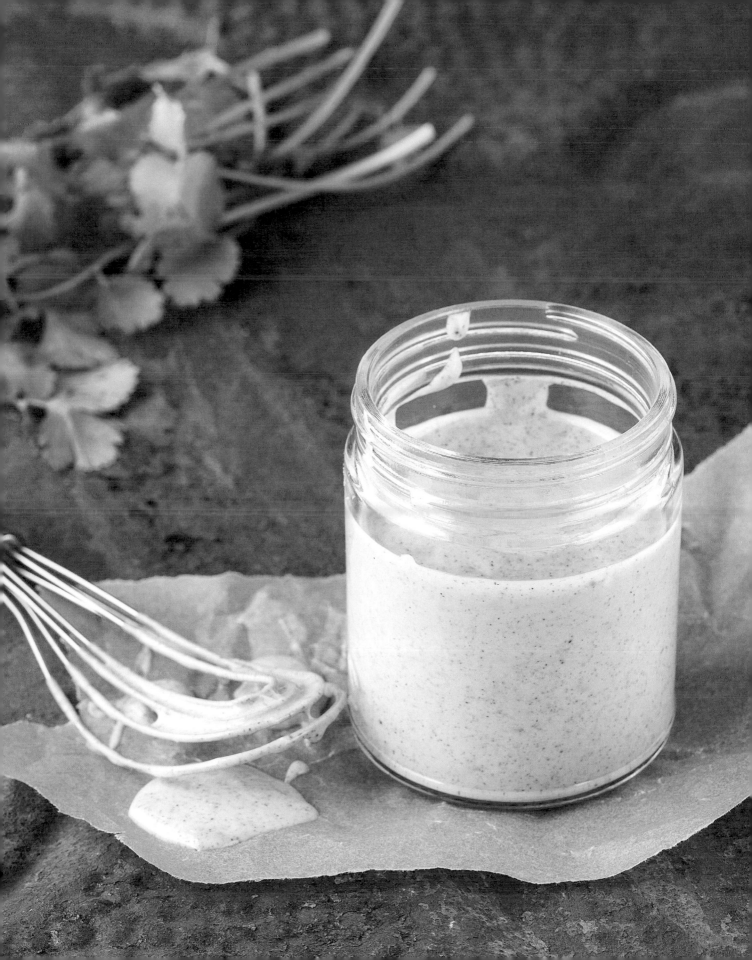

basil-thyme vinaigrette

prep time: 5 minutes   yield: 2 cups

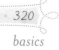
You will never see my fridge (or purse for that matter!) without a bottle of this vinaigrette. We use it almost every night drizzled over a simple green salad, and I often carry a small bottle with me when we go out to eat. Check the label on the balsamic vinegar carefully—there are many imposters sold that include sugar in the ingredients!

ingredients

- ½ cup balsamic vinegar
- 1 tablespoon honey
- 2 teaspoons Dijon mustard
- 3 cloves garlic
- ¼ cup fresh basil leaves
- 2 sprigs fresh thyme
- ⅔ cup extra-virgin olive oil

method

1. Place all the ingredients, except the oil, in a blender or small food processor and purée until smooth.
2. With the blender running, slowly pour in the oil in a steady stream.
3. Continue blending for 15 seconds to fully incorporate the oil.

tidbits:

Alternatively, finely mince the garlic and whisk it together with the vinegar, honey, Dijon mustard, and herbs. Slowly pour in the olive oil, whisking continuously until emulsified.

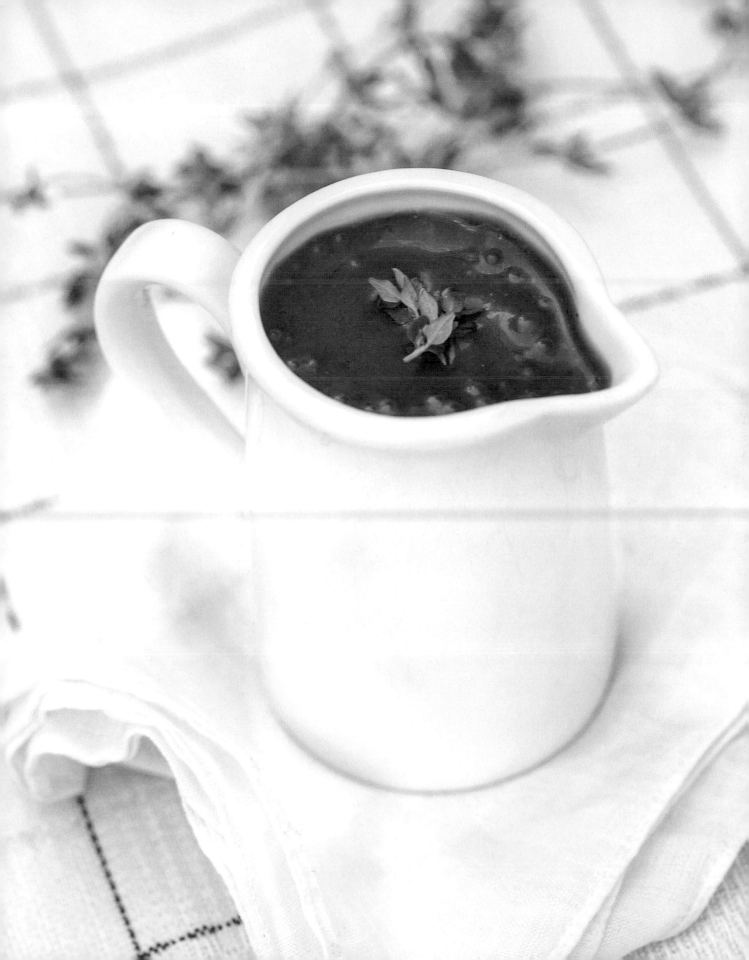

asian pear chutney

prep time: 10 minutes   cooking time: 30 minutes   yield: 3 cups

This condiment was created after an abundant Asian pear harvest from our backyard one fall. I originally paired it with an Indian Spiced Pork Roast (page 178), but it has since been spooned over fish and chicken and has even been added to meatballs to shake the palate up a bit!

ingredients

- 3 large Asian pears, peeled, cored, and chopped
- 1 cup minced yellow onions
- ½ cup raisins
- ½ cup unsweetened apple or pear juice
- 3 tablespoons apple cider vinegar
- 1 tablespoon honey or maple syrup
- 2 teaspoons lemon juice
- 1 teaspoon freshly grated ginger
- ¼ teaspoon garam masala

method

1. Place all the ingredients in a saucepan and simmer for 30 minutes, stirring occasionally.
2. Cool to room temperature then serve, or refrigerate for later use.

tidbits:

Asian pears are closely related in shape and texture to a mild apple. If Asian pears are not available, a mild-flavored apple can stand in.

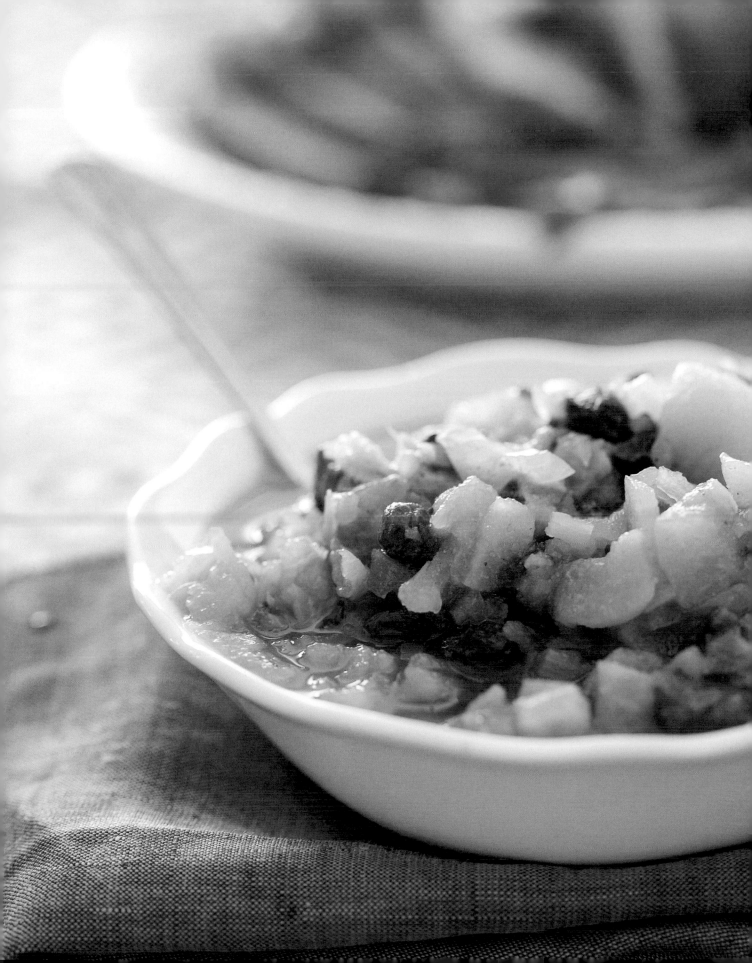

fig jam

prep time: 5 minutes   cooking time: 25 minutes   yield: 3 cups

Homemade fruit preserves simply burst with way more flavor than their store-bought counterparts. This recipe does not use added pectin as most jam recipes do, so it is all natural and only lightly sweetened to enhance the already sweet fruit.

ingredients

- 1 pound black mission figs, stems removed
- 2 tablespoons fresh lemon juice
- 1 teaspoon lemon zest
- ⅓ cup honey

method

1. Place the figs, lemon juice, and lemon zest in a blender or food processor.

2. Process until finely chopped. Pour the chopped fruit into a saucepan and add the honey.

3. Bring to a boil over medium-high heat, then reduce the heat to low and simmer for 20 minutes.

4. Allow the jam to sit at room temperature for 30 minutes, then store in airtight jars in the refrigerator.

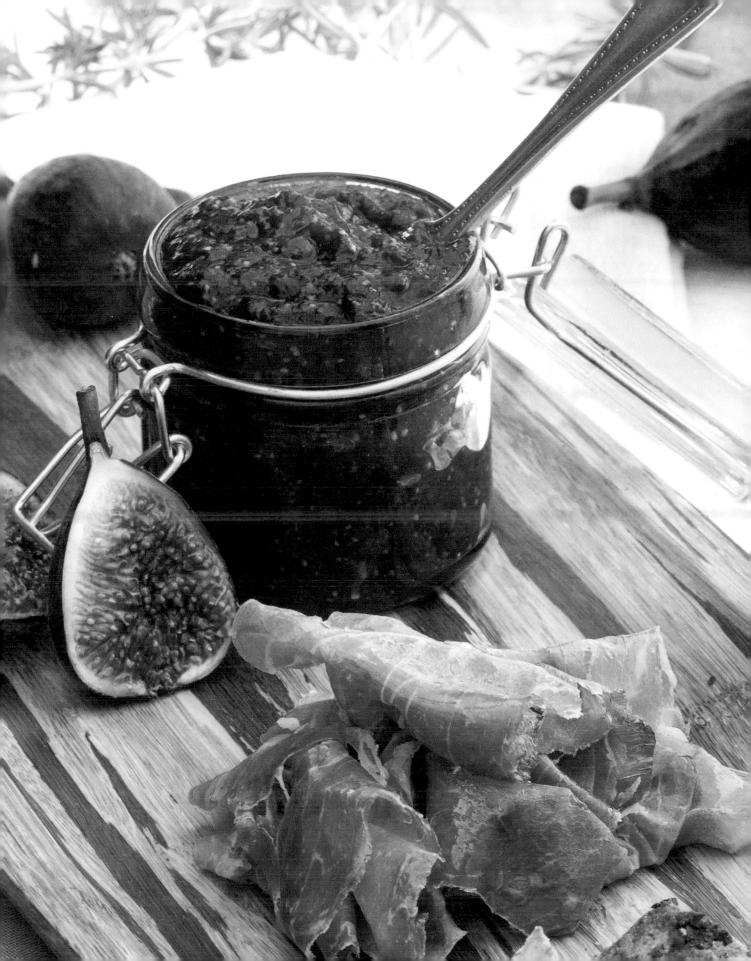

smoky barbecue sauce

prep time: 8 minutes   cooking time: 30 to 40 minutes   yield: 1½ cups

Spicy, tangy, and a little smoky: this barbecue sauce is everything a good barbecue sauce should be. Plus, it has all the flavor complexity of being smoked for hours, but takes only 30 minutes. Whether you are brushing it on some meat for the grill or dunking your Crispy Chicken Tenders (page 206) in it, it will quickly become a staple in your kitchen.

ingredients

- 1 cup tomato puree
- ½ cup honey
- ¼ cup white vinegar
- 2 tablespoons tomato paste
- 1 tablespoon coconut crystals*
- 1 tablespoon coconut aminos
- 1 teaspoon fish sauce
- ¾ teaspoon natural liquid smoke
- ½ teaspoon sea salt
- ½ teaspoon paprika
- ½ teaspoon chili powder
- ½ teaspoon Dijon mustard
- ¼ teaspoon cayenne pepper
- ¼ teaspoon minced garlic
- ¼ teaspoon onion powder
- ¼ teaspoon allspice
- ¼ teaspoon cracked fresh black pepper

*Omit the coconut crystals for SCD.

method

1. Place all the ingredients in a saucepan set over medium-high heat and whisk to combine.

2. Bring to a boil, then reduce the heat and simmer for 30 to 40 minutes, until the sauce has reduced by about half.

3. Bring to room temperature before storing in the refrigerator for later use.

tidbits:

- You can double the recipe and store half in the freezer. Thaw in the refrigerator for a day before using.

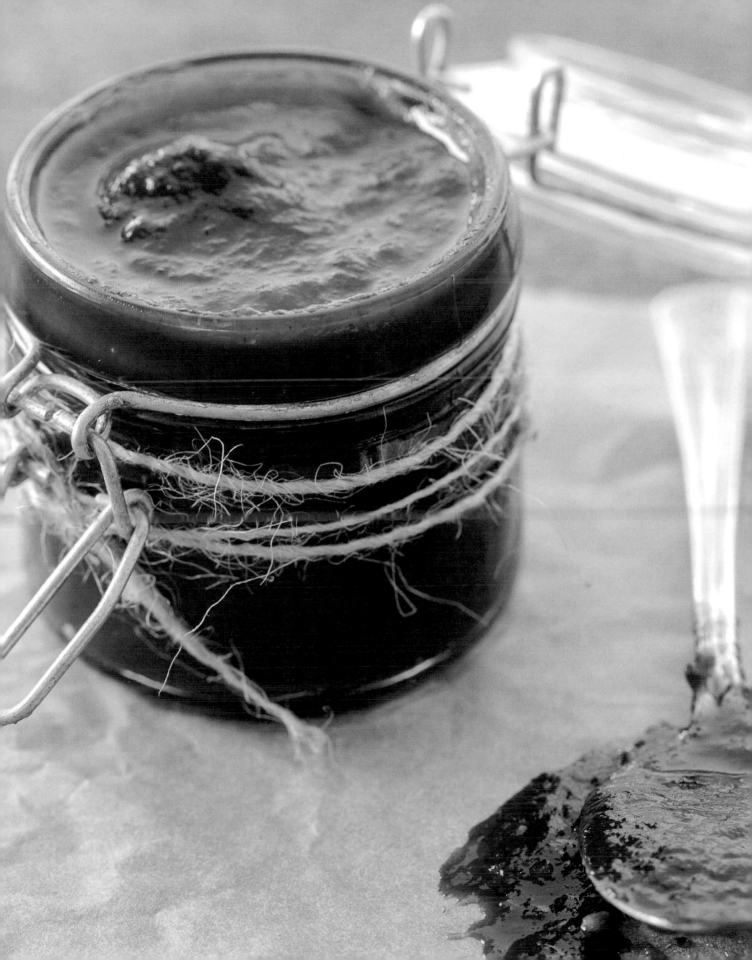

tomato ketchup

prep time: 5 minutes   cooking time: 45 minutes   yield: 2 cups

In my past life, foods like French fries were simply a vehicle for consuming ketchup. When I first swore off refined sugars and processed food, I decided ketchup was just better off forgotten because every recipe I tried for homemade never compared to the store–bought. I have finally come up with one that I proudly keep bottled in my refrigerator and enjoy smeared on all of my old favorites.

ingredients

- 1 tablespoon coconut oil
- ½ yellow onion, halved
- 1 clove garlic, crushed
- 1 26-ounce jar or box tomato puree
- ½ cup honey
- ⅓ cup white vinegar
- 1 tablespoon tomato paste
- ½ teaspoon sea salt
- 8 whole cloves
- 10 whole allspice berries

method

1. Place the oil in a deep skillet or saucepan over medium heat. Add the onion and garlic and sauté for 5 minutes, until fragrant.

2. Add the remaining ingredients and bring to a boil. Reduce heat to medium-low and simmer uncovered for 40 minutes, until the sauce has thickened and reduced by half.

3. Remove the onion, cloves, and allspice.

4. Bring to room temperature before storing in the refrigerator for later use.

tidbits:

You can double the recipe and store half in the freezer. Thaw in the refrigerator for a day before using.

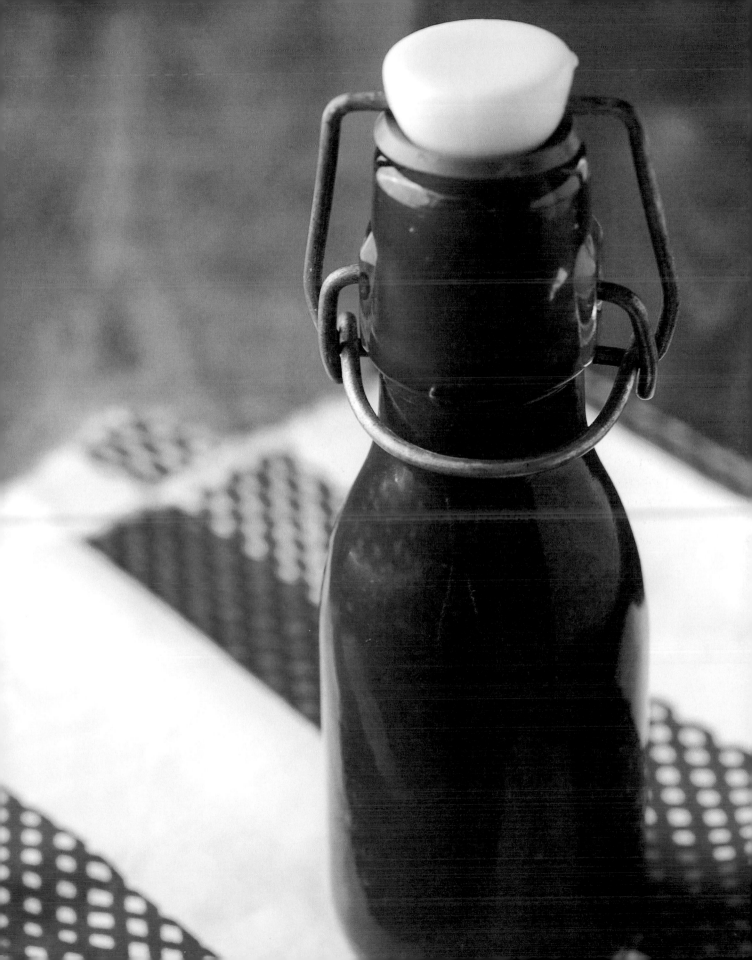

blueberry preserves

prep time: 5 minutes   cooking time: 20 minutes   yield: 2 cups

Most people don't realize how easy it is to make their own jams and are surprised by the lovely flavor and texture of this recipe. Making it homemade eliminates the processed sugars, commercial pectin, and other unhealthy ingredients generally found in store-bought jams.

ingredients

- 3 cups blueberries, frozen and thawed or fresh
- ½ cup honey
- 2 tablespoons fresh lemon juice
- 1 teaspoon finely grated lemon zest

method

1. Place the blueberries in a medium saucepan and crush them with the back of a fork or a potato masher.

2. Add the remaining ingredients and bring to a boil over medium-high heat. Stir frequently while the mixture boils for 15 to 20 minutes and starts to thicken. Test for doneness by placing a spoonful in the freezer for 5 minutes. If the jam solidifies, it's done.

3. Skim off any foam and ladle the jam into a sterilized jar.

4. Cool to room temperature, and then store in covered airtight containers in the fridge for later use.

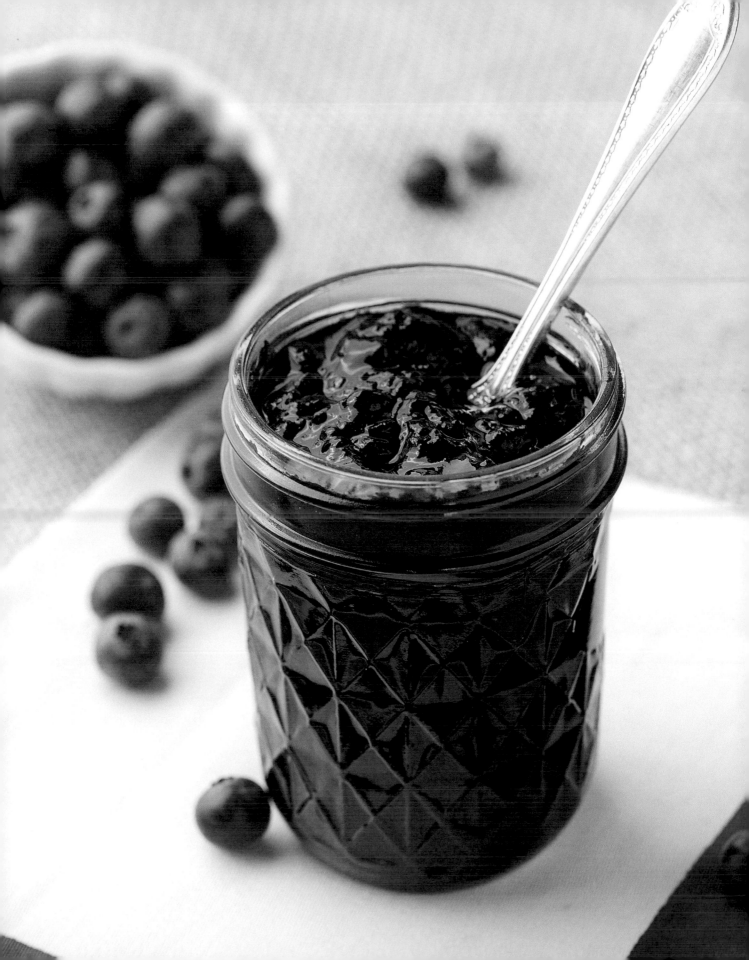

fresh salsas and guacamole

Making salsa is a breeze, and the flavors are bolder when you whip it up fresh at home. Use these salsas and the guacamole to spice up scrambled eggs, as dips for chips (page 80), or to spoon on top of a hamburger.

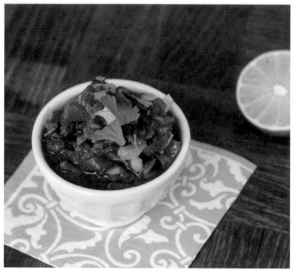

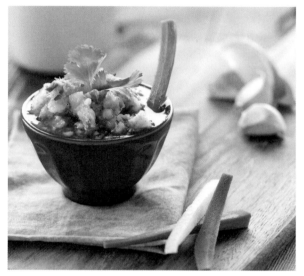

pico de gallo

prep time: 10 minutes   yield: 1 cup

ingredients

- 1 medium tomato, cut into chunks
- ¼ medium red onion, cut into large chunks
- 1 tablespoon chopped fresh cilantro
- 2 cloves garlic cloves
- ½ small jalapeño pepper, seeded
- ½ teaspoon sea salt

method

Place all the ingredients in a food processor and pulse a few times, until everything is roughly chopped. Alternatively, finely chop all the ingredients by hand then combine in a bowl.

pineapple salsa

prep time: 10 minutes   yield: 2 cups

ingredients

- 4 cups diced fresh pineapple
- 1 cup red bell pepper, seeded and chopped
- ½ small serrano pepper, seeded and chopped
- 2 tablespoons chopped green onions
- 2 tablespoons chopped fresh cilantro
- 1 tablespoon fresh lime juice
- 2 teaspoons apple cider vinegar
- 1 teaspoon minced garlic
- ¼ teaspoon sea salt
- ¼ teaspoon chili powder

method

Place all the ingredients in a food processor. Pulse until fruits and vegetables are finely chopped. Chill 1 hour before serving.

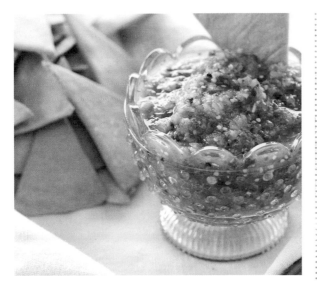

roasted-tomatillo salsa

prep time: 20 minutes   cooking time: 10 minutes
                yield: 2 cups

ingredients

- ½ pound tomatillos, husked and rinsed
- 1 or 2 Serrano chilies, stemmed
- 1 large clove garlic
- ¼ cup chopped fresh cilantro
- ¼ cup diced white onion
- 2 teaspoons fresh lime juice
- ¼ teaspoon sea salt
- ¼ teaspoon cumin

method

1. Preheat the oven to 425°F.

2. Place the tomatillos, chilies, and garlic on a rimmed baking sheet in the top third of the oven, about 6 inches away from the heating element. Roast until black spots bubble up and the vegetables soften, about 5 minutes. Flip them over and roast for an additional 5 minutes.

3. Cool for 5 minutes, then transfer everything to a blender, including all the pan juices. Add the remaining ingredients and blend until smooth. Chill before serving.

guacamole

prep time: 10 minutes   yield: 2 cups

ingredients

- 4 ripe avocados, pitted and diced
- ¼ cup minced red onion
- ½ jalapeño pepper, stemmed, seeded, and diced
- 2 cloves garlic, minced
- 1 tablespoon chopped fresh cilantro
- Juice from 1 lime
- ½ teaspoon sea salt
- Pinch cracked black pepper

method

1. Place the avocado in a bowl and mash until mostly smooth. Alternatively, place in a food processor and pulse.

2. Add the remaining ingredients and stir to combine. If using a food processor, pulse 4 times to combine. Serve immediately.

---

tidbits:

Choose your spice intensity for any of these salsas by adding more or less chilies. They are small but pack a lot of spice, so use sparingly until you have tasted the salsa! For a very mild salsa, remove all the seeds prior to blending.

Danielle Walker

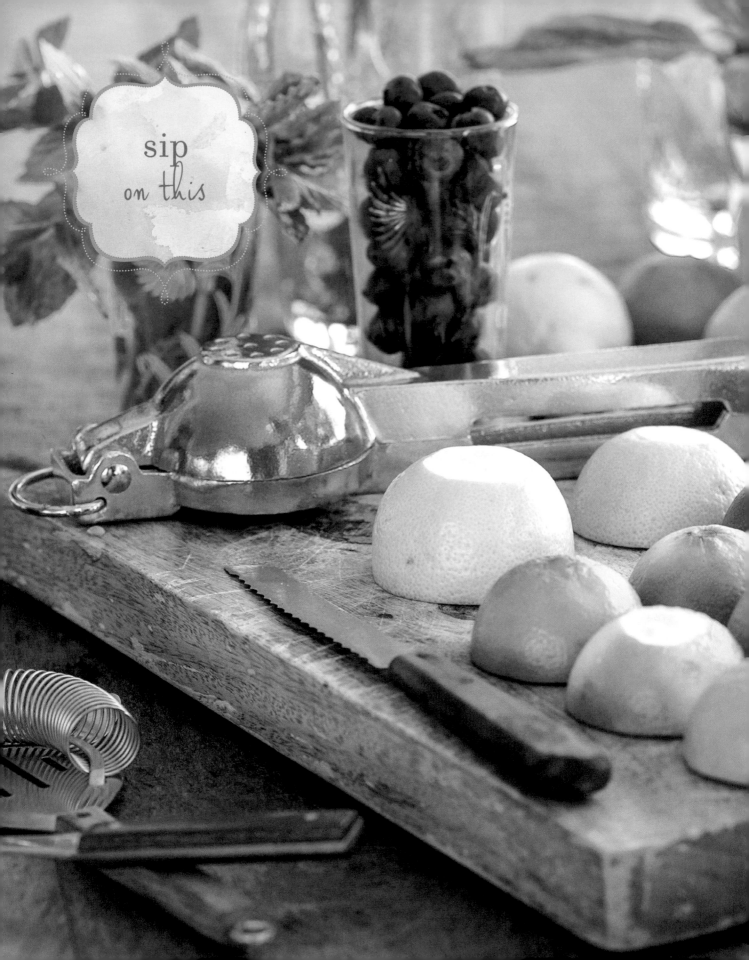

sip
on this

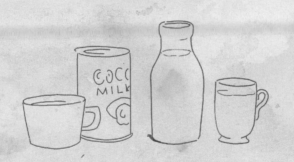

paleo fables

Good times can still be had by those following the Paleo lifestyle. Cocktails are often synonymous with sugary syrups and artificial mixers, but I enlisted the help of my craft cocktail mixing brother, Joel, to create these specialty real food 'mocktails', or 'fables' as he calls them. We also see no problem with adding a few splashes of 100% agave Tequila or Mezcal to any of these beverages! (1.5 ounces should do)

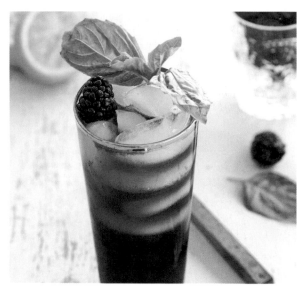

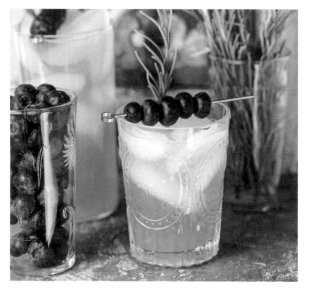

berry-basil spritzer

prep time: 5 minutes yield: 1 serving

ingredients

- 3 blackberries or raspberries
- 3 large basil leaves, torn
- 1 ounce honey syrup*
- 1 ounce fresh lemon juice, strained
- 4 ounces sparkling mineral water
- Ice

method

Gently muddle berries, basil leaves, and honey syrup in the bottom of a cocktail shaker. Add lemon juice and shake, covered, with ice vigorously for 10 seconds. Strain through a mesh strainer into a tall glass of fresh ice. Top with sparkling water and stir to incorporate.

rosemary-blueberry smash

prep time: 5 minutes yield: 1 serving

ingredients

- 7-8 blueberries
- 1 rosemary sprig, stripped
- 1 ounce honey syrup*
- 1 ounce fresh lemon juice, strained
- 4 ounces sparkling mineral water
- Ice

method

Gently muddle berries, rosemary leaves, and honey syrup in the bottom of a cocktail shaker. Add lemon juice and shake, covered, with ice vigorously for 10 seconds. Strain through a mesh strainer into a tall glass of fresh ice. Top with sparkling water and stir to incorporate.

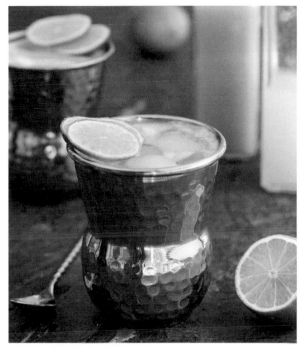

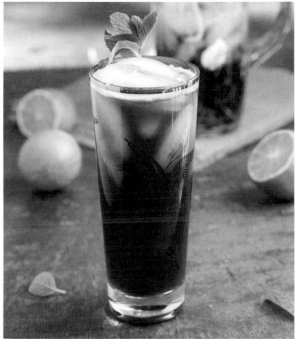

mango mule

prep time: 5 minutes   yield: 1 serving

ingredients

- 4 to 5 slices cucumber
- 1 ounce honey syrup*
- 1½ ounce mango puree
- 1½ ounce fresh lime juice
- 1½ ounce ginger beer
- Ice

method

Muddle cucumber and honey syrup in the bottom of a cocktail shaker. Add the mango purée and lime juice and shake, covered, with ice vigorously for 10 seconds. Strain into a tall glass of fresh ice. Top with ginger beer and stir to incorporate.

cranberry limeade

prep time: 5 minutes   yield: 1 serving

ingredients

- 2 ounces fresh lime juice
- 2 ounces honey syrup*
- ½ ounce cranberry concentrate
- 10 mint leaves
- 4 ounces sparkling mineral water
- Ice

method

Add lime juice, honey syrup, cranberry concentrate, and mint to a cocktail shaker and shake, covered, with ice vigorously for 10 seconds. Strain into a tall glass of fresh ice. Top with sparkling water and stir to incorporate.

tidbits:

*Honey Syrup is our substitution for simple syrup. Take 1 part honey and dissolve it in 1 part hot, but not boiling, water. Store in the refrigerator for 1 month in a sealed bottle and use it in all of your cocktails!

Danielle Walker

mulled apple cider

prep time: 5 minutes   cooking time: 30 minutes   yield: 4 servings

Sipping on warm apple cider, fragrant with mulling spices, in front of a roaring fire is the quintessential expression of fall as far as I'm concerned. You can make this in larger batches and keep it in the refrigerator to enjoy throughout the week.

ingredients

- 6 cups unfiltered apple cider
- Zest from 1 orange
- Zest from 1 lemon juice
- 4 cinnamon sticks
- 3 whole star anise pods
- 2 teaspoons whole cloves
- 2 teaspoons whole allspice berries

method

1. Place all the ingredients in a large saucepan over medium heat. Simmer for 30 minutes. Strain and serve.

tidbits:

Unfiltered cider is raw apple juice that has not undergone a filtration process to remove coarse particles of pulp or sediment. Make your own apple cider at home by juicing a combination of Granny Smith, Gala, Red Delicious, and Fuji apples.

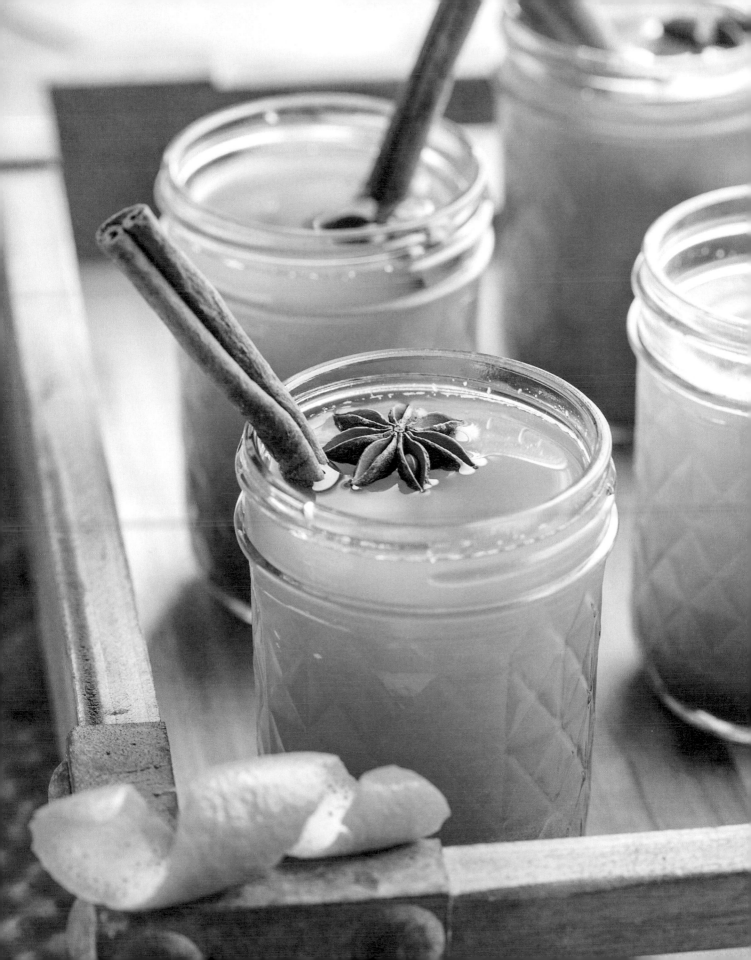

vanilla bean hot cocoa

prep time: 5 minutes   cooking time: 15 minutes   yield: 4 servings

Rich and creamy, this dairy-free hot chocolate warms both the body and soul on a chilly day.

sip on this

ingredients

- 2 cups unsweetened almond milk*
- 1 can coconut milk
- 1 vanilla bean, split lengthwise and seeds scraped
- 3 ounces dark chocolate (80 percent cacao or higher)
- 2 tablespoons unsweetened cocoa powder
- ¼ cup honey

Use all coconut milk for nut-free.

method

1. Place the almond milk, coconut milk, vanilla bean seeds, and the pod in a saucepan over medium-high heat. Bring to a boil, then reduce heat to low and simmer for 10 minutes. Strain the mixture then return to the pan.

2. Whisk in the chocolate, cocoa powder, and honey. Warm for 5 minutes, whisking occasionally, until the chocolate is melted and the hot chocolate is thick and creamy.

tidbits:
Meringue cookies will melt like marshmallows when added to the top of this hot chocolate. You can find recipes for these on my blog.

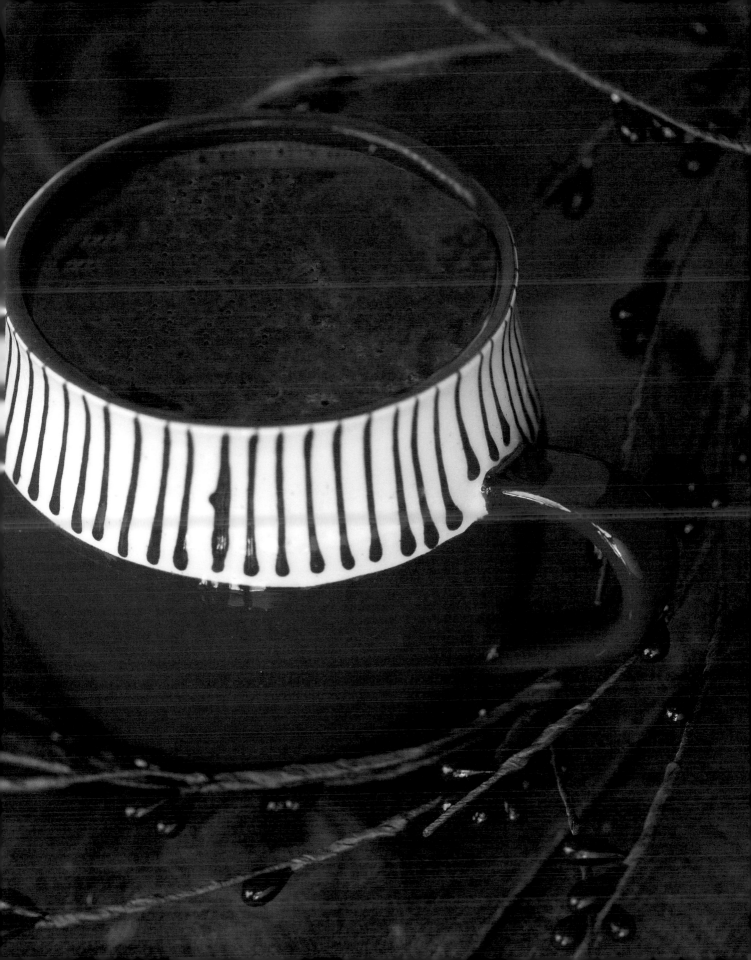

french vanilla coffee creamer

prep time: 5 minutes   cooking time: 35 minutes   yield: 2 cups

I often hear that one of the hardest things for people to give up when they transition to Paleo is their morning coffee with flavored creamers. So I created a homemade coffee creamer without hydrogenated oils or high-fructose corn syrup to help all those people make a sweet and easy transition.

ingredients

- 1 cup almond milk*
- 1 cup coconut milk
- 2 tablespoons honey
- 2 tablespoons maple syrup
- 1 vanilla bean

Use all coconut milk for nut-free.

method

1. Place the first 4 ingredients in a saucepan over medium-high heat. Bring to a low boil, and then remove from heat.

2. Split the vanilla bean down the middle and scrape out the seeds. Place the seeds and bean in the milk, then cover and let steep for 30 minutes.

3. Strain and bring to room temperature before covering and storing in the refrigerator for later use.

tidbits:
You can play with the flavors by using hazelnut milk or adding nutmeg and cinnamon.

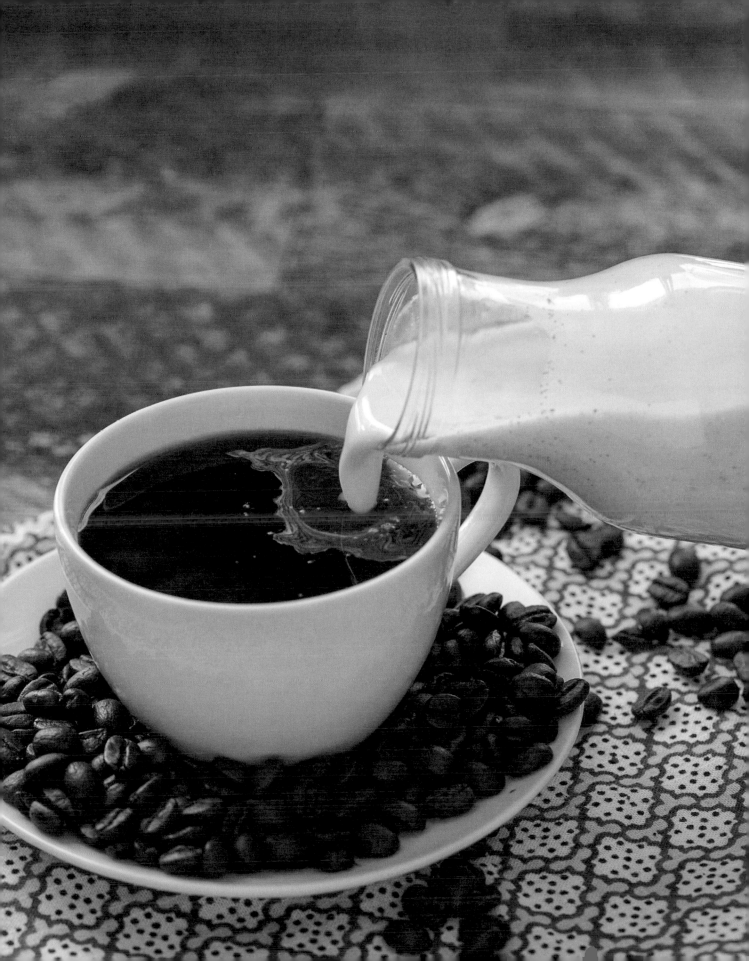

thai iced tea

prep time: 5 minutes + 1 hour for chilling   cooking time: 30 minutes

yield: 4 to 6 servings

My husband, Ryan, loves this sweet, full-bodied beverage that complements the spice and salt of Thai dishes. Generally made with sweetened condensed milk, half-and-half, and loads of white sugar, this rendition is made with coconut milk and honey for an equally enjoyable but healthy drink. Because this tea mixture is very concentrated once it has steeped so long, it shouldn't be used alone but is delicious when combined with milk.

ingredients

- 5 cups water
- ¼ cup honey
- 8 bags Assam tea
- 1 whole star anise
- 2 cardamom pods
- 1 cup coconut milk

method

1. Place the water in a saucepan over high heat and bring to a boil. Stir in the honey, and then add the tea bags, star anise, and cardamom. Remove from the heat, cover, and let steep for 30 minutes.

2. Place the tea in the refrigerator to chill for 1 hour or overnight.

3. Fill glasses with ice and then pour tea over the ice until ¾ full. Top each glass with 2 to 4 tablespoons of the coconut milk and serve immediately.

4. Leftover brewed tea can be stored in the refrigerator for later use.

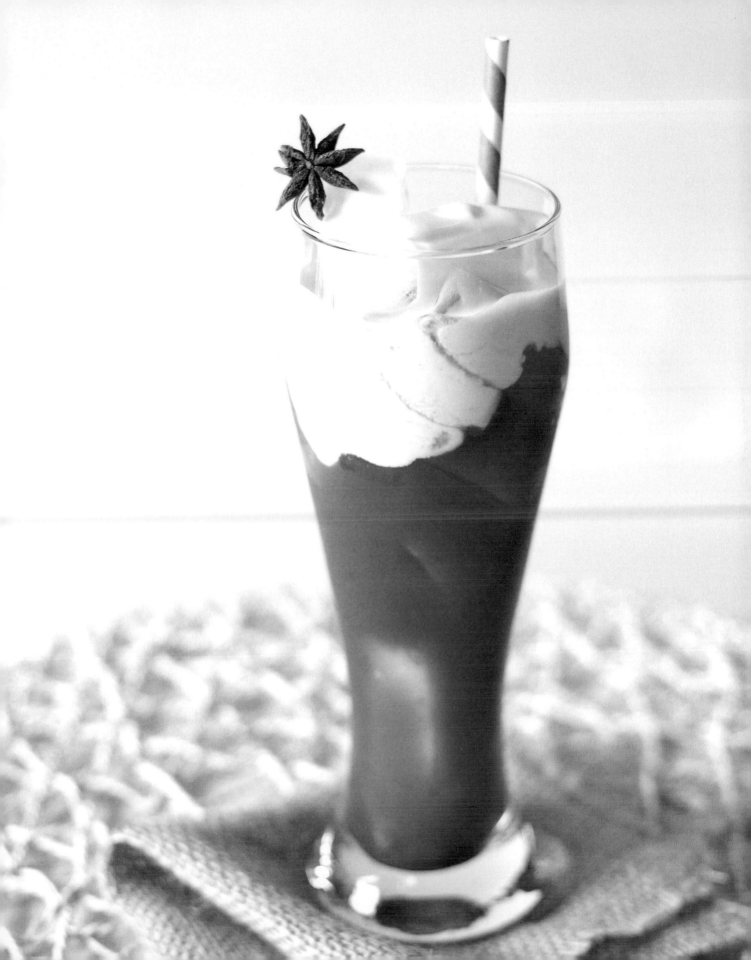

chai latte

prep time: 10 minutes   cooking time: 40 minutes   yield: 4 to 6 servings

One of my favorite things to do with my sister is get a chai latte and walk around our outdoor mall when the weather is brisk. We bundle up and warm our bodies with the comforting spices of chai and reminisce. We've always called it "Christmas in a cup," because no matter what time of the year it is, chai wafts the scents of the holiday season into the air.

ingredients

- 10 cups filtered water
- 18 bags black tea (preferably Darjeeling)
- 4 cinnamon sticks
- 4 whole star anise
- 1 tablespoon whole cloves
- 2 vanilla beans, split
- 3 tablespoons chopped fresh ginger
- 1½ teaspoons whole cardamom pods, smashed with the butt of a knife
- 1½ teaspoons black peppercorns
- 1½ teaspoons nutmeg
- 1 teaspoon fennel seed
- Zest from 1 orange
- 1 cup honey
- ¼ teaspoon fresh lime juice
- Coconut milk or almond milk

method

1. To make the tea concentrate: Place the water and tea bags in a large pot over high heat and bring to a boil. Reduce the heat to a simmer and add the remaining ingredients, except the honey, lime juice, and milk. Simmer uncovered for 20 minutes. Remove the tea bags and continue simmering for an additional 20 minutes. Strain the tea into a large bowl and discard the spices. Stir in the honey and lime juice while the tea is still hot.

2. Bring to room temperature then cover and store in the refrigerator for later use.

3. To serve: Mix 1 part concentrate with 2 parts milk (try using half coconut and half almond milk). Heat, or serve over ice.

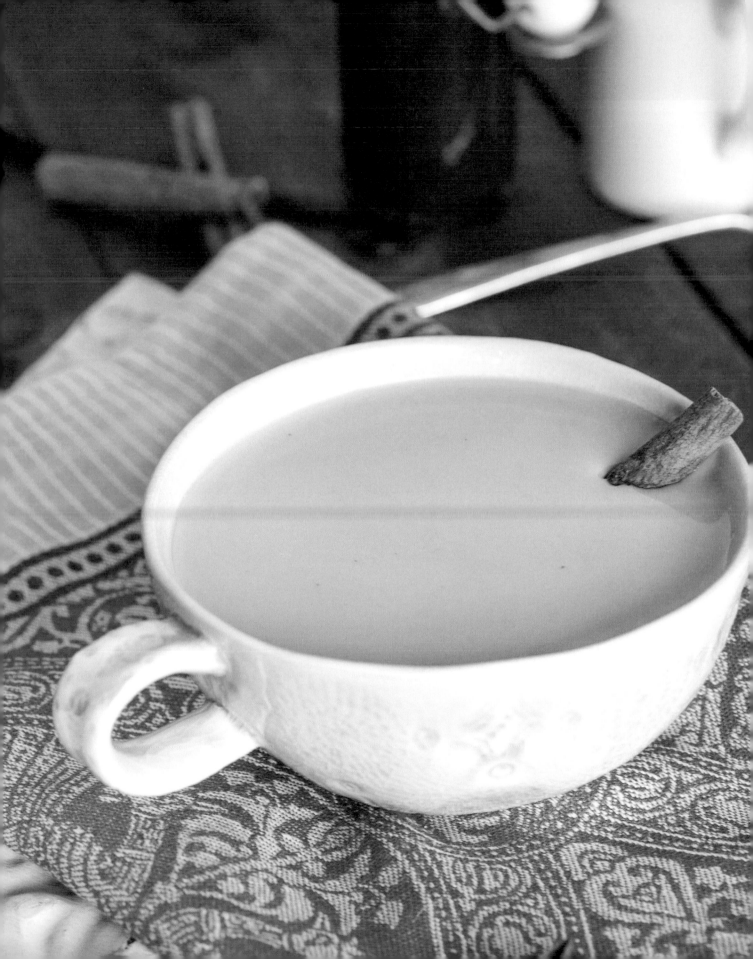

creamy chocolate shake

prep time: 5 minutes   yield: 2 servings

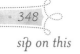

You'd never know there's half an avocado lurking inside this shake: besides making it thick 'n' creamy, it adds some healthy fat and Vitamin E. I drink this shake as a meal replacement on days when I'm running around like crazy. It's rich and filling and completely disguises my daily supplements.

ingredients

- 8 ounces almond milk
- ½ cup crushed ice
- 1 ripe banana
- 2 large pitted dates or 1 tablespoon honey
- ½ avocado (about ¼ cup)
- 2 tablespoons unsweetened cocoa powder
- 2 tablespoons almond butter
- 1 teaspoon ground golden flaxseeds

method

1. Place all the ingredients in a blender. Blend for 30 to 45 seconds, until smooth.

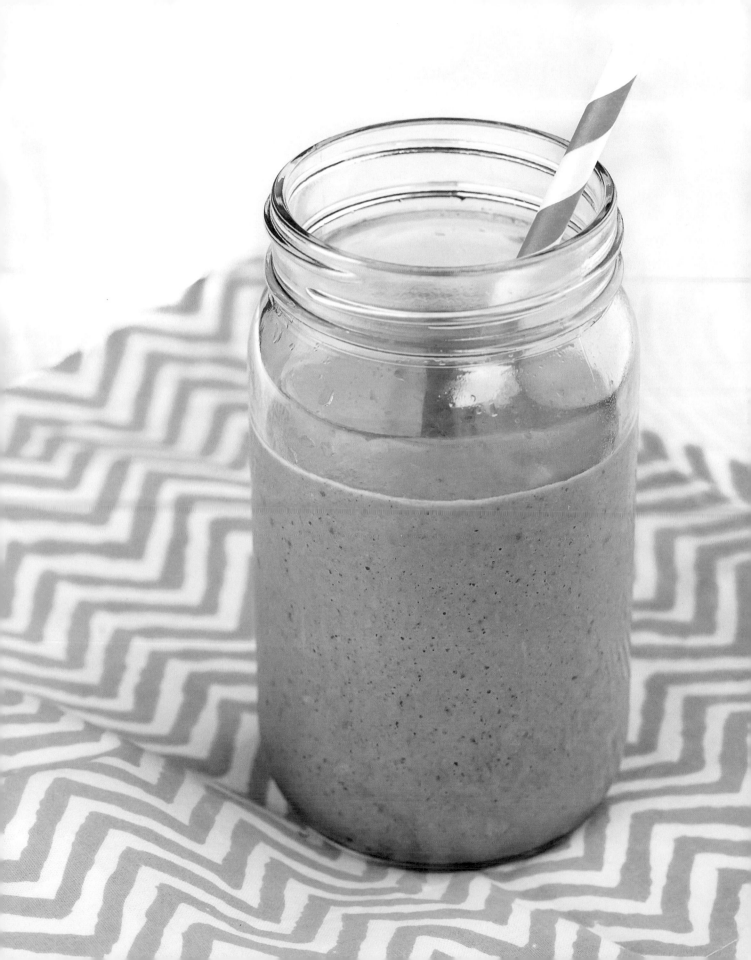

menu suggestions

thai-takeout night

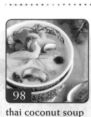
98

thai coconut soup (tom kha gai)

216

toddler-approved vegetable curry

148

thai pad see ew

156

pan-seared salmon in red curry sauce

344

thai iced tea

game day

86

sweet potato chips with creamy cilantro-serrano

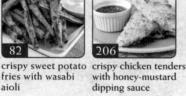
82

crispy sweet potato fries with wasabi aioli

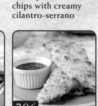
206

crispy chicken tenders with honey-mustard dipping sauce

258

real-deal chocolate-chip cookies

254

dark chocolate cake brownies

classic american comfort food

90

clam chowder

114

grilled artichokes with rémoulade

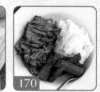
170

slow cooker pot roast

122

mashed cauliflower

274

chocolate cream pie with chocolate-cookie crust

light ladies' luncheon

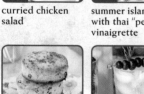
102

curried chicken salad

100

summer island salad with thai "peanut" vinaigrette

232

currant scones

336

rosemary-blueberry smash

island fare

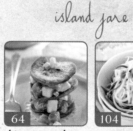
64

ahi mango poke stack

104

green papaya salad

126

coconut-lime rice

152

macadamia-coconut crusted ono with mango coulis

mangia!

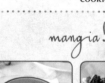
94

roasted butternut squash soup with sausage

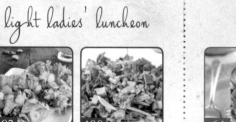
72

fried brussels sprouts and cauliflower

172

granny sarella's spaghetti sauce

238

sun-dried tomato rosemary scones

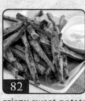
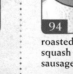

AGAINST *all* GRAIN

cocktail party

70
soaked trail mix

68
chicken satay with "peanut" sauce

86
sweet potato chips with creamy cilantro-serrano dipping sauce

74
korean beef-wrapped asparagus

264
double-chocolate macaroons

336
berry-basil spritzer

337
cranberry limeade

quick and easy

101
arugula, citrus, and bacon salad

158
lemon-basil sea bass en papillote

268
lemon vanilla bean macaroons

meatless monday

216
toddler-approved vegetable curry

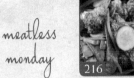

118
basic cauli-rice

116
stir-fried baby bok choy

cold winter night

96
slow-cooker beef chuck chili

108
warm spinach salad with bacon and mushrooms

240
rosemary breadsticks

asian fusion

106
asian mango slaw

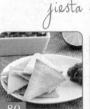

112
ginger-garlic broccoli

74
korean beef-wrapped asparagus

130
slow cooker sesame-orange chicken

sunday brunch

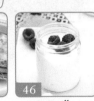

38
sausage quiche with sweet potato crust

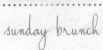

46
coconut milk yogurt

56
vanilla-almond granola

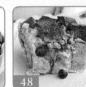

48
french toast casserole

fiesta night

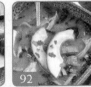

80
chips and salsa

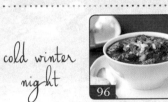

92
mexican chicken chowder

182
carne asada burrito bowls

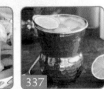

337
mango mule

Danielle Walker

resources

I order a lot of my nonperishables on Amazon.com and frequently purchase my grass-fed beef online. You can find all of my favorite pantry items conveniently in one spot here:

www.againstallgrain.com/shop/

Or search for your local retailers from the sites below:

··

US Wellness Meats
www.uswellnessmeats.com

Tropical Traditions Coconut Products and Organic Foods
www.tropicaltraditions.com

Digestive Wellness Nut Flours
www.digestivewellness.com

Natural Value Coconut Milk
www.naturalvalue.com

Honeyville Farms Almond Flour
www.honeyville.com

Enjoy Life Chocolate Chips
www.enjoylifefoods.com

Artisana Nut Butters
www.artisanafoods.com

Red Boat Fish Sauce
www.redboatfishsauce.com

Navitas Naturals Raw Cacao Powder
www.navitasnaturals.com

Bionaturae Tomato Products
www.bionaturae.com

Coconut Secret Coconut aminos and Coconut crystals
www.coconutsecret.com

Le Creuset Cookware
www.lecreuset.com

Dagoba Organic Chocolate
www.dagobachocolate.com

Shun Cutlery
www.shun.kaiusaltd.com/knives

conversions and substitutions

nuts and flour weight measurements (approx)

Blanched Almond Flour		Coconut Flour		Raw Whole Cashews	
1 TEASPOON	2 g	1 TEASPOON	3 g	1/4 CUP	40 g
1 TABLESPOON	7 g	1 TABLESPOON	7 g	1/3 CUP	49 g
1/4 CUP	24 g	1/4 CUP	26 g	1/2 CUP	79 g
1/3 CUP	32 g	1/2 CUP	54 g	3/4 CUP	118 g
1/2 CUP	48 g	3/4 CUP	80 g	1 CUP	150 g
1 CUP	90 g	1 CUP	112 g		

liquid or volume measures

1 TEASPOON	5 ml
1 TABLESPOON	15 ml
2 TABLESPOONS	30 ml
1/4 CUP	59 ml
1/3 CUP	79 ml
1/2 CUP	118 ml
2/3 CUP	158 ml
3/4 CUP	177 ml
7/8 CUP	207 ml
1 CUP	237 ml
2 CUPS	473 ml
4 CUPS	946 ml
1 PINT	473 ml
2 PINTS	946 ml

oven temperatures

°F	°C
475	240
450	230
425	220
400	200
375	190
350	180
325	160/170
300	150
275	140
250	120/130
225	110

measuring equivalents

1 TABLESPOON	3 TEASPOONS
1/8 CUP	2 TABLESPOONS
1/4 CUP	4 TABLESPOONS
1/3 CUP	5 TABLESPOONS +1 TEASPOON
1/2 CUP	8 TABLESPOONS
2/3 CUP	10 TABLESPOONS +2 TEASPOONS
3/4 CUP	12 TABLESPOONS
1 CUP	48 TEASPOONS
1 CUP	16 TABLESPOONS
8 FLUID OUNCES	1 CUP
1 PINT	2 CUPS
1 QUART	2 PINTS
4 CUPS	1 QUART
1 GALLON	4 QUARTS
16 OUNCES	1 POUND

dry weight measurements

(approx)

1 OZ	28 g
2 OZ	55 g
3 OZ	125 g
4 OZ	125 g
8 OZ	240 g
12 OZ	375 g
16 OZ	454 g
32 OZ	907 g

baking pan substitutions

10" x 3½" BUNDT = two 8" x 2" ROUNDS	10" x 2" ROUND = 9" x 9" x 2" SQUARE
10" x 3½" MUFFIN TIN = 8½" x 4½" x 2½" LOAF = 9" x 1½" ROUND = 8" x 8" x 1½" SQUARE	10" x 3½" ROUND = two 8" x 1½" ROUNDS = 10" x 15" x 1" JELLY ROLL = 8" x 8" x 2" SQUARE

NOTE: baking times will vary depending on pan size. Deeper pans, for example, require longer baking times.

acknowledgments

to Ryan – my love and my best friend:

thank you for your infinite support and for putting up with my neglect during this book process. You push me to surpass my own expectations and always have the utmost faith in my ability to succeed. You were my nurse during my many times of illness and an incredible parent to Asher when I was not able to be one. Thank you for willingly taste-testing every recipe in this book and graciously bringing home dinner on nights when I was simply tired of cooking. Thank you for braving trips to Tahoe alone with Asher so I could work and for always being my most honest and constructive critic.

to Asher,

you won't remember this process by the time you are able to read this, but thank you for putting up with me always saying, "Mommy has to do the dishes" or, "Please don't take the cookie off the plate while I take a picture of it." You are my whole life, and the reason I had no choice but to get well—so I could experience your joy and laughter to its fullest. Some of your most memorable and sweetest first words were, "Cook with Mama?" My greatest delight comes from making something with you in the kitchen and then seeing you enjoy it at the table.

to my parents, Bob and Cindi,

for cheerleading me through this process and for continually believing in me. Thank you for raising me to persevere and see the blessings that God can provide amidst struggles.

to my other parents, Barb and Dwight,

thank you for all your help with Asher during the final weeks before my deadline, eagerly boasting to your friends about me, and for constantly having faith in me.

to Amy,

my cherished friend and Asher's second mommy while I finished the final stages of this book. Thank you from the bottom of my heart for loving him like your own and always assuring me that he was in good hands while I worked. You are such a gift!

to all of Asher's other "friends,"

who played soccer, baseball, or cars with Asher while I was elbow deep in dirty dishes or hovering awkwardly over a new dish with a light reflector in one hand, diffuser in the other, while clicking the capture button with my toe.

to Jennifer Skog,

my dear friend and lifestyle photographer for this book. You saw my vision and made it come to life, even while eight months pregnant. Thank you for climbing onto countertops and photographing in precarious positions in order to capture my essence in the kitchen and my family so perfectly.

to Erich and Michele at Victory Belt Publishing,

thank you for patiently walking a complete rookie through the book writing process and having so much faith in my ability to succeed.

to all of our family members, neighbors, and friends

who gamely ate my experiments and provided feedback for every single dish in this book—not that you didn't enjoy it! Thank you for allowing this book to be the topic of every conversation for the past year and for putting up with me through all of it!

to my recipe testers, especially Rob, Nicole, and Kailee,

your enthusiasm and gratitude fueled me through the recipe-development stages and gave me enormous confidence in my recipes. Thank you for testing everything on your own dime and time, and for always giving me useful critiques (and praise).

to PJ of Milk Glass Rentals

for allowing me to borrow some of your incredible vintage gems and lending your eye to styling a few shoots.

finally, to my Creator,

You have redeemed a very grave illness by blessing me with abundant creativity in the kitchen and the ability to bring joy to others through food. For that, I am eternally grateful.

Danielle Walker

success stories
and gratitude from fans

My blog and social media followers have become like family to me over the years, and they inspire me to push my creative envelope. They motivate me to invent decadent recipes week after week, and always shower me with affirmation and gratitude in return. The emails I receive on a daily basis fill my heart with encouragement and confirm that I am making a difference in the lives of others. I truly have the most gratifying job in the world. I have collected some of the most touching messages from my fans and included them in this book as a memento of my journey and also to share with my readers the kind of healing that can come from adopting this style of eating.

"My son has been a type 1 diabetic since 4 years old. When he was little, we had to choose between allowing him to have birthday cake or his dinner as we were on a strict carb count. Not so yesterday! He was able to have your real-deal chocolate chip cookies and strawberry shortcake cupcakes. Honey is a blood-glucose level stabilizer—unlike other sweeteners. Almond and coconut flours are proteins and not carbohydrates—so your recipes were perfect for a challenging health condition and were definitely 'the icing on the cake' yesterday. THANK YOU for all you do! You have no idea how your efforts in the kitchen are changing the lives of others— for better health and happiness. Who doesn't want to see her child smile on his birthday as he blows out his candles—even if her 'child' is 20 years old? God bless!" —*Moriah*

"I don't often buy cookbooks anymore, but I will be buying yours. Your grain-free bread recipe is outstanding. I bake it for myself and also make and ship loaves to my 92-year-old mother, who likes it so much she stopped eating bagels for breakfast and just wants 'the bread my daughter makes.'" —*Linda*

"I wanted to let you know how much I loved the hot chocolate recipe. Getting diagnosed with celiac a couple of years ago was very difficult to deal with, and one of the hardest things to lose was a Parisian-style hot chocolate. You're changing lives through food. Thank you so much!!" —*Christine*

"Thank you so much, Danielle, for sharing your wonderful recipes! My son was recently diagnosed with Crohn's and we've been on an emotional rollercoaster. Thanks to your SCD legal choc-chip cookies, things aren't looking so gloomy anymore!" —*Susan*

"Thank you so very much for all you do. I have Crohn's and began on the SCD last June and your recipes have made the transition to a life-changing (and lifestyle-challenging) diet so much easier. I'm sure that my continued success with the diet is due in large part to your blog and the recipes you share. It's obvious you put a tremendous amount of time and energy into your cooking and baking. Again, Thank you!!" —*Nitsirk*

"Your cookbook and your blog are helping me be a better mom by keeping my kids healthy. You show 'real meals' and I am grateful for your approach. Thank you for the sacrifices you have made and for helping so many desperate mommies like myself. I am grateful!"—*Megan*

"Thank you for all your wonderful recipes! I found out I have celiac disease in August. Like any autoimmune disease, it has brought many new challenges and required a lot of learning. I honestly had never heard of 'grain-free' or 'Paleo' until a few months ago when I started researching different diets. I have stuck 100% to my gluten-free diet since finding out I have celiac disease, but think I would feel even better by switching to grain-free/Paleo. I just wanted to say that I love your recipes and every single one I've tried makes me feel like I can do this! Almost every morning now my toddler pulls the fry pan out of the pantry and asks for 'nana-cakes,' which are your grain-free banana pancakes! We love them!"—*Erin*

"I am so happy that I found your website and follow you on Facebook. Your recipes are divine. Thank you for your dedication and enthusiasm to share your love of cooking with us. I have been trying your recipes and love them."—*Jessica*

"All of your recipes are fantastic—and I cannot wait for your cookbook to come out!!! Thank you so much for making my Paleo lifestyle sustainable!"—*Niki*

"I am doing the Paleo diet after my 6-month-old daughter has been diagnosed with allergy colitis. I am nursing so the Dr. has had me cut out dairy, wheat and soy. So the recipes and your blog are very much appreciated! They are delicious and take the stress out of trying to find something good to eat. I am lacking time with my busy household of 4 kiddos and hubby! Thank you!!"—*Denyse*

"Everything I have tried of yours is exceptional! It's so helpful and encouraging when you strip your diet of common ingredients to find alternatives with an even better taste! Thank you for taking your time to create recipes for all of us to benefit from. I LOVE your blog and every recipe I have made or tried has been SO good. I trust everything you make. It's nice when you can just try a recipe and know it's going to be good. I hardly ever have that luxury, but I know I can count on your recipes whenever I try a new one."—*Nicole*

"Thank you! Thank you! For so many of your recipes. Our treasured little 5 year old boy who enjoyed good health until last fall when he developed a seizure disorder that 3 different pediatric neurologists have said cannot be controlled with diet (while his body shows amazing signs of healing & seizure management through diet so far) is finally able to have a delicious version of Stuffed French Toast every Sunday like he used to enjoy at our favorite breakfast restaurant. Your pancakes, waffles, real deal choc chip cookies & many other breakfast recipes especially have added back a certain quality to our daily life that restrictive diets can jeopardize. I have shared your blog with the nutritionist we are working with and other functional medicine believers. You are a.m.a.z.i.n.g! Thank you for what you do!"—*Christine*

"I can't thank you enough for your recipes. My niece was diagnosed with autism and my sister had her on a gluten and dairy free diet since. She took a few months to gain the courage to start the SCD, as she was very intimidated by all the restrictions. She finally started early this week and almost gave up because her daughter wasn't liking the bread options that my sister had for her. We are so glad that you put your recipes out there for people to enjoy and in my sister's case rely on—she feels less pressure and more confident that she will be able to do this for her daughter. We can't thank you enough for this."—*Lisa*

"You are such a gift to any food lover who has been limited by a restricted diet! Eight years after my diagnosis of Crohn's disease, I live an extremely active and healthy life with no symptoms. As I read your story, I realized we have been on the same journey for quite some time. You are truly talented in the kitchen and jump-started my passion for a grain-free lifestyle all over again. We have been raving about your talent and your recipes ever since. I think your waffles have been our favorite so far and I'm still amazed by the bread recipe but now I must try them all! Thank you again for sharing your recipes; you have been an inspiration to my family and so many others!"—*Jennifer*

"Thank you for taking the time to do the research, testing and creativity that I don't have time to do myself as a full time, one income family. I am super excited about your bread recipe on your blog. Can't wait to try it. I have Rheumatoid Arthritis. I am following the Paleo/Primal diet right now. I am hoping to not have to cut out eggs and nightshades. I am trying it this way at first; if I don't get results I will go stricter. Thanks again! You and a couple of other bloggers are making my life so much easier!!"—*Terry*

"You are my Ina Garten/Cooks Illustrated of the Paleo world. I can make one of your recipes for the first time and feel confident enough to serve it to guests. You are a culinary magician!"—*Maggie*

"From the Netherlands I want to say thank you. I really love cooking (and eating) so at first my world fell apart when I started the SCD because there was so much I couldn't eat anymore. But then I thought it would be a challenge to still cook and eat good and delicious food. In Holland there is not much to find, but then I found your website!!! I was so happy and thrilled. It actually made me cry. It was such a relief to see such beautiful pictures and recipes. Suddenly I felt I could do this. Recover and still be happy with cooking and eating delicious foods. So thank you so much for sharing your recipes and your story!! When I have some difficult and sad days, your website and your recipes give me the power to go on. Thank you so much for being inspirational and motivating!"—*Janine*

"I discovered your blog and I quit my medication and have been cooking your recipes. I have never felt so good as I do now compared to the past 11 years since being diagnosed with ulcerative colitis at 21. You have saved my life! I felt like crying when I first read about the SC diet because it seemed hopeless to follow. Luckily I found your website and I now eat delicious SCD legal food! You are my hero! I actually feel grateful for ulcerative colitis since it has forced me to eat healthy. I am definitely still learning about controlling my UC with diet, but with your help, I know it is possible. Thank you, thank you! Thanks so much for sharing your talents."—*Amy*

"I sent your treats to a birthday party with my 7-year-old daughter so that she would have a special treat to eat while her friends ate cake and ice cream. No tears, no begging for sugar—just pure elation over her 'healthy dessert.' Our family is also grain/dairy/sugar free. YOU, Danielle, made life on Sunday a lot easier for this girl. Thank you for being born."—*Heather*

recipe index

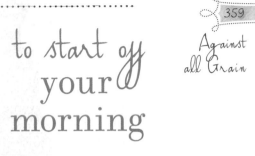 to start of your morning

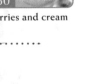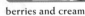
small bites

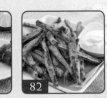

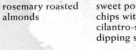
Danielle Walker

soups, salads, and sides

90
clam chowder

92
mexican chicken chowder

94
roasted butternut squash soup with sausage

96
slow-cooker beef chuck chili

98
thai coconut soup (tom kha gai)

100
bibb lettuce with d'anjou pears, shaved fennel, avocado, and toasted walnuts

100
summer island salad with thai "peanut" vinaigrette

101
arugula, citrus, and bacon salad

101
winter salad with roasted beets and butternut squash with champagne vinaigrette

102
curried chicken salad

104
green papaya salad

106
asian mango slaw

108
warm spinach salad with bacon and mushrooms

110
roasted-garlic mashed faux-tatoes

112
ginger-garlic broccoli

114
grilled artichokes with rémoulade

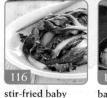
116
stir-fried baby bok choy

118
basic cauli-rice

120
shaved brussels sprouts with bacon, leeks, and pomegranate seeds

122
mashed cauliflower

124
grilled lemon-garlic zucchini

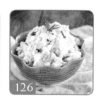
126
coconut-lime rice

the main event

130
slow cooker sesame-orange chicken

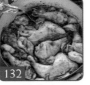
132
braised chicken in artichoke-mushroom sauce

134
"fettuccine" alfredo with blackened chicken

136
chicken cobb salad

138
slow cooker chicken tacos

140
pulled barbecue chicken sandwiches with coleslaw

142
citrus-cumin chicken

144
club sandwich wraps

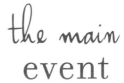
146
lemon herb-roasted chicken and vegetables

148
thai pad see ew

150
petrale sole with lemon-caper sauce

152
macadamia-coconut crusted ono with mango coulis

154
seafood, chorizo, and chicken paella

156
pan-seared salmon in red curry sauce

158
lemon-basil sea bass en papillote

160
prawn and pumpkin yellow curry

162
honey-lime salmon tostadas

164
sausage and butternut squash stuffed tomatoes

166
greek gyro pasta with lamb meatballs

168
spinach sausage lasagna

170
slow cooker pot roast

172
granny sarella's spaghetti sauce

174
curried short ribs

176
barbecue bacon burgers with rosemary-garlic mushrooms

178
indian-spiced pork roast with cumin-curry carrots

180
london broil with rosemary vegetables

182
carne asada burrito bowls

184
korean beef noodle bowls

Danielle Walker

for the kid in all of us

188 not-a-grain bars ("cereal" breakfast bars)

190 banana mouse pancakes

192 spaghetti squash boats with mini-meatballs

194 hidden-veggie muffins

196 cutout cookies with frosting

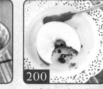
198 chicken-zoodle soup

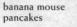
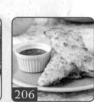
200 apple sandwiches

202 trail mix granola bars

204 fruit roll-ups

206 crispy chicken tenders with honey-mustard dipping sauce

208 cinnamon applesauce

210 mini-meatloaf muffins

212 chewy honey graham crackers

214 fruit juice gelatin shapes

216 toddler-approved vegetable curry

218 almond crisps

muffins, loaves, and morning cakes

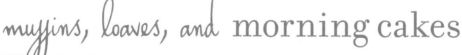

222 cinnamon-raisin coffee cake

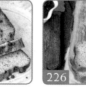
224 banana bread

226 world-famous sandwich bread

228 spiced pumpkin muffins

230 orange-cranberry muffins

232 currant scones

234 glazed lemon poppy seed pound cake

236 zucchini bread

238 sun-dried tomato rosemary scones

240 rosemary breadsticks

242 hamburger buns

244 peach streusel coffee cake

sweets and treats

248 chocolate layer cake

250 snickerdoodle cupcakes

252 strawberry cake with lemon cream filling

254 dark chocolate cake brownies

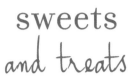

256 pumpkin donuts (with maple-bacon glaze or chocolate frosting)

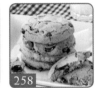
258 real-deal chocolate-chip cookies

260 n'oatmeal raisin cookies

262 "peanut butter" cookies

264 double-chocolate macaroons

266 seven-layer bars

268 lemon vanilla bean macaroons

270 honey graham piecrust

272 black-bottom banana cream pie

274 chocolate cream pie with chocolate-cookie crust

276 meyer lemon meringue pie

278 double-chocolate frozen yogurt with "peanut" butter fudge swirl

280 french vanilla ice cream

282 mint-chip ice cream

284 ganache tart with toasted hazelnuts

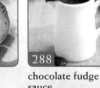
286 lemon curd

288 chocolate fudge sauce

290 caramel sauce

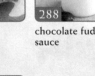

292 coconut milk whipped cream

294 italian meringue frosting

296 chocolate swiss meringue buttercream

298 vanilla frosting

Danielle Walker

basics

302
crepes

304
basic nut cheese

306
marinara sauce

308
mayonnaise

310
pastry crust

312
pizza crust

314
almond milk

316
chicken broth

318
thai 'peanut' vinaigrette

320
basil-thyme vinaigrette

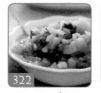
322
asian pear chutney

324
fig jam

326
smoky barbecue sauce

328
tomato ketchup

330
blueberry preserves

332
pico de gallo

332
pineapple salsa

333
roasted-tomatillo salsa

333
guacamole

sip
on this

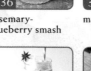
336
berry-basil spritzer

336
rosemary-blueberry smash

337
mango mule

337
cranberry limeade

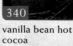
338
mulled apple cider

340
vanilla bean hot cocoa

342
french vanilla coffee creamer

344
thai iced tea

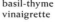

346
chai latte

348
creamy chocolate shake

index

Danielle Walker